THE SURGERY OF THE SKULL AND BRAIN

THE SURGERY OF THE SKULL AND BRAIN

L. BATHE RAWLING, F.R.C.S.

GYAN

Published by

Gyan Publishing House
5, Ansari Road
Daryaganj, New Delhi-110002
Phone: 011-47034999, 9811692060
E-mail: books@gyanbooks.com

Distribution Network
gyanbooks.com
India, USA, Canada, UK, Australia, France

ISBN : 978-81-212-9162-0 (PB)
First Published, 1912

2nd Impression 2023

Printed at: Gyan Press, Delhi.

THE SURGERY OF THE SKULL AND BRAIN
Author: L. BATHE RAWLING

OXFORD MEDICAL PUBLICATIONS

THE SURGERY OF
THE SKULL AND BRAIN

OXFORD MEDICAL PUBLICATIONS

THE SURGERY OF THE SKULL AND BRAIN

BY

L. BATHE RAWLING, F.R.C.S.

SURGEON, WITH CHARGE OF OUT-PATIENTS, SENIOR DEMONSTRATOR OF PRACTICAL SURGERY
DEMONSTRATOR OF OPERATIVE SURGERY, ST. BARTHOLOMEW'S HOSPITAL
LATE HUNTERIAN PROFESSOR, ETC.

LONDON

HENRY FROWDE
OXFORD UNIVERSITY PRESS

HODDER & STOUGHTON
WARWICK SQUARE, E.C.

1912

PREFACE

THIS work on the Surgery of the Skull and Brain is based on experience derived, and on research carried out, during the past ten years.

Cranio-Cerebral Surgery, though still in its infancy, has progressed with leaps and bounds during the past few years. This book represents the most modern aspects of the case and is brought up to date by means of a recent visit to some of the leading surgical clinics of the United States of America.

I have realized to the full the difficulties of the task which I have undertaken, but have every confidence that they have been overcome and that a reasonable measure of success has been obtained. With this anticipation, this work on the Surgery of the Skull and Brain is offered to the Profession.

L. BATHE RAWLING.

April 1912.

CONTENTS

PAGE

CHAPTER VIII

CHAPTER IX

CHAPTER X

CHAPTER XI

LIST OF ILLUSTRATIONS

THE SURGERY OF THE SKULL AND BRAIN

CHAPTER I

CRANIO-CEREBRAL TOPOGRAPHY

THE surgeon who is called upon to carry out operations on the skull and brain must possess an accurate knowledge of the anatomy of the parts involved. Added to this, he must have at his command some simple method of depicting on the surface of the skull the more important structures.

The more complicated systems of cranio-cerebral topography are of little practical value to the surgeon. Simplicity is essential, and the following outline will be found to furnish an adequate practical guide.

Firstly, the skull can be divided into two lateral halves by the surface-marking of the superior longitudinal venous sinus.

The superior longitudinal sinus. This sinus originates at the crista galli and, passing backwards along the attached margin of the falx cerebri, terminates at the internal occipital protuberance. It may be represented by a line drawn from the base of the nose (the nasion), over the vertex of the skull, to the external occipital protuberance (the inion)—this line corresponding in its course to the occasionally persistent metopic suture between the two halves of the frontal bone, to the sagittal suture between the parietal bones, and to the middle line of the upper or tabular portion of the occipital bone.

Secondly, each lateral half of the skull can be subdivided into supra- and infratentorial regions by a line which marks the external attachment of the tentorium cerebelli; in other words, by the line of the lateral sinus.

The lateral sinus. This sinus is represented by a line presenting a slight upward convexity, which is drawn from the external

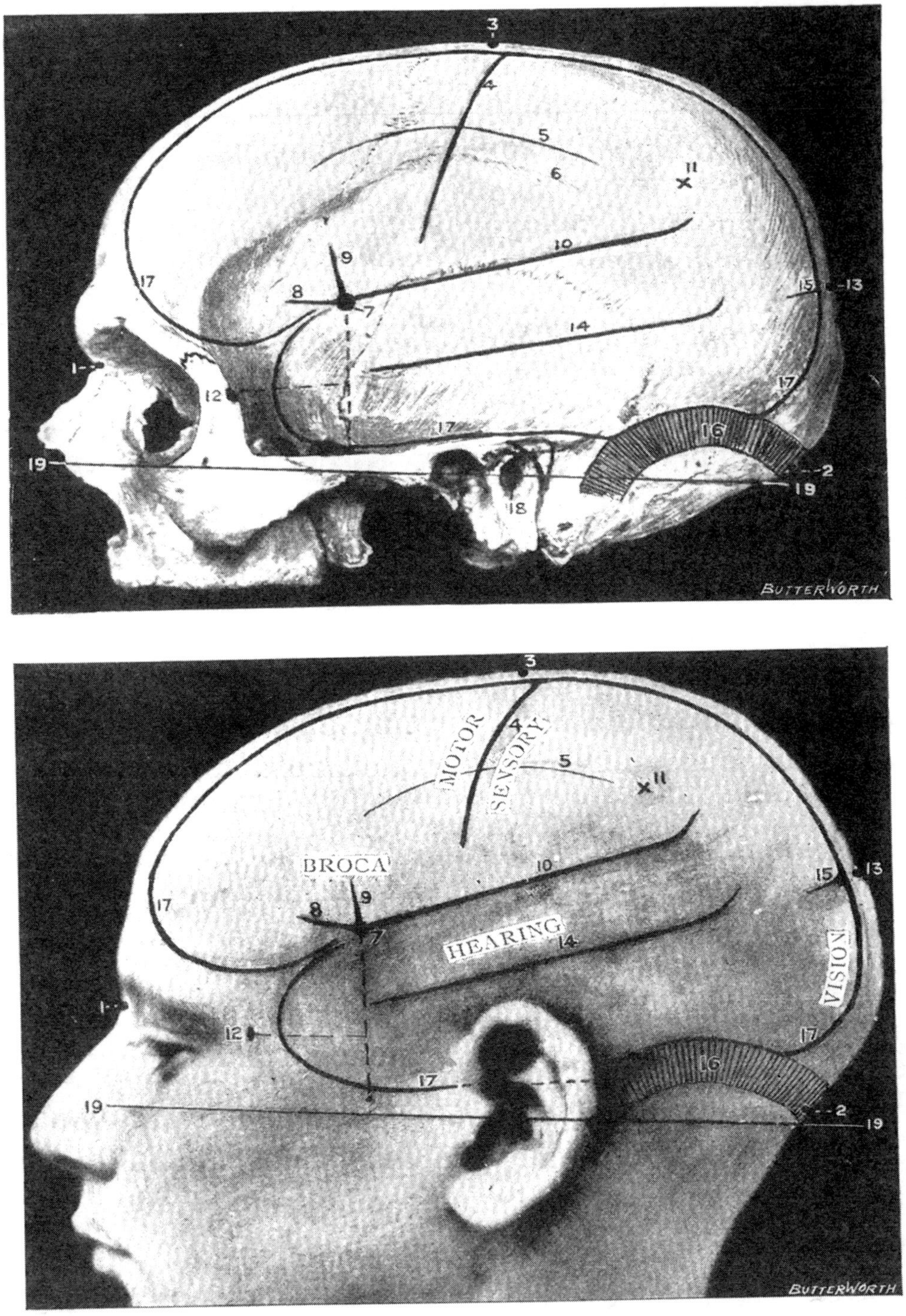

FIG. 1. CRANIO-CEREBRAL TOPOGRAPHY. 1, The nasion; 2, The inion; 3, The mid-point between nasion and inion; 4, The Rolandic fissure; 5, The superior temporal crest; 6, The inferior temporal crest; 7, The Sylvian point; 8, The anterior horizontal limb of the Sylvian fissure; 9, The vertical limb of the Sylvian fissure; 10, The posterior horizontal limb of the Sylvian fissure; 11, The parietal prominence; 12, The malar tubercle; 13, The lambda; 14, The first temporo-sphenoidal sulcus; 15, The external parieto-occipital sulcus; 16, The lateral sinus; 17, 17, 17, The level of the base of the cerebrum; 18, The external auditory meatus; 19, 19, Reid's base-line. (*Reproduced, by the permission of Mr. H. K. Lewis, from the author's work on 'Landmarks and Surface-markings'.*)

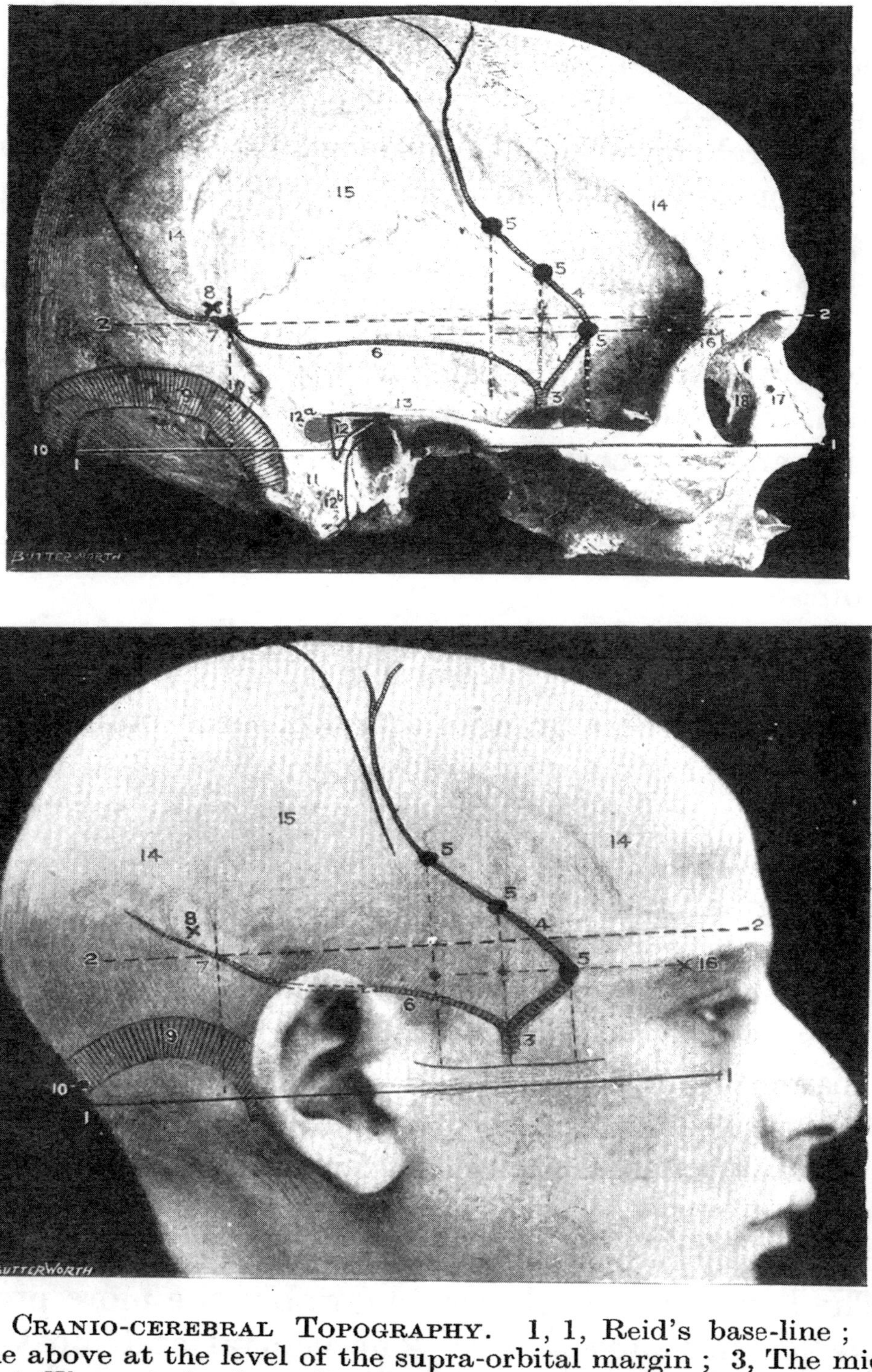

FIG. 2. CRANIO-CEREBRAL TOPOGRAPHY. 1, 1, Reid's base-line; 2, 2, A line parallel to the above at the level of the supra-orbital margin; 3, The middle meningeal artery; 4, The anterior branch; 5, 5, 5, The three sites for trephining; 6, The posterior branch; 7, The site for trephining; 8, The point for trephining to reach the descending horn of the lateral ventricle; 9, The lateral sinus; 10, The inion; 11, The mastoid process; 12, Macewen's suprameatal triangle; 12*a*, The mastoid antrum; 12*b*, The facial nerve; 13, The suprameatal and supramastoid crests; 14, 14, The temporal crest; 15, The temporal fossa; 16, The external angular frontal process; 17, The tendo-oculi attachment; 18, The lachrymal groove. (*Reproduced, by the permission of Mr. H. K. Lewis, from the author's work on 'Landmarks and Surface-markings'.*)

occipital protuberance to the upper and posterior part of the mastoid process of the temporal bone.

The infratentorial region. The cerebellum lies wholly beneath the tentorium cerebelli, and it is obvious that, in operations carried out over this portion of the brain, the surgeon is limited in his field of exposure, above by the line of the lateral sinus, and on either side by the posterior border of the mastoid process. The division between the halves of the cerebellum may be represented by a line drawn vertically downwards from the external occipital protuberance to the nuchal region. This line also represents the surface-marking of the occipital sinus and falx cerebelli.

The supratentorial region. Brief allusion must be made to certain landmarks that aid in the representation of structures situated in this region:—

(*a*) *The external angular frontal process.* The suture between the external angular frontal process and the corresponding process of the malar bone lies immediately above the central point of the outer border of the orbital cavity.

(*b*) *The malar tubercle.* A slight prominence on the posterior border of the frontal process of the malar bone, about $\frac{1}{4}$ inch below the external angular frontal process.

(*c*) *The temporal crest.* A prominent ridge that is directed upwards and backwards from the external angular frontal process. The crest cuts across the lower portion of the parietal bone, passing below the parietal prominence, and curves downwards towards the upper and posterior portion of the mastoid process. It terminates by becoming continuous with the upper root of the zygomatic process. The crest consists of two parts, the upper and lower temporal crests. To the upper is attached the temporal fascia, to the lower the temporal muscle. The lower crest is almost invariably the more prominent.

(*d*) *The parietal prominence.* The central and most prominent part of the parietal bone. It indicates the point at which ossification commenced, and lies about $\frac{3}{4}$ inch above the termination of the posterior horizontal limb of the fissure of Sylvius.

(*e*) *The zygoma.* When traced in the backward direction, the zygoma is found to divide immediately in front of the ear into three roots, of which the anterior, merging into the eminentia articularis, and the middle, aiding in the formation of the post-glenoid process, are of no practical utility in surface-marking. The upper or posterior root sweeps backwards above the external auditory meatus to become continuous with the suprameatal and supramastoid crests, the former of which forms the upper boundary of *Macewen's suprameatal triangle*, a triangular depression at the upper and posterior border of the external auditory meatus. This triangle may be taken as representing the opening of the mastoid antrum into the middle ear.

These landmarks having been determined, the following structures may be mapped out on the surface of the skull.

The middle menigeal artery. This artery is given off from the internal maxillary ; after a short extra-cranial course it enters the skull through the foramen spinosum, and soon divides into two main terminal branches. The site of division corresponds to a point situated just above the centre of the zygoma.

The *anterior branch* passes at first in a forward and upward direction towards the anterior inferior angle of the parietal bone, and then turns upwards and backwards towards the vertex of the skull. The main ‘ danger zone ’ in the course of this vessel may be mapped out by taking points which lie respectively 1, $1\frac{1}{2}$, and 2 inches behind the external angular frontal process and an equal distance above the upper border of the zygoma. A line uniting these three points represents that part of the anterior division of the middle meningeal artery which is most liable to injury and which therefore most frequently requires exposure.

The uppermost point may, however, be regarded as the ‘ site of election ’ for exposure of the artery, as, in trephining over either of the two lower points, difficulty may be experienced in the removal of the disk of bone, since the posterior border of the great wing of the sphenoid tails off on to the anterior inferior angle of the parietal bone in such a manner that to effect a clean removal of the disk is often impossible. Another disadvantage to trephining low down lies in the fact that in about 30 to 40 per cent. of cases the artery occupies, in that situation, a canal in the bone.

The *posterior branch* passes almost horizontally backwards, parallel to the zygoma and supramastoid crest, towards the posterior inferior angle of the parietal bone. The vessel can readily be exposed by trephining over the point at which a line drawn backwards from the upper border of the orbit, parallel to Reid's base-line,[1] cuts another line directed vertically upwards from the posterior border of the mastoid process.

Both branches of the middle meningeal artery possess important relations to the cortex cerebri, the anterior branch passing upwards in relation to the precentral or motor area, traversing, from below upwards, the motor speech area (on the left side of the head), the centres for the movements of the face, upper extremity, trunk, and lower extremity. The posterior branch, on the other hand, passes backwards in relation to the temporo-sphenoidal lobe, one of the so-called 'silent areas' of the brain. Throughout their course the middle meningeal vessels lie between the dura mater and the bone.

The lower limit of the cerebrum. The lower limit of the cerebrum can be mapped out in the following manner: From a point situated about ½ inch above the nasion a line is drawn outwards which follows the curve of the upper border of the orbit as far as the external angular frontal process, thence curving upwards and backwards to the Sylvian point (see below). The temporo-sphenoidal lobe sweeps forwards to the posterior border of the malar bone, and its lower limit lies practically flush with the upper margin of the zygoma. At and behind the ear the lower limit of the cerebrum corresponds to the suprameatal and supramastoid crests, subsequently following the curve of the lateral sinus from the mastoid process to the external occipital protuberance.

The Sylvian point and fissure. The Sylvian point represents the site of divergence of the three limbs of the Sylvian fissure. It lies 1¼ inches behind the malar tubercle and 1½ inches above the upper border of the zygoma. The main posterior horizontal limb passes backwards and upwards to a second point situated ¾ inch below the parietal prominence.

The vertical limb is directed upwards for about 1 inch, whilst the anterior horizontal limb passes forwards for about the same distance.

The fissure of Rolando. This, from a surgical point of view,

[1] Reid's base-line is a line drawn around the skull, starting in front at the lower border of the orbit and passing through the central point of the external auditory meatus.

the most important fissure of the brain, is represented as follows: A point is taken in the median antero-posterior line which lies ½ inch behind the mid-point between nasion and inion, and from this point a line is drawn, for 3½ to 4 inches, towards the mid-point of the zygoma. This line is inclined to the median antero-posterior line at an angle of 67½° (three-quarters of a right angle).

The parieto-occipital and first temporo-sphenoidal fissures. In the representation of these two fissures, two points require to be determined—the malar tubercle and the lambda. Allusion has already been made to the former; the latter is usually readily located as the point of intersection of the sagittal and lambdoid sutures. A line uniting these two points corresponds in its middle third to the temporo-sphenoidal fissure, and in its posterior inch or so to the external parieto-occipital sulcus, a fissure separating the occipital and parietal lobes of the brain.

The cortical motor and sensory areas. The researches of Sherrington and Grünbaum,[1] Campbell,[2] and others tend to show that the *cortical motor areas* are situated entirely anterior to the central fissure or fissure of Rolando, extending above well over on to the mesial aspect of the brain, though not so far as the calloso-marginal fissure, and in the downward direction to within a short distance of the fissure of Sylvius. In the posterior direction the motor area includes the anterior boundary and part of the bottom of the fissure of Rolando, whilst in front it spreads, by means of gyri annectantes, on to that part of the brain which lies anterior to the precentral sulcus. The anterior termination is indefinite, but the motor strip is, on an average, not more than ¾ inch in breadth.

The genua of the Rolandic fissure are said to bear a more or less definite relation to the motor areas. In my experience, however, they are too variable, and any importance which might obtain is further diminished by the fact that the surgeon should never rest content with that limited exposure of the brain which was so much in vogue till recent years. The suspected region is widely exposed by osteoplastic flap, and if doubt exists as to the particular part of cortex exposed the question is accurately settled by faradization.

[1] *Proceedings and Philosophic Transactions of the Roy. Soc.*, 1901.

[2] *Localization of Cerebral Function.* Camb. Univ. Press, 1905.

This motor strip corresponds, from above downwards, to the movements of the contralateral lower extremity (toe to hip), trunk, upper extremity (shoulder to fingers), neck and face. It is a point of some general utility to bear in mind that the temporal crest intervenes approximately between the regions responsible for the

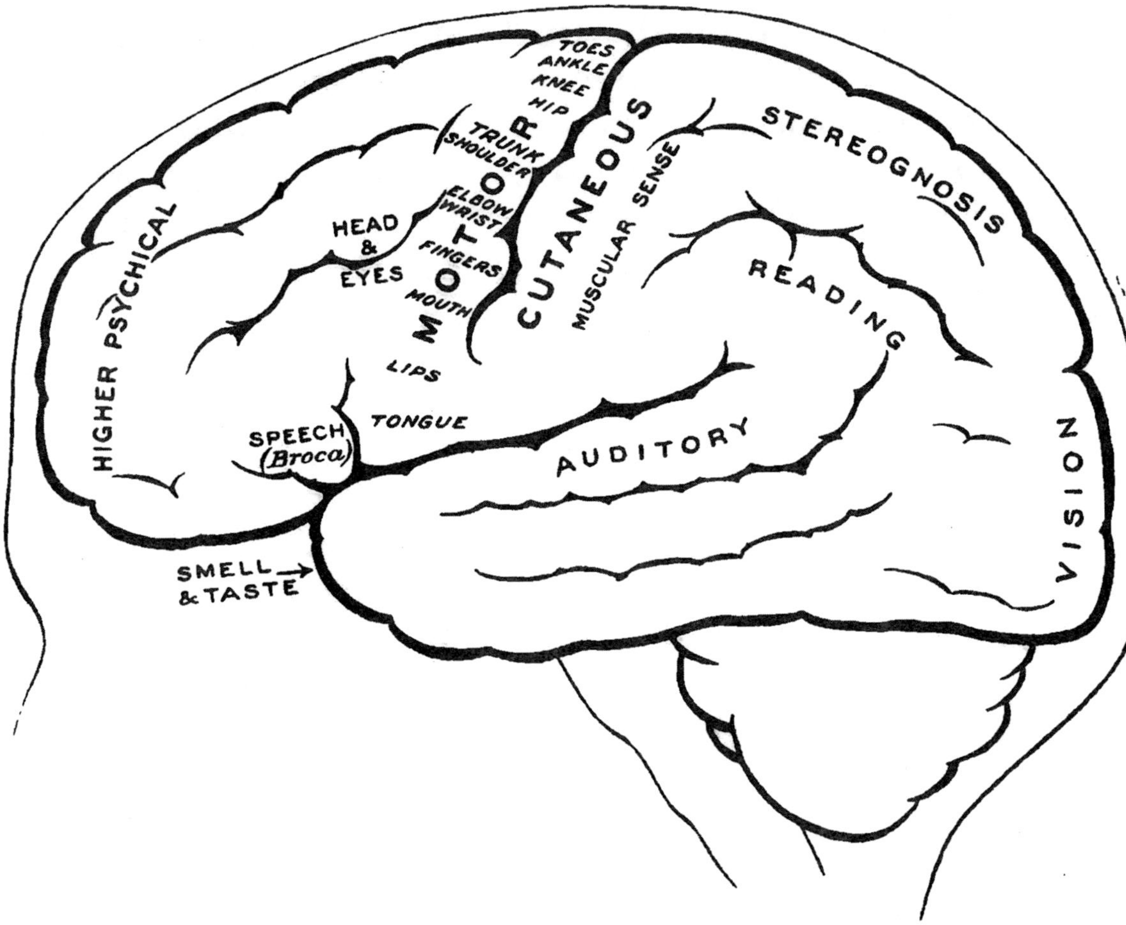

FIG. 3. THE CORTICAL MOTOR AND SENSORY AREAS.

movements of the upper extremity (above the crest) and those for the movements of the head and face (below the crest).

On the left side of the head—in normal right-handed individuals —the *motor speech area of Broca* corresponds to the third left frontal convolution, in the angle between the anterior and posterior horizontal limbs of the Sylvian fissure.

The ' primary registration ' of ' *common sensation* ' occurs in the post-central gyrus, immediately posterior to the fissure of Rolando. This tactile area occupies a position behind the fissure of Rolando similar in extent to that occupied by the motor area in front. It commences at the bottom of the fissure of Rolando and extends backwards over rather more than half the exposed area of the post-central convolution. It reaches down to near the Sylvian fissure and extends over on to the mesial aspect of the brain. Furthermore, it is probable that sensation in any given part lies on more or less the same level as the corresponding motor area.

Immediately posterior to the tactile area and occupying the posterior and upper part of the post-central convolution, the area responsible for *muscle-sense* is situated.

Stereognosis—memory pictures, object perception, &c.—is referred to the superior parietal lobe.

Primary visual impressions are received in the occipital lobe, more especially on the mesial aspect thereof.

Finally, the four areas concerned in **speech**—motor speech, writing, reading, and hearing—are anatomically separated from one another and yet closely associated, so much so that one can hardly be involved without the other. The motor speech centre of Broca has already been mentioned as occupying—in right-handed individuals—the posterior part of the third left frontal convolution. Writing lies immediately above and in front, in the posterior part of the middle frontal gyrus, auditory impressions are received in the posterior and upper part of the first temporo-sphenoidal lobe, whilst the power of reading is dependent on the integrity of the supra-marginal and angular gyri (see also Fig. 57).

Smell and Taste lie in close relation to the anterior pole of the temporo-sphenoidal lobes.

CHAPTER II

THE SPECIAL TECHNIQUE IN OPERATIONS ON THE SKULL AND BRAIN

Preparatory treatment. Where possible at least two or three days should elapse between the admission of the patient and the day of operation. During this period the patient should be confined to bed with all possible cheerful surroundings. The bowels are regulated and the diet restricted.

The extent to which the scalp should be shaved and the time at which this procedure should be carried out vary according to the circumstances of the case. Much depends on the sex and age of the patient and the nature of the proposed operation. Insomuch, however, as it is always inadvisable to prolong the period of anæsthesia, it follows that the shaving should be carried out previous to the operation. With regard to extent, each case must be judged on its own merits. For instance, considerable concession must be made in the case of a young woman on whom the surgeon proposes to carry out a subtemporal decompression operation, and in the case of a neurotic or elderly patient who is the subject of trigeminal neuralgia. There can, however, be no question that the limitation of operative field advocated by some surgeons is fraught with considerable risk from the point of view of wound infection.

If the question be discussed with the patient the surgeon will find the ground cut away from beneath his feet, and that he has to make considerable and inadvisable concessions. Taking everything into consideration, although it is seldom necessary to shave the whole head, I am accustomed to order such preparation as will allow of a very wide margin. To shave the whole head is not only unnecessary but is also exceedingly distasteful to the patient. The front, back, or side of the head should be prepared only—on the morning of the operation, so as to allow of a comfortable night's rest. After shaving, the scalp is thoroughly cleansed with soap and water, and the head surrounded by a sterilized towel. The final skin sterilization is carried out when the patient is under the anæsthetic.

The iodine method has always given satisfactory results, the skin being painted, half an hour previous to operation, with a 2½ per cent. solution of iodine, and again after the administration of the anæsthetic. Still, I cannot avoid a certain penchant for the older method—sponging with ether to remove the fats, washing with a 1 in 500 spirit solution of biniodide of mercury, and finally douching with a weaker mercury solution.

Precautions against the development of shock. It is almost inevitable that all serious head-operations should be associated with some degree of shock, though, from my experience, I am convinced that, with due precautions, it is far less serious than is generally supposed. The development of shock is very largely dependent on the amount of blood lost during the operative procedures. The various methods adopted to control hæmorrhage are enumerated later. In addition, attention should be paid to the following details :—

1. Half an hour before the operation an injection of a quarter of a grain of morphia should be given hypodermically. The addition of one-hundredth of a grain of atropin, recommended by some surgeons, interferes somewhat, by its action on the pupil, with the data deemed necessary for the administration of the anæsthetic.

2. The theatre should be maintained at a temperature between 65 and 75 degrees Fahrenheit. The table should be suitably warmed.

3. The patient's body should be covered with warm blankets, and, in the more serious cases, the lower extremities may be bandaged, from below upwards.

It has been recommended that the brain, if exposed, should be protected from the cooling effects of the atmosphere by irrigation with saline solution at a temperature between 110 and 115 degrees Fahrenheit. Personally I prefer to keep the operative field as dry as possible.

An assistant should be told off, whose duty lies in keeping a record both of blood-pressure and pulse-rate. The lowering of blood-pressure is the surest guide to the surgeon of approaching danger.

It is often considered that rapidity of operation is essential. There can be no greater error. To ensure success the utmost care must be taken to control the loss of blood, for which it is essential that each step of the operation should be carried out deliberately and carefully.

The anæsthetic. Needless to say, it is essential that the surgeon should have at his disposal an anæsthetist of great experience in head operations.

Ether is regarded with favour in the United States, and in other countries, but we prefer chloroform on the ground that, by its lowering effect on the blood-pressure, there is less venous oozing, and added to this there is probably less tendency to post-operative vomiting. I have recently had the opportunity of seeing the open ether method as carried out in the States, on one occasion for an operation lasting four hours, and in this and in other cases the patient left the operation table in excellent condition, recovering also rapidly from the effects of the anæsthetic.

The lowering of blood-pressure as produced by chloroform might be advanced as an argument against the use of that drug, shock being the greatest danger to be feared in these operations. Still, I must say that I prefer chloroform so long as it is administered by a skilled anæsthetist.

In any case, it is advisable to have oxygen ready to hand.

The position of the patient. Special tables have been invented and special positions advised. Thus, the dental-chair position is recommended for operations on the Gasserian ganglion, and, in cerebellar operations, it is urged that the patient should be turned on his face, the forehead resting on a tripod, the shoulders on supports fastened to the head of the table. Personally, I do not consider that any special arrangements are required in the majority of cases. Much can be done with sand-bags and firm pillows. Even in the exposure of one cerebellar hemisphere I prefer to utilize the semi-prone position.

In bilateral cerebellar exposure, however, the patient must be placed on his face, the forehead resting on special supports, and the shoulders on props or pillows so as to allow of free entry of air into the chest. In such cases the anæsthetic is administered from below.

I am not enthusiastic over the so-called dental-chair position, but the operating table should be constructed in such a manner that the head and shoulders of the patient can be well raised, the body being inclined to the floor at an angle of about 30–40 degrees.

Preparation of the operative field. When the patient is fully under the anæsthetic, the final cleansing of the scalp is carried out and the operative field cut off from all possible sources of infection. In the States, in Cushing's clinic, the anæsthetist is completely covered with a large sterilized sheet, which is fastened to the head of the patient. In this country we prefer that our anæsthetist should have full knowledge of the progress of the operation, and I think that the advantages are with us. In any case, the whole head is enveloped in gauze, two or three layers thick and about 18 inches square. This sheet is thrown over the patient's head and maintained in position by means of the scalp-tourniquet (see pp. 14, 15). Around this sterilized towels are arranged, either fastened to one another or stitched to the scalp. When the operation is conducted in the temporal region the towels, unless fastened to the skin by means of a few sutures or safety-pins, tend to become displaced, and by so doing add to the risk of wound infection.

THE CONTROL OF HÆMORRHAGE

Hæmorrhage from vessels of the scalp. All surgeons must have appreciated the difficulty attendant on the application of forceps to, and the ligature of, divided scalp-vessels. The patient may lose a considerable quantity of blood, and much valuable time will be wasted before the more essential part of the operation is commenced. All this can, under ordinary circumstances, be avoided by the use of the scalp-tourniquet. As used by Cushing it consists of a rubber ring fashioned after the style of an Esmarch's tourniquet, encircling the head and passing from the lower frontal region in front, above the ears, to the lower occipital region behind. A median tape, passing from glabella to occiput, prevents any tendency for the tourniquet to slip down over the eyes, at the same time acting as a convenient landmark for the superior longitudinal sinus.

The tourniquet, when applied with the correct pressure, should, under ordinary circumstances, completely control all hæmorrhage from the divided scalp-vessels. It should be noted, however, that bleeding will be rather increased than otherwise if the tourniquet be so loosely applied as to impede the venous return without compressing the scalp arteries. A little experience will soon enable the operator to gauge the requisite pressure.

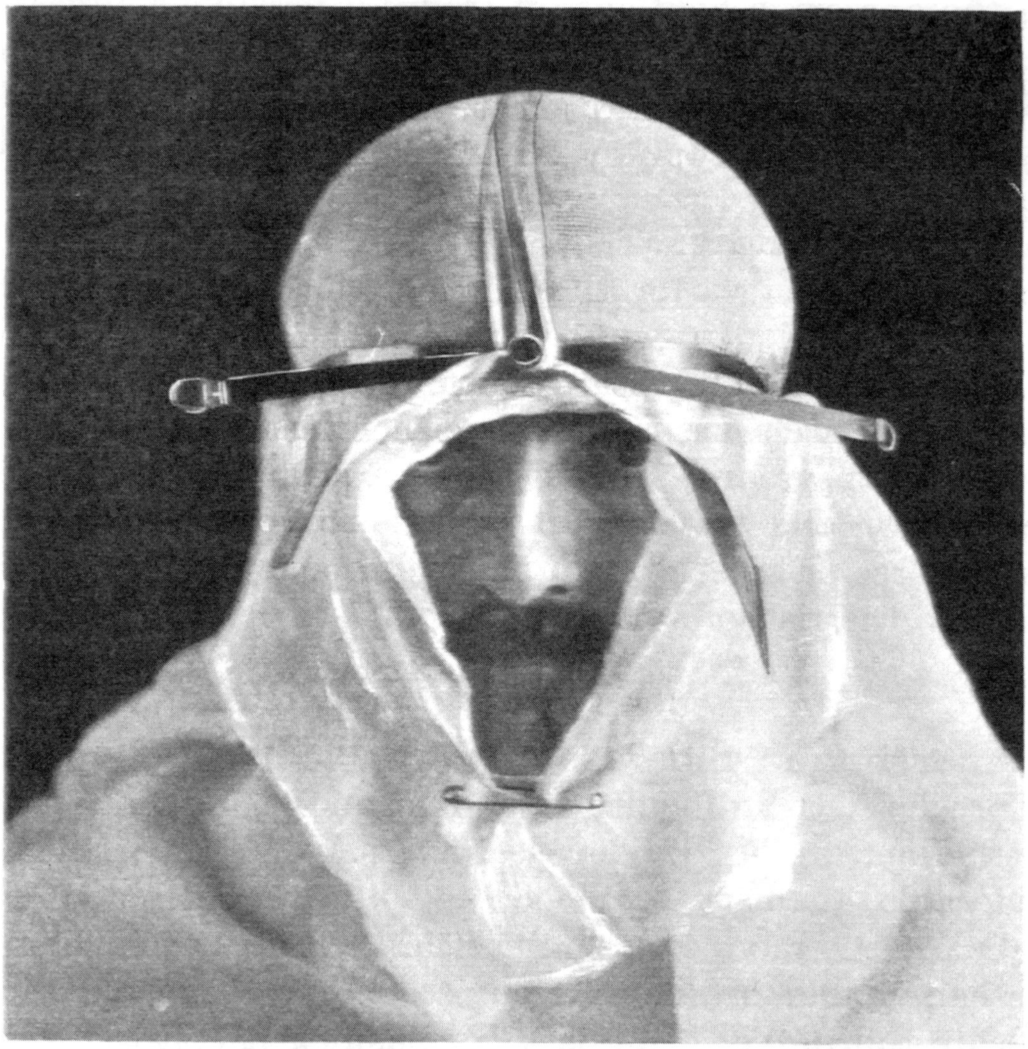

FIG. 4. THE SCALP-TOURNIQUET. *Front View.*

There is one other exception to the satisfactory working of the scalp-tourniquet. In the presence of a superficial cerebral tumour, especially when of a malignant nature, the normal communication between the intra- and extra-cranial vascular systems may be so exaggerated that those scalp-vessels which receive diploic and emissary venous communications will give rise to some trouble. This difficulty should be overcome—not by rapidity in the formation and turning down of the flap—but by clipping each vessel as exposed or divided, by the application of pressure and by foraminal occlusion (see also p. 17).

I found Cushing's tourniquet rather inconvenient in its application, and, after various modifications, am accustomed to use the one depicted in the illustration. It consists of two flat metal bands

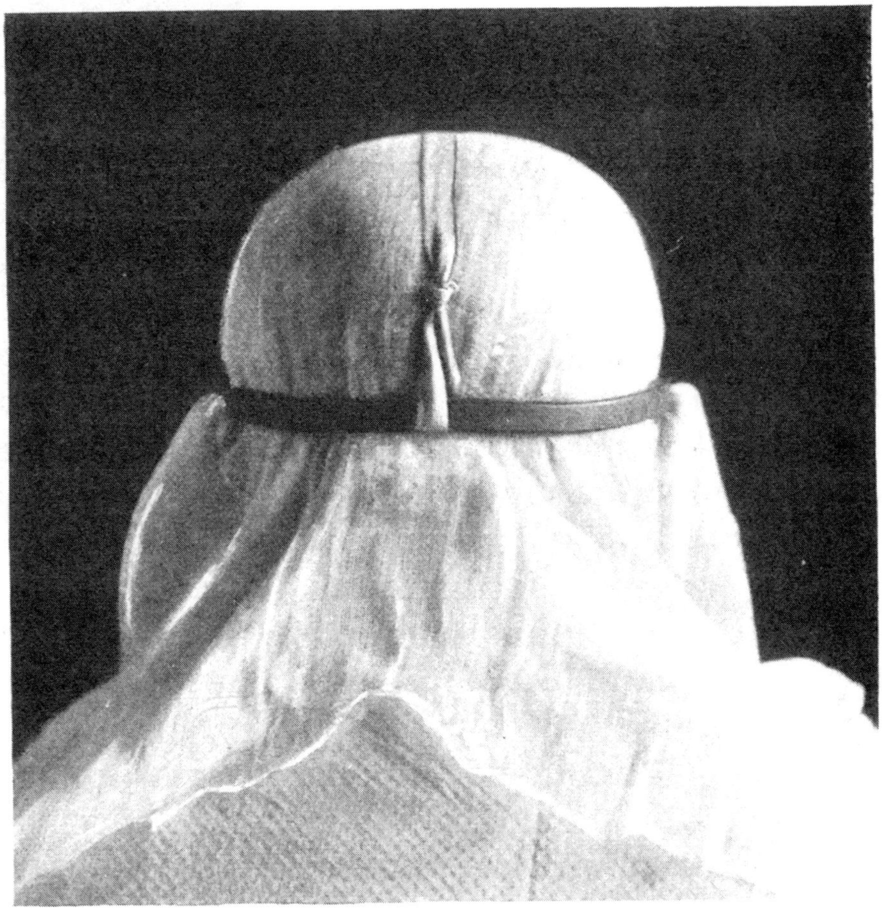

FIG. 5. THE SCALP-TOURNIQUET. *Back View.*

connected posteriorly by a strong rubber connecting link, the two bands passing in front through a metal fixation piece possessing a screw which, when tightened up, allows of the maintenance of the desired pressure. The median tape, previously mentioned, helps to keep the tourniquet in position.

The tourniquet is applied as follows: the whole head is enveloped in gauze—two or three layers thick, and cut to the size and shape of a large handkerchief. The tourniquet is slipped over the head, as low down as possible, and then tightened up. The median tape, having a loop behind through which the tourniquet passes, is laid in the middle line and tied round the screw on the fixation piece.

The gauze should then be moistened with saline solution or some mild antiseptic, so that it clings tightly to the underlying scalp and becomes sufficiently translucent to allow of the recognition of any underlying landmarks that may have been previously mapped out with the scalpel, iodine, silver nitrate, or aniline pencil.

The scalp-flap is then framed by incisions carried down to the bone, through gauze and scalp, in one sweep. The flap is turned down and covered with gauze. By the adoption of this method hæmorrhage from scalp-vessels is efficiently controlled and the risk of wound infection is reduced to a minimum.

After the completion of the operation, the scalp-flap is approximated and sewn into position, first by numerous buried fine silk sutures bringing together the aponeurotic layer of the scalp, and finally by a few silk or salmon-gut sutures passed through the skin itself. Gauze dressings are applied, the tourniquet loosened, and a roll-gauze bandage quickly applied circumferentially around the head, low down over the forehead and occipital region. This roll bandage in reality takes the place of the tourniquet, but is, of course, applied with moderate pressure only.

If the wool and bandage now applied over all should include the ears, these two organs should be well covered with vaseline. Few things are more uncomfortable to the patient than the contact of wool and bandage to the ears.

The tourniquet should be utilized whenever possible. In operations, however, that are conducted near the base of the skull—subtemporal decompression, cerebellar exploration, &c.—the surgeon, in his effort at hæmostasis, must rely on the application of digital pressure on either side of the incision, the more careful exposure of the vessels, and the application of forceps as soon as they are seen or divided, or by the utilization of Vorschütz's hæmostatic safety-pins.

Other methods of controlling scalp-bleeding are as follows :—

1. Kredel's hæmostatic sutures, passed with a large curved needle which slides along the bone and emerges about 5 to 7 cm. from the

point of introduction. The silk ligatures are then tied over metal plates, so curved as to lie flush with the surface of the skull in the particular region involved. Four of these plates would be used in the formation of an osteoplastic flap, one on the distal side of each of the three scalp incisions, and one along the base of the flap.

2. The enclosure of the proposed incision by a running suture which, passing down to the bone, emerges about 1 inch further on, then so to speak repeating itself in part until the whole region is surrounded. The ligatures are then tightened up. This method takes some time in its application, and presents no advantages over the scalp-tourniquet.

3. The blocking of the main arterial supply—temporal, occipital, and supra-orbital vessels—by modified safety-pins, mass ligatures, &c. Arterial compression by means of the modified safety-pin as suggested by Vorschütz will be found most useful in those operations in which the scalp-tourniquet cannot be utilized—subtemporal decompression, &c.

Hæmorrhage from the bone. Severe bleeding may take place from the mastoid and other emissary veins, and from the open mouths of those abnormally dilated diploic and emissary veins so often encountered in the exposure of an underlying dural or superficial cerebral tumour. The foramina in the bone, when exposed, must be occluded as quickly as possible. For this purpose we have the following methods at our disposal—plugging with small bone or wooden pegs, blockage with minute plugs of cotton-wool, and the utilization of Horsley's wax, smeared over the part and well pressed home.

Hæmorrhage may also occur from the bone during trephining, more especially when the operation is conducted over that part of the anterior division of the middle meningeal artery which runs through a channel in the spheno-parietal region. Here the disk of bone should be removed as quickly as possible and the channel plugged with pegs, cotton-wool, or wax.

Oozing from the raw surface of the cut bone is controlled by rubbing in aseptic wax, or by the crushing together of the inner and outer tables.

Hæmorrhage from the dural vessels. In this case the bleeding may occur from three sources, meningeal veins—often of considerable size when related to neighbouring tumour-formation—the middle meningeal artery, and the venous sinuses of the brain.

Hæmorrhage from meningeal veins may be arrested by one or other of the following methods :—

1. Gentle pressure as applied either by dry gauze, or wet gauze soaked in saline solution at a temperature between 110 and 115 degrees Fahrenheit.

2. The application of a piece of muscle to the bleeding-point. This method was, I believe, first introduced by Sir Victor Horsley.

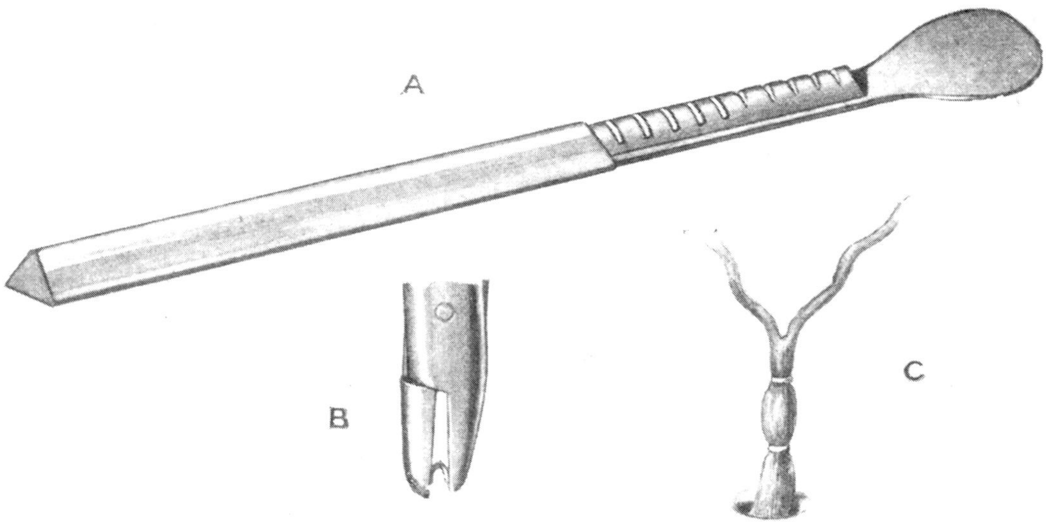

FIG. 6. CUSHING'S CLIPS. A, The holder of the clips ; B, A clip ready to be applied ; C, Two clips applied to the middle meningeal artery.

Some muscle is usually available for the purpose, usually the temporal muscle. A small portion of muscle is snipped off, spread out as a flat muscular pad, the bleeding area dried, and the graft quickly applied. It soon adheres, and usually arrests the hæmorrhage.

3. The application of a ligature. This method is placed last, being the most difficult. It is usually necessary to underrun the bleeding-point with a fine needle threaded with the finest of silk. It presents the disadvantage in that the needle may perforate the dura mater and puncture one of the superficial cerebral veins.

Hæmorrhage from the middle meningeal artery may be controlled by ligature or torsion, and added to these methods we have one other, recently introduced by Cushing—silver wire 'clips'. These clips are U-shaped, loaded on a magazine, picked up as required in the jaws of a specially indented forceps, and clipped on to the vessel—usually one on either side of the bleeding-point.

Hæmorrhage from venous sinuses is dealt with on p. 150.

Hæmorrhage from the superficial vessels of the brain. This form of hæmorrhage, one of the most troublesome complications arising in head-operations, most commonly results from hasty or careless opening of the dura mater. Thus, when the dura is incised in a case of greatly increased intracranial pressure, the brain herniates suddenly outwards, and the incautious use of the knife will damage one of the dilated superficial cortical veins. The dura should always be opened with the greatest care, the knife being passed lightly over the membrane till the pia-arachnoid is exposed, when the dural margins are lifted up with small tenaculum forceps and the membrane slit up with blunt-pointed scissors or on a grooved director.

In the event of injury, the bleeding may often be controlled by light pressure with dry gauze, or wet gauze wrung out in hot saline solution as described above. If this fails, a very fine silk ligature may be passed beneath the vessel on either side of the site of bleeding. This procedure is not easy to accomplish, the tissues are so soft and friable. However, every effort must be made to arrest the bleeding, for not only does the hæmorrhage obscure the field of operation, but the presence of a blood-clot beneath the dura mater will lead at a later date to the formation of adhesions between the various membranes of the brain—a potent cause of headache, epilepsy, &c.

THE OPENING OF THE SKULL

Two methods are adopted in the exposure of meninges and brain—craniectomy and craniotomy.

Craniectomy implies the formation of a scalp-flap, exposure of the bone, trephining of the skull, and enlargement of the gap to the required size and shape.

Craniotomy implies the formation of a flap of scalp and bone in one, and the exposure of an area of dura and brain directly proportionate to the size of the bone-flap.

Craniectomy. After the application of protective gauze and tourniquet, the scalp-flap is framed according to the requirements of the case. If the tourniquet is used, the knife is entered at one extremity of the proposed flap, carried down to the bone—through gauze and scalp in one—and the incision completed in a single sweep. Under other circumstances, digital pressure is applied to the main flap-supplying vessel, e. g. the temporal artery over the base of the zygoma, or else Kredel's clamps or Vorschütz's hæmostatic safety-pins are passed in such a manner as to control bleeding from the main supplying vessel. In the event of bleeding, the surgeon goes along quietly, deepening his incision and seizing each vessel as exposed.

In turning down the scalp-flap it is usually recommended that the pericranium should be included. This is quite unnecessary, and,

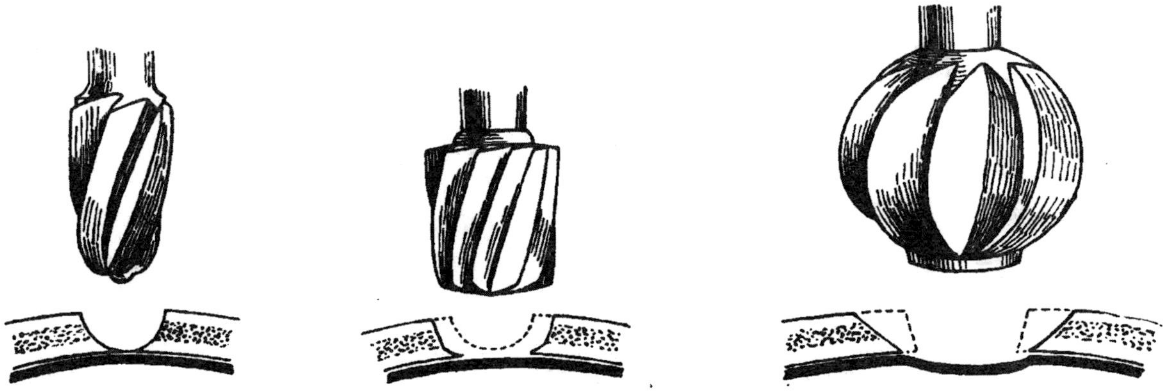

Fig. 7. Hudson's Trephine. Showing the usual method of using the spiral perforator, spiral follower, and enlarging burr.

under certain circumstances, should certainly be omitted (see p. 129). It should be stripped away from the underlying bone as required.

The trephining may be carried out with the hand-trephine, or by means of saws, burrs, and trephines driven by electricity. With the exception of a few words on Hudson's trephine, I do not propose to discuss the relative advantages and disadvantages of these mechanically-driven instruments. I hold the opinion that the hand-driven instrument is sufficiently rapid in its work, that it is infinitely safer, and that the surgeon should accustom and perfect himself with those instruments which are to him most convenient and most portable. He will not always be conducting his operations in a perfectly equipped hospital, much of his work will be carried out in the nursing home or in the country. Whatever method be adopted, the operator should use those instruments to which he is most accustomed.

Hudson's trephine is shaped after the style of the carpenter's brace and is fitted with three cutting heads—the perforator, the follower, and the enlarging burr. It is claimed that injury to the dura and brain is impossible, the instrument becoming automatically locked so soon as the resistance of the internal table is overcome, a thin film of bone being pushed in front of the advancing head. I have had the opportunity of using this instrument, and so far as my experience goes it answers all requirements. Still, I prefer the ordinary hand-trephine so long as it satisfies certain requirements. It must be of simple mechanism and strong, the handle of good size and shaped to fit the hand, the shaft and head so interlocked as to allow of no independent movement, and the hollow head sharply toothed and bevelled externally, in continuity with the teeth, for a distance of half an inch. The bevelling is so arranged that the actual cutting process is only effected during supination of the hand and forearm. The pin of the trephine should not project beyond the cutting edge for a greater distance than about ·2 cm. This pin should be readily removable.

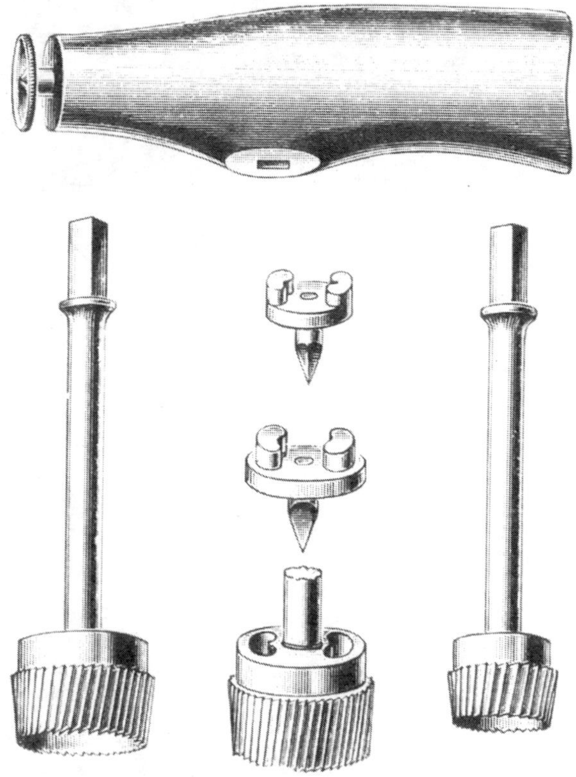

FIG. 8. THE HAND-TREPHINE.

The pattern which I am accustomed to use is depicted in Fig. 8. The trephines are kept in three sizes—diameter $\frac{1}{2}$, 1, and $1\frac{1}{2}$ inches. The intermediate size is used for ordinary trephining, the small one for the formation of the osteoplastic flap, the large for the removal of a disk of bone which includes within its circumference the area involved in some depressed and punctured fractures (see p. 133).

The site of trephining may be fixed by the introduction of a bradawl through the scalp, so indenting the external table that the spot can be verified on turning down the scalp-flap. The pin of the trephine is there applied, and the trephine directed at right angles to

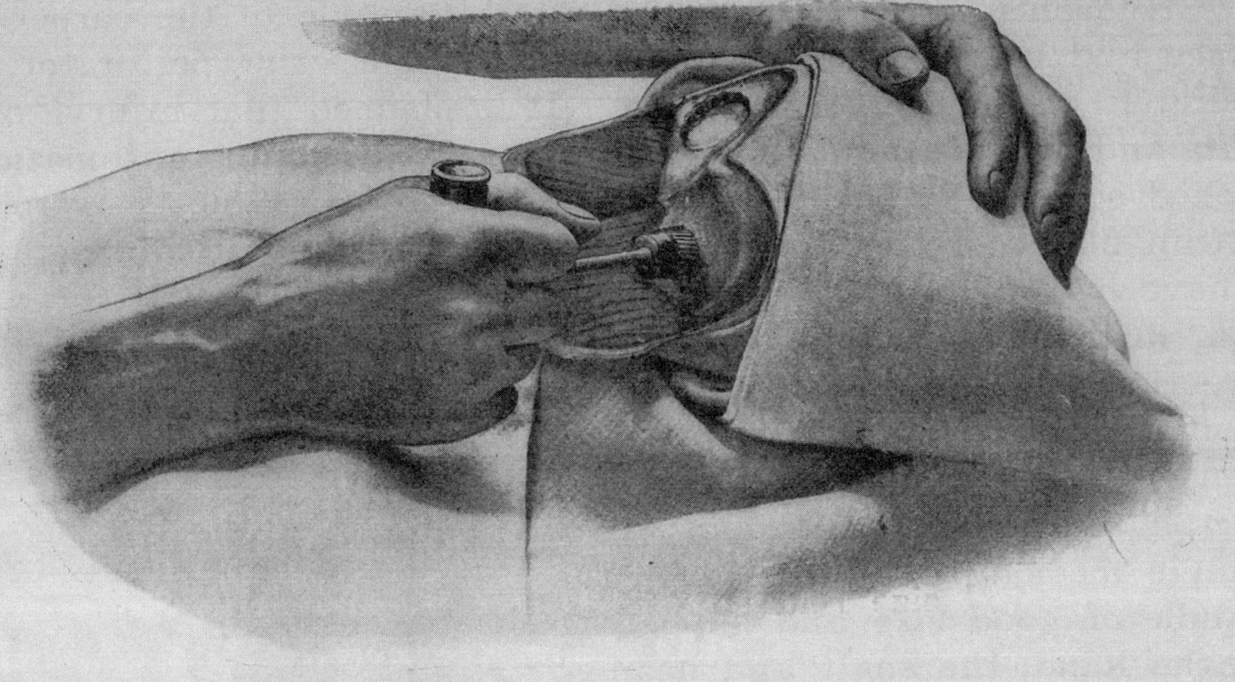

Fig. 9.

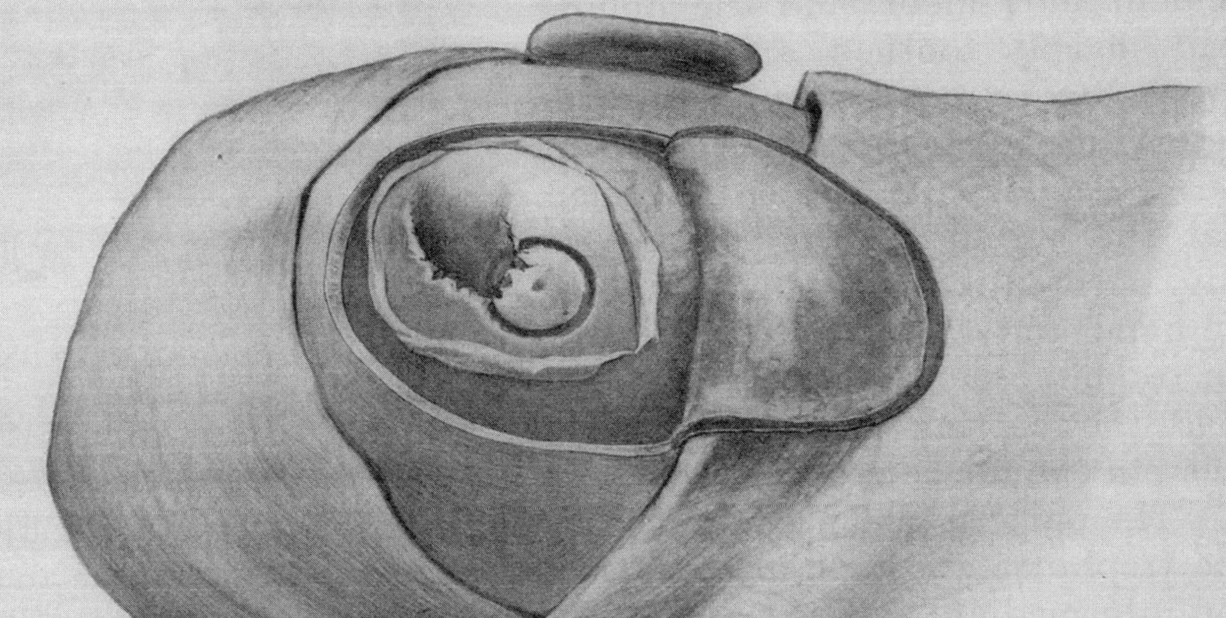

Fig. 10.

To show the Technique of Trephining. Fig. 9 illustrates the act of trephining for cerebellar exposure. Fig. 10 shows a trephine-disk to one side of a depressed fracture.

the surface of the skull, or at that angle which is suited to the region attacked. The pin is discarded when a sufficient groove has been attained. The trephine must be kept under perfect control, muscular effort only being required during the act of supination.

The firm nature of the external table will be readily appreciated ; so soon as this resistance is overcome the trephine will be felt to

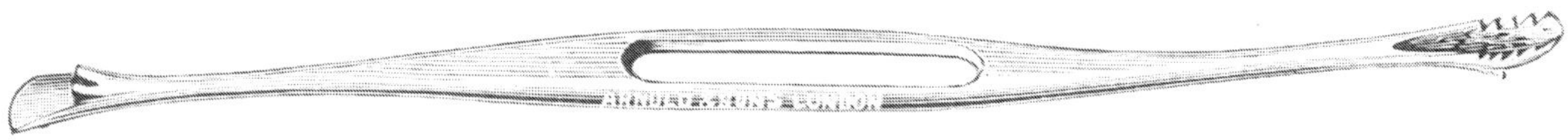

FIG. 11. HORSLEY'S DISK OR BONE ELEVATOR.

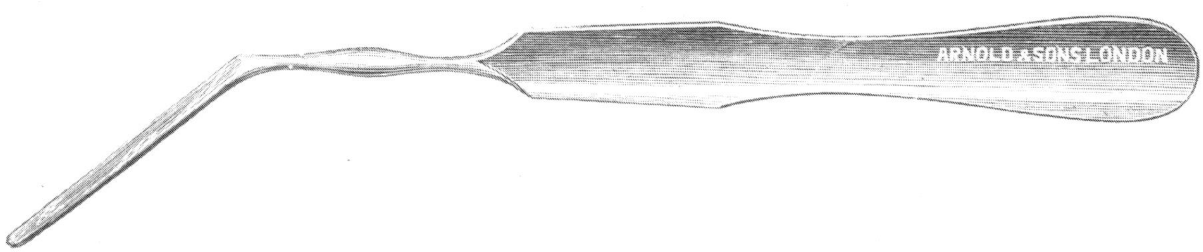

FIG. 12. HORSLEY'S DURAL SEPARATOR.

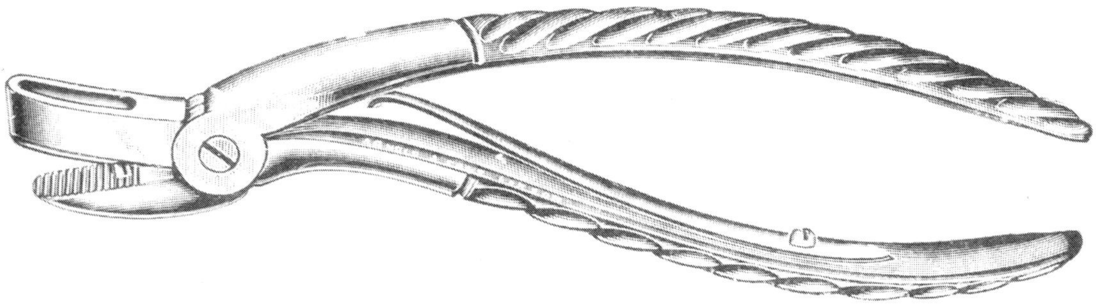

FIG. 13. KEEN-HOFFMANN'S CRANIECTOMY FORCEPS.

be cutting its way through a softer structure, whilst the increased bone-dust and venous oozing will make it evident that the instrument is biting its way through the diploic tissue. Greater resistance is again encountered on meeting the internal table, warning the operator that the time has come when greater care must be exercised. The bone-dust must be wiped away, the teeth of the trephine cleansed with nail-brush or sponge, and the depth of the groove estimated. The groove should be of the same depth throughout its circumference, or of that depth which is suited to the part involved.

The readiness of the disk for removal is best demonstrated

by digital pressure. When it gives to that pressure, whether in whole or in part, the elevator may be applied and the fragment removed.

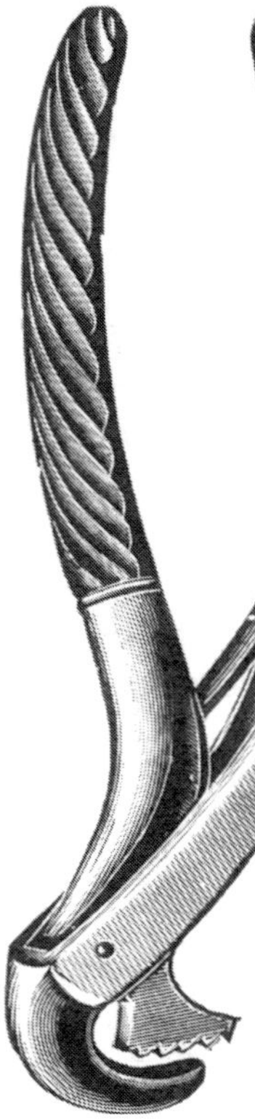

FIG. 14.
LANE'S FULCRUM CRANIECTOMY FORCEPS.

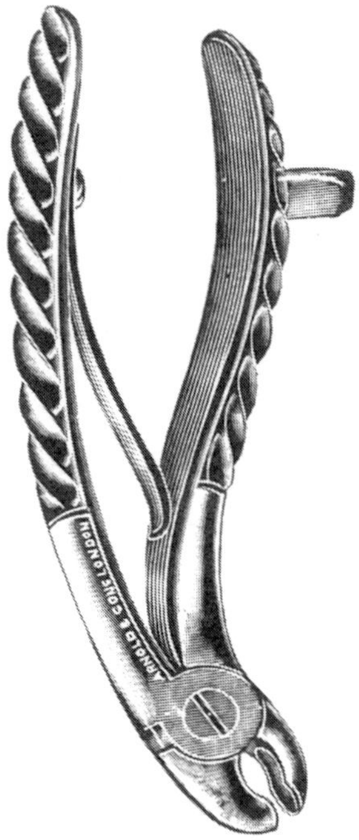

FIG. 15.
HORSLEY'S GOUGE FORCEPS.

In the temporal and cerebellar regions special care is required by reason of the absence of diploic tissue.

It is impossible to lay too much stress on the necessity of avoiding injury to underlying dura and meningeal vessels. Injury to these structures not infrequently upsets the whole plan of campaign.

The enlargement of the trephine hole to the required size and shape. Previous to any attempt at enlargement of the trephine hole, the dura mater must be separated from the bone with the aid of Horsley's dural separator or other suitable instrument. Of the many patterns of craniectomy forceps, the following will be found to suit all requirements :—

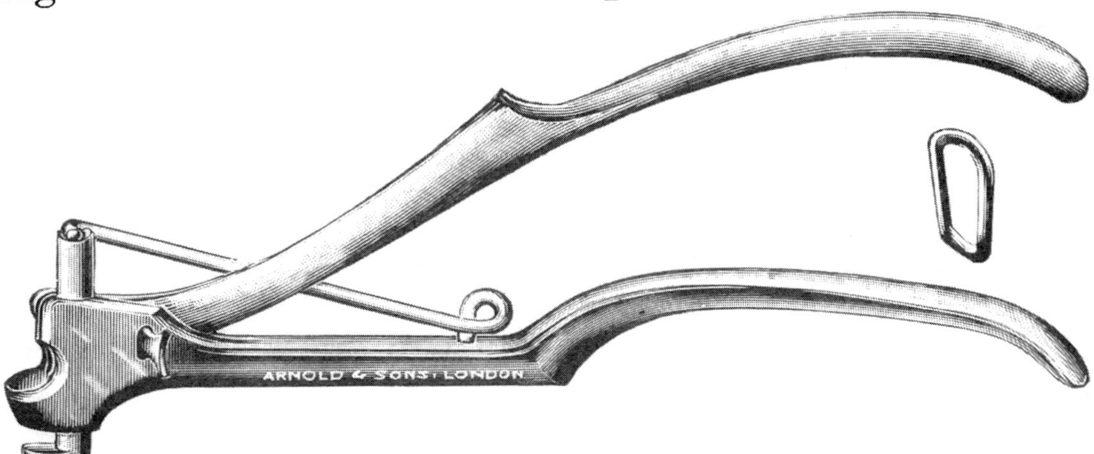

FIG. 16. DE VILBISS'S CRANIECTOMY FORCEPS.

Keen-Hoffmann. The visceral blade is introduced between the dura and the bone and 'morcellement' carried out. It is essential that the surgeon should not be too greedy, resting content with the removal of small fragments at a time.

Lane's fulcrum forceps. They possess great mechanical advantage and are mainly suited for the rapid removal of large portions of bone.

Horsley's nibbling or rongeur forceps. This instrument is mainly utilized in the smoothing and refreshing of sharp edges of bone, and in the 'morcellement' of the thinner portions of the skull—temporal and cerebellar regions.

De Vilbiss's forceps. A clever contrivance whereby the operator is enabled to cut a narrow channel in the bone. Mainly utilized in the formation of the osteoplastic flap.

Craniotomy. Craniotomy, or osteoplastic resection of the skull, was first carried out by Wagner. It is proposed to describe that method only which, by experience, has been found to meet all requirements—the formation of the osteoplastic flap by means of the hand-trephine, Gigli's saw, and de Vilbiss's forceps.

The protective gauze dressing and scalp-tourniquet are applied as before. A large ▽-shaped incision is made in such a manner as to include the area which it is desired to expose. The two vertical limbs of the incision should converge to such a degree as to allow of the subsequent ready fracture of the flap along its base. The knife is entered at one extremity, carried down to the bone, and the three incisions rapidly made, one after the other. Along the line of each of the three incisions, the pericranium is stripped away from the bone so as to allow of adequate exposure. At the anterior and posterior angles of the flap the tissues are retracted a little more, permitting the application of a half-inch diameter trephine. Here the two trephine-holes are bored—with the usual precautions against damage to the dura mater—and the two disks of bone elevated and removed.

Between these two trephine-holes the dura mater is separated from the bone and the special director introduced, entering at the one hole, emerging at the other, and lying throughout between the dura and the bone. The saw is now passed along the groove of the director, the handles affixed, and the bone intervening between the two trephine-holes divided, not straight out to the surface, but bevelled or cut in such an oblique manner that the bone-flap, when replaced, rests on a ledge (see Figs. 17–19). The sawing process generates considerable heat, and the assistant should be instructed to keep up irrigation with saline solution or sterilized water. The sawing is carried out by steady side-to-side traction, without jerks;

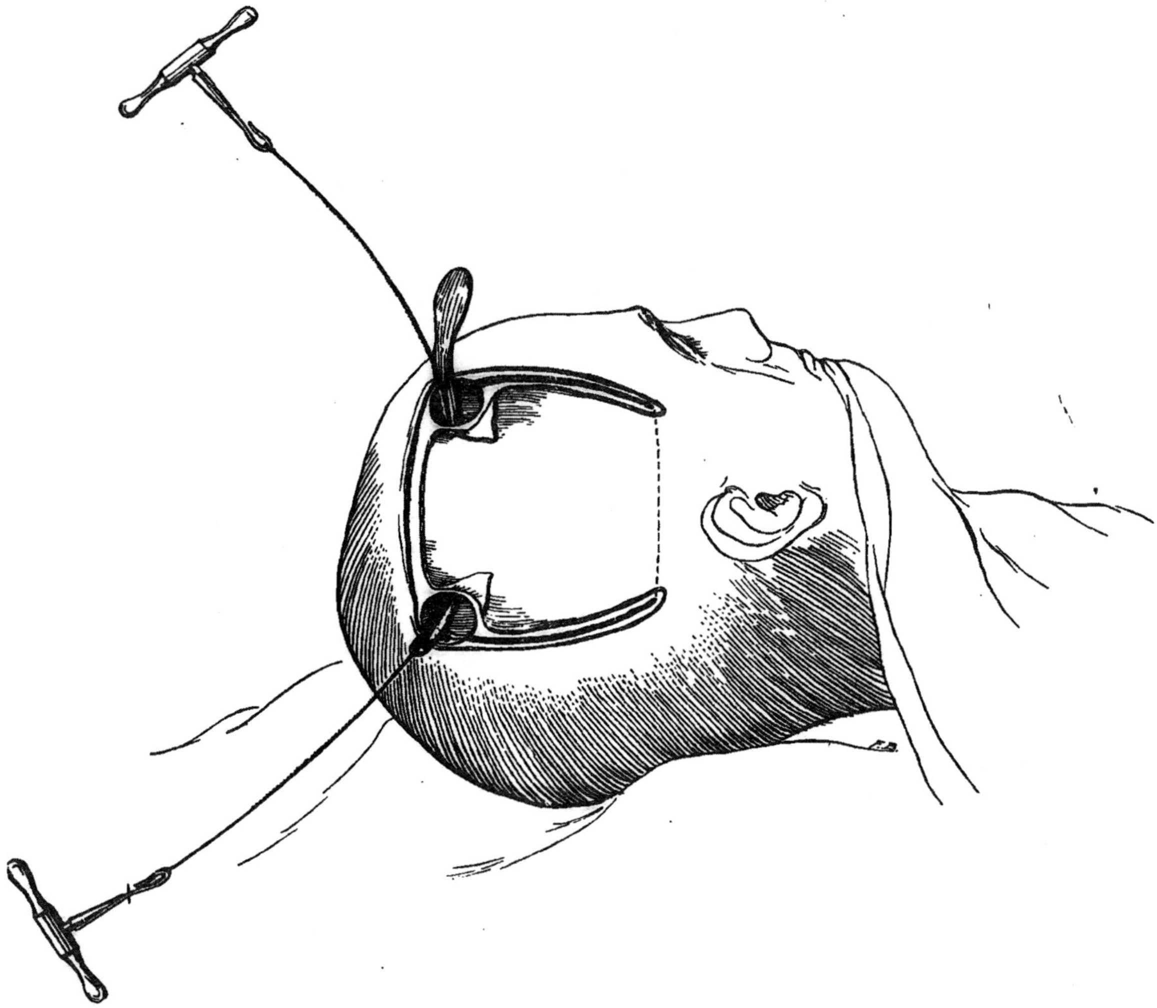

FIG. 17. FIRST STAGE IN THE FORMATION OF AN OSTEOPLASTIC FLAP. Gigli's saw, protected from the dura mater by the special director, passing between the two trephine-holes. For further description, see text.

if the saw breaks, the special handle may be attached, thus obviating the necessity of introducing a new saw.

The dura is now separated from the bone along the line of the two vertical incisions, and the visceral blade of de Vilbiss's forceps insinuated beneath the bone, starting at one trephine-hole and working downwards to the lower limit of the incision. It is essential that the operator should be satisfied with the ' morcellement ' of small portions of bone at each bite of the instrument. At the lower end of each

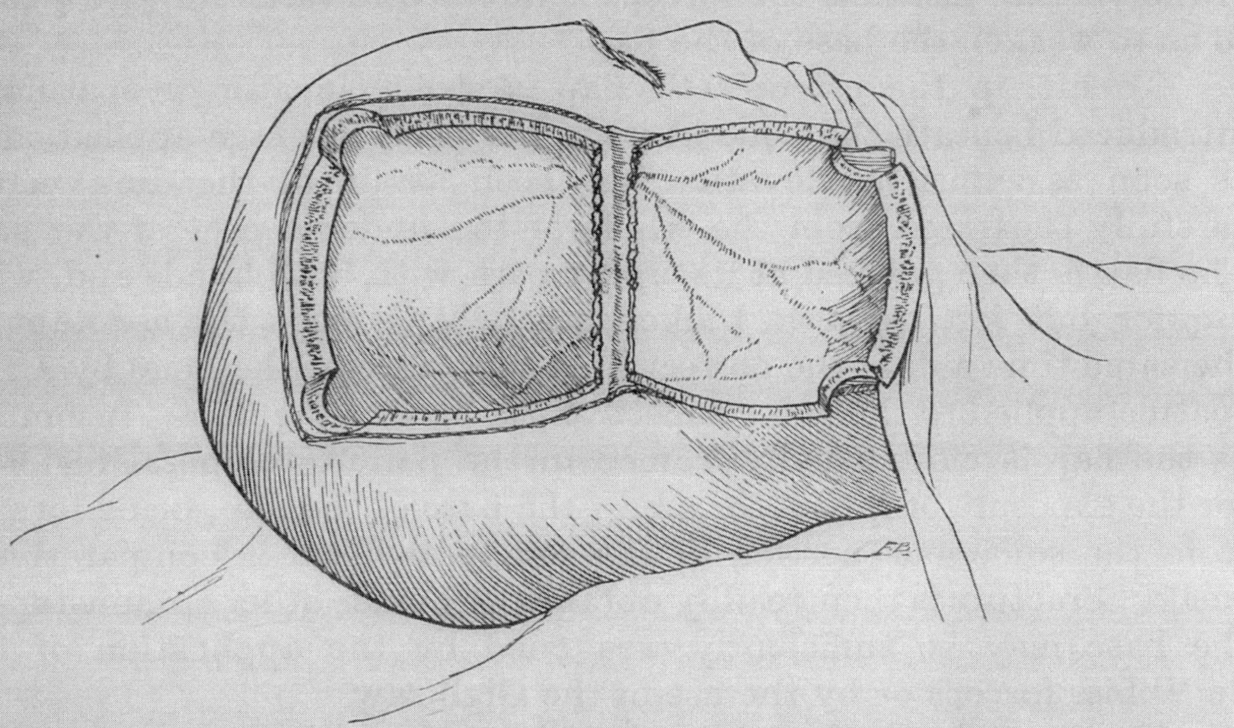

FIG. 18. SECOND STAGE IN THE FORMATION OF AN OSTEOPLASTIC FLAP. The bone-flap turned down and the dura mater exposed.

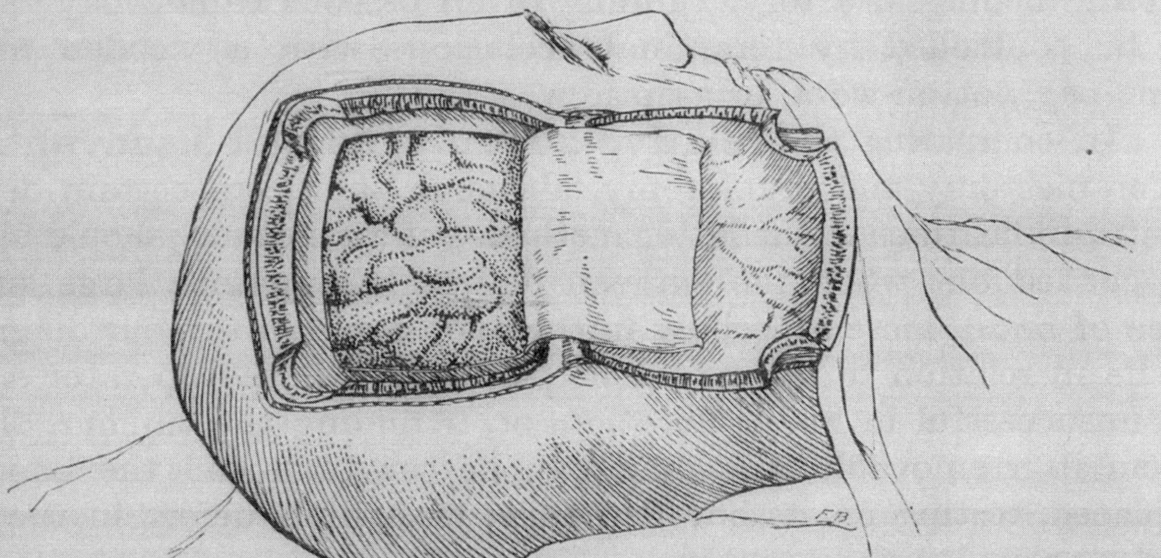

FIG. 19. THIRD STAGE IN THE FORMATION OF AN OSTEOPLASTIC FLAP. The dural flap turned down and the brain exposed. Note the relation of the scalp, bone, and dural incisions to one another.

of the vertical incisions the forceps is directed inwards for $\frac{1}{4}$ to $\frac{1}{2}$ inch so as to weaken the base of the flap.

To lift up the osteoplastic flap, a stout elevator or spatula is introduced beneath the bone at its upper part, leverage applied, and, as soon as sufficient elevation has been attained, the dura mater carefully separated from the whole of the under aspect of the flap. The flap is then grasped at its upper part with both hands and, with a quick but forcible jerk, broken across at its base, the assistant at the same time aiding the correct linear fracture of the bone by a flat spatula applied to the outer aspect of the base of the flap. Insomuch as the flap is most usually framed in the parieto-temporal region—for the exposure of the motor area—the base of the flap, being formed from the squamous portion of the temporal bone, is comparatively weak. Fracture is then readily obtained. Under other circumstances the base may be sufficiently weakened by the application of the de Vilbiss forceps or by the use of the Gigli saw.

The bone-flap is thrown back and enveloped in gauze. Its basal region is examined for a possible injury to meningeal vessels. In the event of such complications the bleeding vessel is clipped, ligatured, or underrun. Possibly some branch of the anterior division of the middle meningeal artery, running in an osseous canal, may require to be controlled by foraminal occlusion—with a wooden match, bone peg, cotton-wool, or aseptic wax.

In comparing the **relative advantages and disadvantages** of craniectomy and craniotomy, although there are certain definite contra-indications to the latter method, yet craniotomy should always be carried out when the surgeon desires to expose a large surface area of brain, more especially in the exposure of a tumour diagnosed to lie in relation to the motor cortex. Even if the operator should be unsuccessful in his exploration, or, if finding the tumour, should deem it irremovable, the dura can be sewn up and the bone-flap replaced, resting on its bevelled edge, with little defect in the skull and a normal surface contour.

The three main disadvantages to craniotomy are as follows:—(1) the operation can seldom be done under much less than thirty minutes; (2) there is some slight risk of complication through injury to the middle meningeal artery; and (3) the dura mater may be so adherent to the bone as to be torn in the process of flap-elevation. Time, however, is usually of little importance; bleeding from the middle meningeal artery may be controlled, and dural lesions may be avoided by careful technique. In general, the advantages of osteoplastic resection greatly outweigh the disadvantages.

The more definite contra-indications to the formation of the bone-flap are as follows :—

1. This operation is unnecessarily severe in most cases of intracranial hæmorrhage, e. g. from the middle meningeal artery. It is also usually impracticable by reason of the associated damage to the bones of the vault and base.

2. It is contra-indicated in operations conducted for the exposure of the Gasserian ganglion, its root and its branches (trigeminal neuralgia). In these operations it is essential that the operator should get down as low as possible towards the base of the skull.

3. It is contra-indicated in operations conducted in the cerebellar region. Even after cerebellar exposure by craniectomy, the surgeon is working in a sufficiently confined space. The presence of a bone-flap only adds further difficulty and complication. Added to this is the fact that the thin wall of the cerebellar fossa is not adapted to osteoplastic flap-formation.

Opening the dura mater. Reference has already been made to the great importance of opening the dura in such a manner as to avoid injury to the underlying superficial cerebral vessels (see p. 19). It may be incised in a crucial manner or by flap-formation. Flaps are usually to be preferred if the surgeon desires to have the widest possible view of the brain surface. In the formation of the flap, advantage should be taken of the vessels that minister to its vitality. Thus, in the lateral region of the head, the base lies below, the middle meningeal artery supplying the flap. Under special circumstances, the blood-supply may be disregarded ; the flap never sloughs, so far as my experience goes.

Sewing up the dura mater. Considerable difficulty may be experienced in sewing up the dura—by reason of the bulging of the brain. How these difficulties may be overcome is dealt with on p. 236. The edges should be united by numerous fine silk sutures.

Replacement of the osteoplastic flap and sewing up. The

flap is replaced, care being taken that its lower or fractured edge does not injure the dura mater. The aponeurotic and subcutaneous tissues of the scalp-flap are sewn up in the manner stated on p. 16.

After-treatment. Whether the operation be carried out by craniectomy or craniotomy, the patient is put back to bed in the so-called head-down position, the lower end of the bed being raised at least a foot above the level of the head. In the event of shock, a hypodermic injection of a $\frac{1}{4}$ gr. of morphia should be given, the lower extremities may be bandaged firmly from below upwards, and saline infusions administered, preferably per rectum.

CHAPTER III

CEPHALOCELES. BIRTH-HÆMORRHAGES. BIRTH-FRACTURES. DERMOIDS. HYDROCEPHALUS

CEPHALOCELES

The term 'Cephalocele' has been applied to all those tumours which project through a gap or deficiency in the bones of the vault and base of the skull. The tumour may be congenital or traumatic in origin: the membranes of the brain may alone protrude (meningocele), or the tumour may be composed of normal or altered brain-substance: all the varying conditions, however, are included under one term—**cephalocele.** Congenital and traumatic cephaloceles differ, however, so markedly from one another, both with regard to their pathology and treatment, that they must be considered separately.

Congenital cephaloceles. Billroth and the late Professor von Bergmann were the first to narrate cases in which this deformity was present, Lyssenkow [1] added much to the previous records, and de Quèrvain,[2] by prolonged researches, drew further attention to the subject.

Lyssenkow divided the congenital variety into two main groups—exencephaly and cephalocele—the former resulting from a general error in development (the 'Acrania' of Muscatelle), the latter a partial or local developmental failure. In **exencephaly** there is an extensive gap in the vault of the skull, the remainder of the skull being microcephalic in nature, the brain projecting outwards in a varying degree, and the ventricular spaces distended with fluid. In **cephaloceles** the hole in the skull is usually circumscribed, although the sutures may be widely separated and the ventricles

[1] *Der Hirnbruch und seine Behandlung.* Moscow, 1896.

[2] *De la céphalhydrocèle traumatique* (*Travaux de Neur. Chir.*, iii. 1898).

distended with fluid, yet both skull and brain may be normally developed in all other respects.

Exencephaly presents but few points of surgical interest, insomuch as the condition is barely compatible with life.

Cephaloceles occupy a very different position. The condition is by no means confined to man, and many instances are recorded as occurring throughout the animal kingdom. Norsa Gurrieri,[1] for instance, records a case occurring in the embryo of Mus decumanus vel albinus. The same writer insists that the developmental error involves bones of either cartilaginous or membranous origin, and that the atrophic condition of the bone is the primary cause and the ectopia of the brain a secondary result.

Lyssenkow,[2] after careful investigation of tumours removed by operation and after death, found scattered nerve-fibres, fat-cells, striated muscle and vessels—the products, therefore, of both ectoderm and mesoderm. He also observed the frequent occurrence of an intimate union or fusion between the cephalocele and the overlying integument, and, in consequence, the theory was formulated that the greater number of cephaloceles were in reality cephalomata or true teratoid tumours.

It would appear, therefore, that a cephalocele results from the incomplete cutting off of the neural canal in the head region of the embryo from the overlying epiblast, with consequent fusion between the primary neural tube (from which the brain is developed) with the primordial mesoblastic membranous cranium (from which the membranes are developed), and with the overlying epiblastic layer (from which the epidermal portion of the scalp is developed). In consequence of this localized fusion of layers, the outer dermic coat (from which the membranous skull is developed) fails to form. Bony defects therefore exist through which brain-matter protrudes, the projecting portion often being intimately attached to the skin, and containing not only epiblastic elements, but also mesoblastic tissue from irregular occlusion of the same. The mesoblastic involvement is proved by the presence in the tumour of muscle tissue, vessels, &c.

Position of the tumour. The tumour may project through the

[1] *Archives Italiennes de Biologie*, vol. xxxviii, p. 444.

[2] *Der Hirnbruch und seine Behandlung.* Moscow, 1896.

vault or base of the skull. In the former case, it is almost invariably situated in close relation to the middle line of the skull, from nasion to below the inion.

1. *Occipital cephaloceles*—the commonest variety—occupy, anatomically, two positions (1) between the two lower segments of the

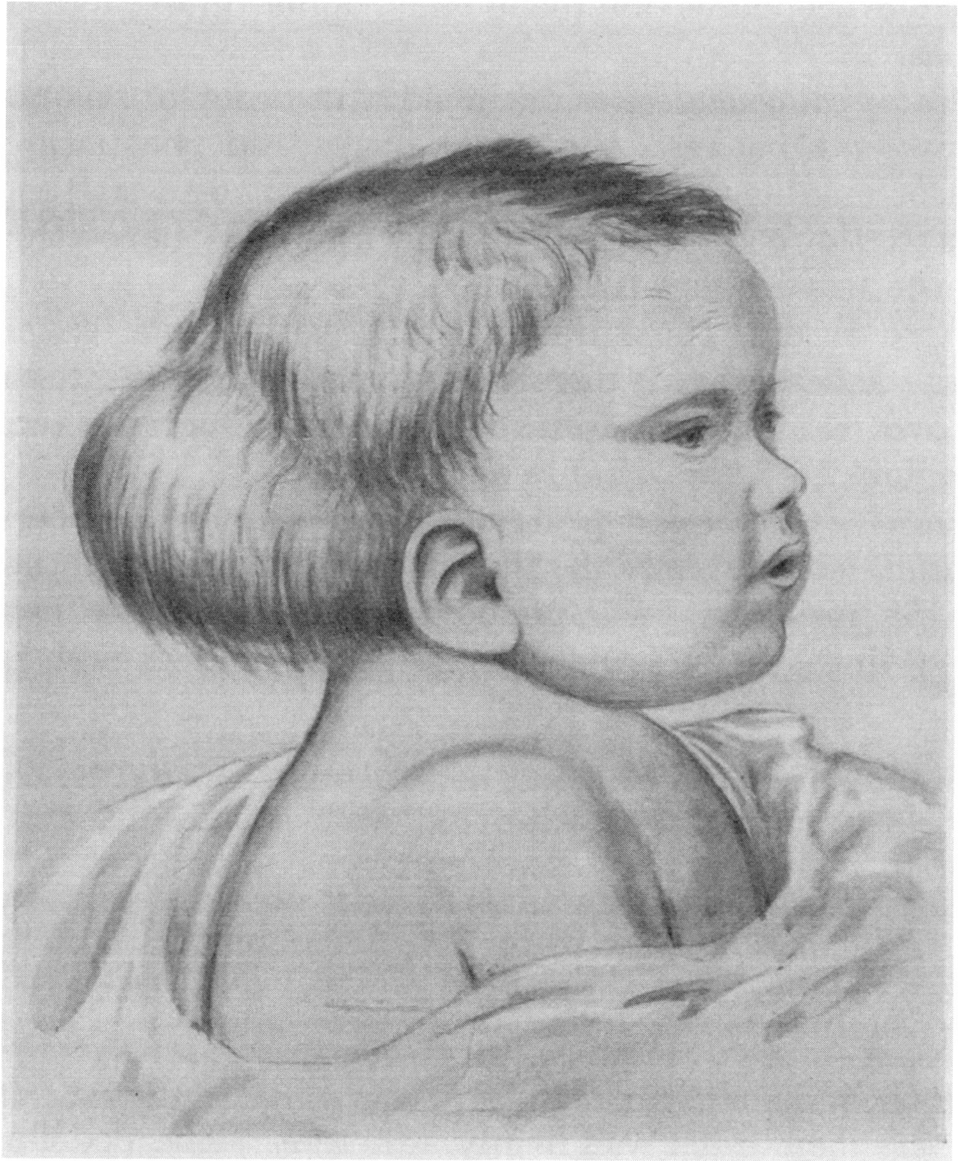

Fig. 20. An Occipital Cephalocele. (For further description, see text.)

occipital bone (inferior occipital cephaloceles), often involving the foramen magnum and sometimes complicated by a condition of cervical spina bifida, and (2) between the two upper segments of the occipital bone (superior occipital cephaloceles), occasionally involving the posterior fontanelle.

The tumour may possess a broad base or may be definitely pedunculated. In the former instance the gap in the bone may be of considerable size and the margins everted : in the latter case, the hole may be quite small.

The deformity is frequently associated with other congenital defects—hydrocephalus, microcephalus, spina bifida, hare lip, hernia, and talipes.

2. *Sincipital cephaloceles* occur next in order of frequency. The tumour projects between the nasal bones and the nasal process of the superior maxilla (naso-frontal), between the nasal process of the maxilla and the orbital plates of the ethmoid (naso-ethmoidal), or between the nasal bones (nasal).

3. More rarely, the tumour overlies the *anterior or posterior fontanelle*. A case of this nature is depicted in Fig. 21, the tumour, situated over the anterior fontanelle, bulging over the temporal and frontal regions to a remarkable extent.

4. *Basal cephaloceles* protrude through the cartilaginous base of the skull, either through the cribriform plate of the ethmoid, between the pre- and basi-sphenoid, or between the basi-sphenoid and basi-occiput, often projecting as a polypoid growth in the nose or naso-pharynx.

An interesting case of basal hernia was reported by von Mayer.[1] The child, 3 days old, was admitted with a tumour projecting into the right nostril, covered with mucous membrane, translucent, encrusted with scabs, pedunculated, and closely resembling a nasal polypus. The possibilities were fully recognized and all necessary precautions taken. The right half of the nose was turned back as a flap, the tumour isolated, ligatured, and removed. Death occurred after six weeks. An oval hole was found in the left half of the cribriform plate through which the dura mater projected and to the margins of which the membrane was firmly adherent. The pedicle contained ganglion-cells and nerve-fibres, whilst the parts removed showed, from without inwards, mucous membrane, dura mater, arachnoid, pia, and glial tissue.

Size, structure, and contents. Sincipital cephaloceles are usually quite small, but the occipital variety and those situated in

[1] *Beitr. zur klin. Chir.*, vol. iii, p. 228.

the region of the anterior fontanelle frequently attain a great size (see Figs. 20–22).

It is not always possible to determine whether the tumour consists of a mere outward protrusion of membranes (meningocele), or whether brain-matter enters into the formation of the tumour (meningo-encephalocele). Fluctuation, translucency, and pulsation

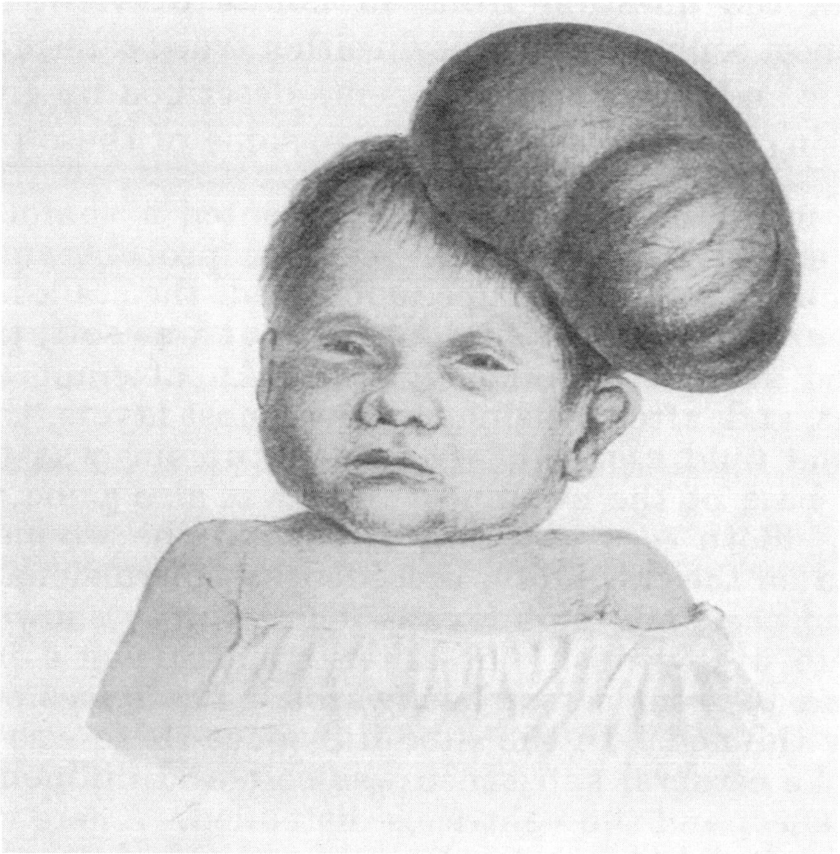

FIG. 21. A CEPHALOCELE OVER THE ANTERIOR FONTANELLE.
(For further description, see text.)

are all points to be investigated. All these features are, however, deceptive, and several cases are on record in which operative measures were carried out under the impression that the surgeon had to deal with a pure meningocele, and in which it was afterwards found that brain-matter formed the basis of the swelling.

When the tumour is large, the skin adherent, when no pedicle is present, when fluctuation and pulsation are absent, and when the tumour is of firm consistency, then it is practically certain that brain-matter shares largely in the formation of the tumour. On the other hand, it is not unusual to find that the brain projects markedly outwards without resulting in any symptoms of brain irritation: fluctuation and pulsation are also not infallible signs, since the brain may occupy the base of the tumour, 'corking-up' the gap in the bone, or the brain may be so thinned by ventricular distension that a mere shell of cerebral matter lies beneath the scalp-covering.

Looking at the question from all points of view, it may be accepted that most cephaloceles contain either true brain-matter or the mixed epiblastic and mesoblastic elements described by Lyssenkow.

The following case serves to illustrate some of these facts: [1]—

The child was 3 months old, and presented a tumour, the size of an orange, situated between the occipital protuberance and the nape of the neck. The mass was pedunculated, the stalk being about the size of a four-shilling piece in diameter. It was soft, translucent, irreducible, and swelled up on coughing. An attempt at removal was carried out, and, after incising the outermost layers, three ounces of cerebro-spinal fluid escaped. A second tumour was then found occupying the base of the swelling. This was also punctured, more fluid escaping. Both sacs were cut away and the wound sewn up. Death occurred on the third day, preceded by convulsions, retraction of the head and neck, and high fever. The autopsy showed that the fontanelles were widely open, the anterior measuring 4 inches from side to side and $2\frac{1}{2}$ from before backwards. The bones of the vault were markedly thinned. In the subdural space there was a quantity of fluid, and the cerebral substance was soft and diffluent, the convolutions flattened, and the ventricles distended. There was a broad gap in the occipital bone, extending downwards into the foramen magnum, and in this situation the cerebellum had bulged backwards into the protruding mass. (See Fig. 22).

For *differential diagnosis, see* p. 57.

Treatment. In considering the question of treatment, the late Professor von Bergmann [2] divided the cases into two groups :—

1. *Inoperable cases.* When associated with premature synostosis and microcephaly.

When associated with hydrocephalus or marked deformity.

When the tumour is situated below the occipital protuberance.

[1] *St. Bart. Hosp. Reports.* Lawrence Ward. May 5, 1896.

[2] *Beitr. zur klin. Chir.*, vol. vii, p. 228.

2. *Operable cases.* Limited protrusions with none of the above defects and disadvantages.

This classification undoubtedly forms a practical basis on which to estimate the feasibility of operative measures, and it would appear

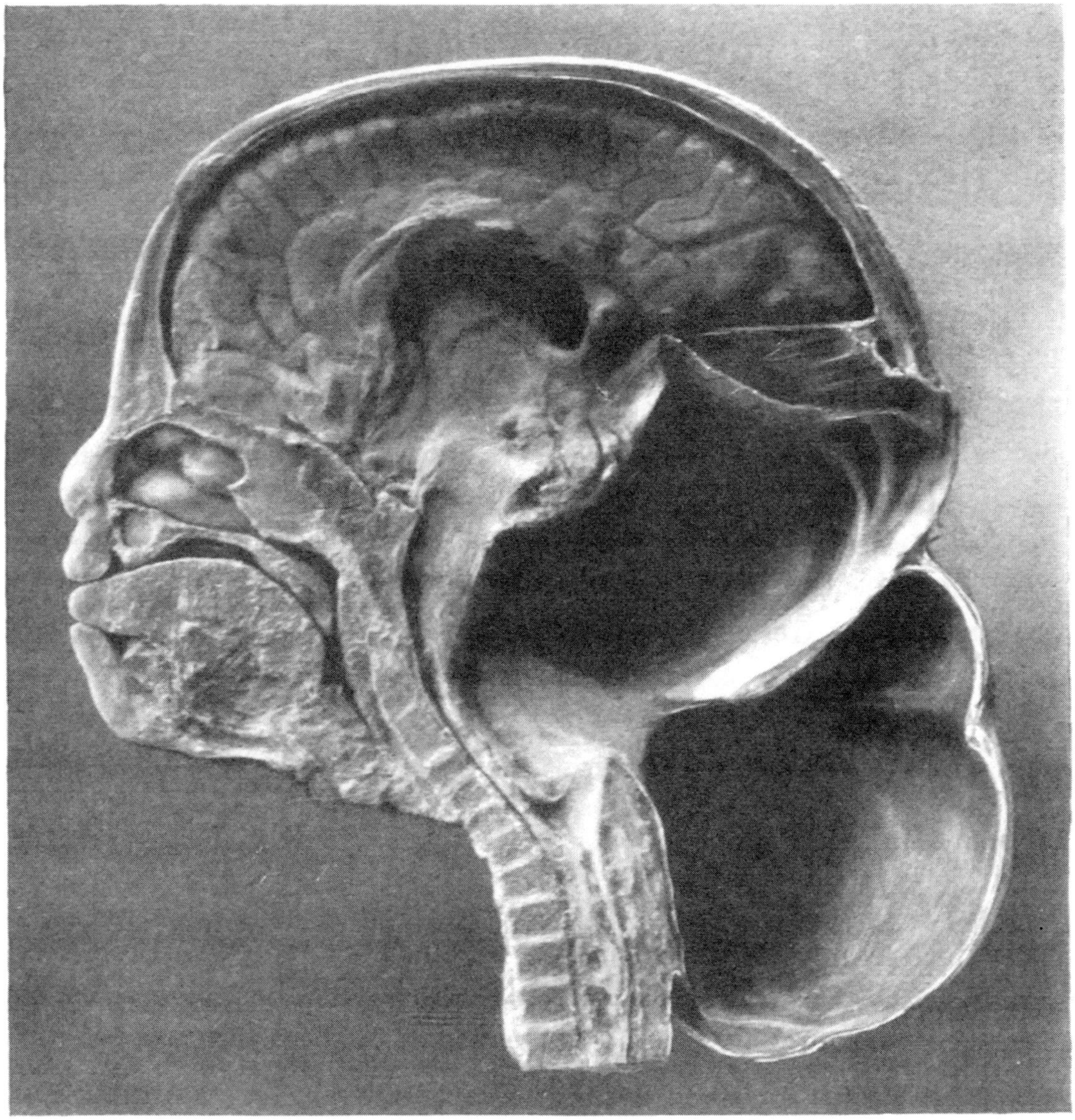

FIG. 22. AN OCCIPITAL CEPHALOCELE. (For further description, see text.)

that sincipital and small occipital cephaloceles are the only cases that come within the realms of operative treatment. In estimating the possibility of operation, however, due consideration must be paid to the fact that, in the very great majority of cases, the tumour tends to increase in size, the bones become further thinned, the margins of the gap more everted, and the development of the brain suffers correspondingly. Again, in spite of the fact that some few cases have survived to adult age, yet it is the general rule for the patient to die within a few weeks or months of birth. For desperate ills, corresponding measures must be undertaken, and in the consideration of the more serious cases the surgeon should be biased in favour of operation unless the general condition of the child shows clearly that no success is possible. The best results have been attained in cases of pure meningocele.

Operation. The unhealthy condition of the overlying integument, especially at the apex of the tumour, prohibits any extensive preparatory cleansing, this process being carried out for the most part when the child is under the anæsthetic.

Scalp-flaps are framed from the region of the base of the tumour, advantage being taken of the more healthy parts. These flaps must be so sized and framed that accurate approximation and complete covering to the gap will be attained at the termination of the operation. The flaps are dissected back to their base. The pedicle of the tumour is defined and an endeavour made to detach it completely from the margins of the osseous defect. This is often a matter requiring considerable patience. The sac of the tumour should then be tapped with trocar and cannula, and the fluid contents allowed to escape slowly, after which the opening into the sac is enlarged and the membranes slit up towards the base of the protrusion.

When dealing with a pure meningocele, the membranous protrusion is cut away in such a manner that sufficient tissue is left to allow of closure of the dural gap. This closure can be carried out either by means of a purse-string suture or by the union of two lateral flaps. In either case, accurate approximation is essential in order to prevent as far as possible the further escape of cerebrospinal fluid.

If the sac should contain an irregular mass of neuroblastic and mesoblastic tissue, apparently not true cerebral or cerebellar substance, this material can be dissected from the membranous sac, ligatured at its base, and freely cut away.

If the sac should contain true brain substance, the possibility of excision can be raised. In the cerebellar region such measures are contra-indicated, and the surgeon must remain content with an attempt at replacing the cerebellar substance within the cranial cavity. This attempt at reposition will be aided by elevation of the head and, occasionally, by lumbar puncture. If the protrusion corresponds to a region which has no known important function, it may be ligatured and cut away flush with the surface of the gap. Hæmorrhage may be considerable, but can be controlled by ligature, pressure, and irrigation with hot water at a temperature between 110 and 115 degrees Fahrenheit. The degree of shock attendant on the operation may be severe, necessitating the most complete attention to preliminary, operative, and post-operative details (see Chap. I).

To *remedy the defect of the bone* Lyssenkow recommends an osteoplastic operation, a flap composed of pericranium, together with the external table of the skull, being framed from the bone above the defect.

The flap is then turned down in such a way that the pericranial surface faces towards the dura, and the fragment is suspended by the continuity of the pericranium. He reports 72 cases so treated, with 37 recoveries and 35 deaths.

König and von Bergmann oppose this osteoplastic operation on the ground that the extreme thinness of the bone seldom permits of the necessary splitting off of the external table of the skull, and that, even when such a course is feasible, the fragment undergoes necrosis.

Transplantation of decalcified and calcined bone, silver and celluloid plates, have all been tried, with no great amount of success. Ssamoylenko proposes paraffin and vaseline injections, especially for the sincipital variety of cephalocele.

When the surrounding bone is of such a nature that it is possible to form an osteoplastic flap, that course should be adopted. Under other circumstances, it would appear preferable to postpone any attempt to close in or protect the gap in the bone in the hope that nature will remedy the defect in part, the surgeon stepping in at a later date with one of the measures advocated for the protection of gaps in the skull (see p. 196).

TRAUMATIC CEPHALOCELES

Many cases have been recorded in which a cephalocele developed after an injury to the skull. In such conditions it is necessary that a comminuted or fissured fracture of the vault should be present, that the underlying dura mater should be torn, and that the adjacent brain substance should be severely contused or lacerated. Cerebro-spinal fluid may alone escape through the gap in the skull to the subaponeurotic and subcutaneous regions, leading to the formation of a *false traumatic meningocele.* When the brain shares in the outward protrusion the condition is known as *false traumatic meningo-encephalocele.* This protrusion of the brain is dependent on the fact that the injury—necessarily a severe one—leads to considerable brain lesion, with subsequent œdema and localized or general increase in the intracranial pressure.

Occasionally, the external accumulation of cerebro-spinal fluid communicates with one of the horns of the lateral ventricle. A meningo-encephalocele, having such connexions, is produced in the following manner :—the protruded brain includes that part of the cerebral substance which bounds one of the horns of the lateral ventricle, usually the descending cornu. The ventricular channel becomes elongated in the outward direction, towards and through the gap in the skull, whilst the increased intraventricular tension gradually dilates up the new channel, and, in course of time, still further spreads out and thins that part of its cerebral boundary which lies external to the skull deficiency.

There can be no question that after the patient has reached the age of three years traumatic cephaloceles are of exceedingly rare occurrence. This special liability in quite young children has been ascribed to the greater elasticity of the infant skull, and to the supposed greater adherence of the dura mater. Though these factors may exercise some influence on the production of the tumour, it seems more probable that the development of a cephalocele is dependent to a greater degree on the general vitality of the child. Thus, a blow that produces in the adult a comminuted or widely fissured fracture of the skull, with laceration of the dura mater and injury to the underlying brain, frequently leads to a fatal result, whilst the child often recovers. Again, in the adult, the force required to produce such a lesion usually suffices to lacerate the integument. Consequently a compound comminuted fracture of the vault with hernia cerebri is relatively more common in the adult than in the infant.

The right side of the head is more frequently affected than the left, and, of all bones in the skull, the parietal is the one most constantly involved.

Symptoms. During the first few days subsequent to the injury the child merely suffers from the symptoms common to all severe head-injuries—concussion and brain irritation. The osseous lesion is obscured by the presence of a well-marked cephalhæmatoma. After the lapse of a short time—usually one to two weeks—the partial resolution of the hæmatoma allows one to observe, for the first time, that a definite tumour remains. This tumour is irreducible, pulsates freely, and may be translucent. If the protruding brain substance includes the precentral region—the motor area—definite weakness or paralysis of the opposite face and extremities may be observed. Usually, however, no such symptoms are forthcoming, and the child appears but little the worse for the accident. Shortly afterwards the tumour becomes more defined in outline, and careful palpation will reveal the defined margins of an osseous deficiency. Compression of the protruded mass will often throw the child into general convulsions, or induce a state of compression with dilated pupils, slow pulse, and stertorous respiration. Compression, however, seldom results in any marked diminution in the size of the tumour. The conditions may remain stationary, but, as a general rule, the hernial protrusion slowly increases in size and the child dies in general convulsions, preceded by symptoms of brain irritation or compression.

Treatment. Three courses are available in the treatment of this condition :—

1. Expectant treatment, combined with the application of pressure.
2. Aspiration and puncture.
3. Free exposure and further treatment according to the conditions found.

In the majority of cases the local conditions preclude any attempt at radical cure—the gap in the skull is large, the margins of the deficiency are thinned and everted, and the brain enters largely into the formation of the projecting mass. Furthermore, the dura mater is torn and in a tag-like condition. Only in the most favourable cases—when the tumour is small and the gap narrow—can radical treatment be advocated.

The application of pressure—without previous aspiration—exercises but little effect on the size of the tumour and, under such treatment, the danger of brain-compression is always present.

Aspiration with the object of removing the fluid constituents of the tumour, and thus of reducing its size, has occasionally been followed by disastrous results. Still, many cases were so treated in the pre-aseptic days, and the modern methods of cleanliness should allow of better results. One or more aspirations may be carried out, this treatment to be followed by the application of steady and uniform pressure, preferably with the aid of elastic bandages, the degree of compression depending on the size and constituents of the tumour. The patient must be watched most carefully, in order to guard against the development of symptoms pointing to cerebral compression. Irritating injections should never be used.

One must acknowledge that this mode of treatment has—except in a few isolated cases—not produced very satisfactory results. Still, since an open operation is usually out of the question, no other course remains.

The after-history of these cases is not very encouraging. In one of Weinlecher's cases the child was living 5 years later, but pulsation was still present. In Lucas's case the patient died 21 months later from meningitis. In Sir T. Smith's case, pulsation was present 3 years after the accident, and in Silcock's there was no marked change for the better after 11 years. On the other hand, a case reported by Golding Bird steadily improved, and a second case reported by the same writer gave every promise of a permanent cure. The two following cases have come under my own observation :—

1. A female child, 11 months old, was knocked down by a van, and, on admission, a large hæmatoma was seen situated over the right temporo-parietal region. The child was semi-comatose, but recovered consciousness next day. The hæmatoma softening, a gap in the bone was felt, one-third of an inch wide, and extending from

the occipital bone upwards and inwards to the middle line. The swelling increased in size when the child cried. Pulsation was present and translucency was obtained. The tumour increased in size for some days, but no untoward symptoms developed. For over one month pressure was applied, but without much benefit, though the general condition of the child was good. The edges of the gap became thickened. The child was then removed from the hospital.

2. A male child fell 19 feet on to his head. He was concussed, and, on admission, presented a hæmatoma over the right fronto-parietal region, and subconjunctival hæmorrhage in the left orbit. Four days later he was apathetic and there was some paresis of the left arm and leg. As the hæmatoma became softer, pulsation was noticed over a small area, and, in this situation, the swelling increased in size on straining. A fracture was detected later, one-third of an inch in diameter, and extending across the left frontal bone to the right temporal region. Pressure was applied, the tumour steadily decreased in size, and eventually the gap was completely closed.

Synopsis of 38 cases of traumatic cephalocele.

Sex. Males, 16. Females, 13. Sex not stated, 9.

Age at time of accident.

2 cases at birth.
9 in the first 6 months.
9 in the second 6 months.
14 between 1 and 2 years of age.
1 between 3 and 10.
1 between 10 and 15.
1 between 15 and 20.
1 between 20 and 30.

Region affected.

Right parietal, 17 cases.
Left parietal, 4 cases.
Other bones, right and left, 8 cases.
Parietal with others, 9 cases.
Parietal bone involved in 30 out of 38 cases.
Right side involved in 27 out of 38 cases.

Date of appearance of tumour.

7 cases in the first week.
11 cases in the second week.
4 cases in the third week.
4 cases between 2 and 18 months.
In the remainder, date uncertain.

Fractures of the skull resulting from injuries received at or shortly after birth. In the consideration of injuries to the skull and brain in babies the following points should be noted :—

1. The bones of the skull are elastic and pliable, and consequently a blow may lead to a 'bending-in', either temporary or permanent. Slight depressions may exist without any associated fracture, but all major depressions are accompanied by a fracture of the bone, especially evident on examination of the internal table.

2. The fibrous tissue intervening between the component parts of the vault tends to cause a limitation of the fracture to the particular bone affected. Downward extension to the base is of infrequent occurrence, but, when that region is involved, the fracture usually follows the transbasic lines described in the section dealing with fracture of the base of the skull (p. 82).

3. The dura is said to be more adherent to the inner table of the skull than in adults. The relative infrequency in the young of extradural hæmorrhage has been ascribed to this peculiarity. It would appear, however, more probable that the rarity of such hæmorrhages results from the bending-in, *without splintering*, of the bone.

4. The brain of the infant is equally—if not more—liable to bruising and laceration, but the results are far less definite than in adults. There can be no question that extensive cerebral injury may exist in the child without leading to the development of any definite localizing symptoms.

FRACTURES OF THE VAULT

(*a*) **Depressed fractures.** Depressed fractures either result from injury received during the birth of the child—whether from forceps delivery or from the pressure exerted on the head by a contracted pelvis—or from blows received shortly after birth.

The depression, varying greatly in depth and extent, may be situated over any part of the skull, but commonly involves the fronto-parietal region. It is often obscured in the early stages by the presence of an overlying hæmatoma, the condition perhaps only being discovered after the absorption of the blood-clot. In many cases no symptoms result, partly owing to the shallowness of the depression and partly due to the situation of the lesion over one of the so-called 'silent' areas of the brain. Under other circumstances the child may evidence the general increase in the intracranial pressure by cyanosis, difficulty in respiration, unconsciousness, and slow pulse. The anterior fontanelle will be tense, and pulsation will be absent or greatly diminished—a feature of the greatest diagnostic value. Localizing symptoms ensue when an extensive depression is situated over the motor area, the extremities of the opposite side being flaccid, or evidencing irritation by twitchings and convulsions.

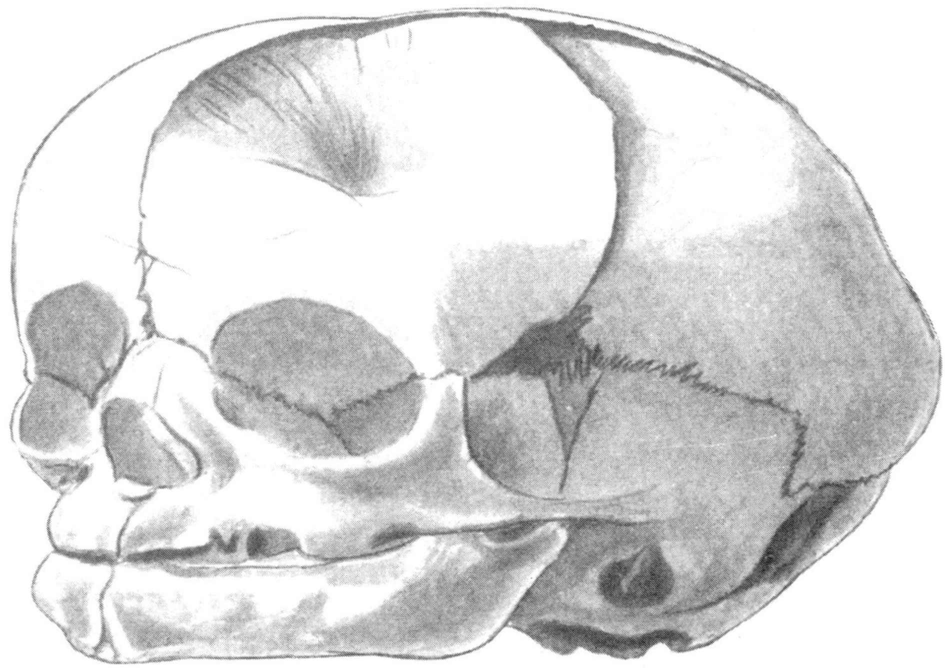

FIG. 23. A DEPRESSED BIRTH-FRACTURE.

The ready response of the infant to cortical irritation frequently results in the early transformation of local twitchings into general convulsions.

Course and treatment. It is often stated that these depressed fractures remedy themselves in the course of time, the development of the underlying cortex curing the depression by the outward leverage exerted. In the minor degrees of depression there may be some chance of such spontaneous cure. I am, however, entirely opposed to the view that spontaneous cure is the rule, and there can be no question that the more severe types of depression remain as permanent defects unless surgical remedies are adopted. Furthermore, even if the deformity should cure itself in time, the intermediate dangers are not to be disregarded, for, during the process of spontaneous cure, there is a decided liability for the depressed cortex to lag behind in the process of development, or to undergo degenerative changes as the result of the pressure exerted—with disastrous results on the parts supplied by the region compressed. Mental deficiency, paralyses, and contractures will result, and there is every reason to believe that some cases of infantile paralysis are dependent on this lesion.

The following case, recently under my care, adds further proof to the statement that spontaneous cure is usually out of the question:—

The child, 10 weeks old, was admitted with a depressed fracture over the parieto-frontal region, oval in shape, and about 3½ inches in its long antero-posterior diameter. The centre of the depression lay about 1½ inches below a normal surface. The injury was produced at birth (contracted pelvis), and frequent convulsions were observed during the first few days of life. The fits then ceased, but the depression became, if anything, more marked day by day. The child was then brought up to see me. The depression was exposed by a suitable scalp-flap and a small trephine hole made immediately posterior to the depression. The dura mater was stripped away from the under surface of the bone and every effort made to remedy the depression. No impression was thus made on the defect. The whole depressed area was then cut out with a pair of scissors, the segment removed, wrapped up in a piece of gauze, and forcibly manipulated in the hope that the depression could be overcome and the segment placed back in the normal position. This attempt was also greeted with failure. The segment was then placed back in the inverted position, the dural surface external and vice versa. The segment required some trimming with the scissors before it fitted accurately in position. The scalp-flap was then replaced. The child suffered but very slightly from the operation, firm union was present in two weeks, and, six months later, examination of the skull showed that the two sides were absolutely symmetrical.

It should be noted that, although the child was only 10 weeks old, and in spite of the fact that the depression was fully exposed, it was quite impossible to lever up the depressed bone. This hardly coincides with the views of those who maintain that birth-depressions undergo spontaneous cure.

Taking all these facts into consideration, it would appear advisable to adopt the following course:—slight depressions, situated in the region of ‘silent’ areas of the brain, may be left for one or two

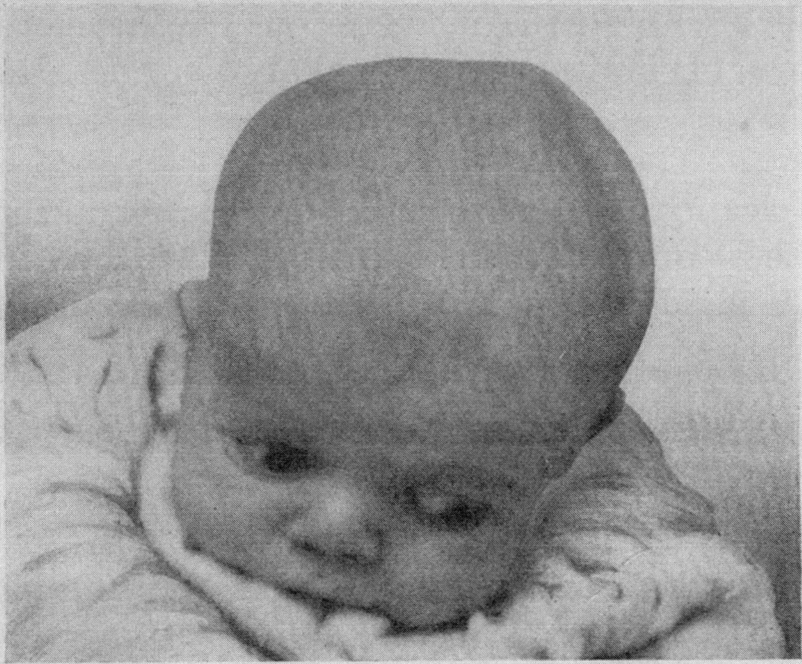

A

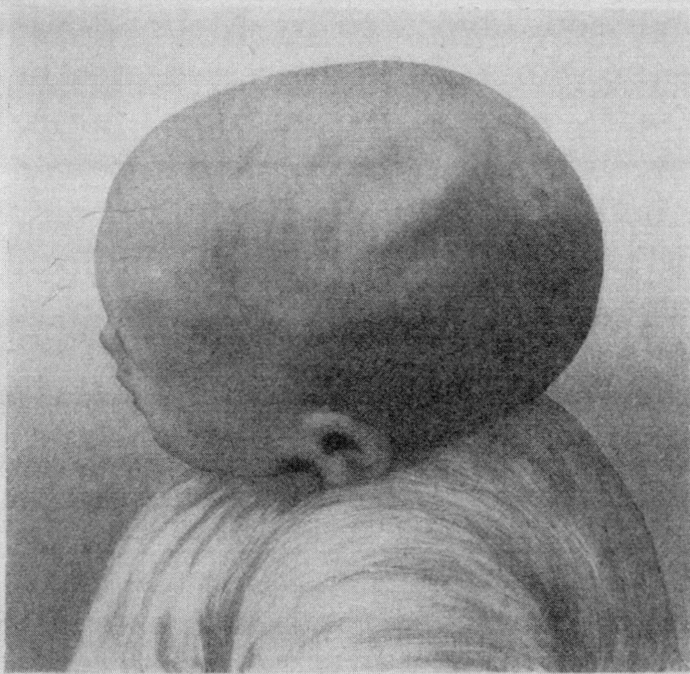

B

FIG. 24. A CASE OF DEPRESSED BIRTH-FRACTURE. A, Before operation; B, After operation. (For further description, see text.)

weeks, and, in the event of failure at spontaneous cure, the depression must be elevated. In all the more serious cases, whether associated with symptoms of brain-pressure or not, surgical interference is imperative.

Operation. The baby would be well wrapped up and, after shaving and cleansing of the scalp, the scalp-tourniquet applied. Babies stand these operations exceedingly well so long as hæmorrhage is but slight. A scalp-flap is turned down and a small trephine ($\frac{1}{2}$-inch diameter) applied immediately to one side of the depression, the trephine circle including the outer margin of the depressed area. The dura is stripped away and a flat periosteal elevator introduced so that its apex corresponds to the apex of the depression. An attempt is then made to lever the depressed area in the outward direction. If that result be attained, well and good. The flap is replaced and dressings applied. In many cases, however, the elevated region promptly assumes its original depressed position as soon as the elevator is removed, and, in other cases, all attempts at rectification of the deformity are of no avail. Under these circumstances, it is advisable to carry out the method advocated by Nicholl—adopted in the case described above—the whole of the depressed area being cut out with blunt-pointed scissors, reduced to a more normal curvature by manipulation between layers of gauze, and replaced in the inverted position, the original dural surface becoming now external. This inversion is requisite, as it is usually quite impossible—even under considerable pressure—to reduce the depression to a permanently satisfactory degree.

Nicholl reports on 23 cases, the ages of the patients varying from 3 weeks to 8 years. The first 13 cases were treated by elevation. The results obtained were most unsatisfactory, complete reduction of the deformity seldom being attained, whilst recurrence, of a greater or lesser degree, was the rule.

In the last 10 cases the inversion method was carried out, with, in all cases, satisfactory results. Bony union was present in 10 days.

Four cases of depressed birth-fractures have come under my own care. In two cases the depression was elevated—in both cases with considerable difficulty—whilst in the other two cases, after failure of leverage, Nicholl's method was carried out, in both cases with eminently satisfactory results.

(*b*) **Fissured fractures.** Fissured fractures are especially prone to involve the parietal bone, and, in their direction, to follow the lines of ossification. Thus, in the case of the parietal bone, the fissures will radiate from the parietal prominence. There is also a certain tendency for the fracture to remain limited to the particular bone affected.

The presence and extent of the fracture is commonly obscured by the overlying hæmatoma, which is either subpericranial or subaponeurotic. On the other hand, the hæmatoma may, from its size and shape, supply evidence as to the nature of the underlying lesion. Thus, when confined to the parietal bone, it may be inferred that the fracture is also limited to that region. Again, when linear, the presumption is that the fracture is of a similar nature. A definite diagnosis may be impossible without aspiration or till after absorption of the hæmatoma. The fissure will then be found to vary in extent from a mere crack in the bone to a wide gap as broad or broader than the width of the finger. In a case recently under my care the fissure, over half an inch in breadth, extended from the vertex to the base, whilst throughout the whole extent of the gap pulsation was readily obtained.

Fissured fractures in the very young possess another point of interest in that the cleft often tends to increase, this being notably the case when the fracture is associated with injury to underlying dura and brain. The local and general increase of intracranial pressure not only widens the gap, but also leads to thinning and eversion of the margins of the deficiency with possible herniation of brain-matter—traumatic cephalocele.

Symptoms. In many cases—in spite of the severity of the lesion—there are no symptoms, the child appearing but little the worse for the accident. In most cases, however, the child evidences symptoms of brain-concussion, irritation, or compression, for which conditions reference should be made to the sections dealing with those subjects.

It should be noted, however, that the anterior fontanelle supplies evidence as to increase or decrease of intracranial pressure. In concussion the fontanelle is depressed, in compression it is tense and pulsation is absent or diminished. Irritation of the brain is evidenced by irritability and general convulsions.

Treatment. In the absence of symptoms, or when the fracture is associated with concussion or irritation, operative measures are contra-indicated, the patient being treated after the general principles laid down for those conditions.

When associated with symptoms of brain-compression, exploration is almost always advisable, the scalp-tourniquet being applied and the injured region exposed by a suitable scalp-flap. Depressed bone is elevated, or the trephine applied so as to fully expose the underlying dura mater. A bulging, non-pulsatile, and plum-coloured membrane points to the existence of a subdural hæmatoma. The membrane is then incised and the clot evacuated. Whenever possible the dura mater should be sewn up and the scalp-flap replaced without drainage.

Operative measures are also indicated when a linear fracture gapes widely—especially when the gap shows a tendency to increase in width. The steps of such an operation are as follows :—

1. Expose the fracture throughout its whole length.
2. Cut away all pericranium or fibrous tissue that intervenes between the margins of the cleft.
3. Separate the dura mater from the bone on either side of the cleft for a distance of about ½ inch, at the same time sewing up any rents in the membrane.
4. Bore a few holes through the skull—using an ordinary bradawl—on either side of the cleft, the holes being placed about ½ inch apart.
5. Approximate and lace the margins of the cleft by means of fine silver wire or strong catgut.
6. Sew up the flap without drainage.

BIRTH-HÆMORRHAGES

Extracranial hæmorrhages. As the result of injury sustained during protracted labour, hæmatomata may develop beneath the aponeurosis of the occipito-frontalis or underneath the pericranium, the latter being the more common situation. The right side of the head is the more frequently involved, and the parietal region is the part usually affected. Occasionally these hæmatomata are bilateral and symmetrical.

The two varieties of cephalhæmatoma—subaponeurotic and subpericranial—possess certain peculiarities that aid materially in their differential diagnosis.

Subaponeurotic hœmatomata. The blood, though spreading widely throughout the subaponeurotic space, tends to gravitate towards the lower confines of that space, and, from the position assumed by the patient, is most evident in the occipital region. The presence of the blood is evidenced by œdema, doughiness, and ecchymosis.

Subpericranial hœmatomata. The blood is confined to the region of the particular bone affected, usually the right parietal bone. This is due to the fact that the pericranium blends at the margins of the bone with the tissue intervening between that bone and the neighbouring parts of the skull.

Subpericranial hæmatomata present further peculiarities. The tumour is usually more or less circular in outline, and fluctuates freely. It may arise immediately after the birth of the child, but, more commonly, some two or three days elapse before attention is drawn to its existence. Within a few days clotting occurs at the periphery of the hæmatoma with the formation of a circumferential ridge. The central portion of the clot remains soft but tense, so much so that firm pressure is required before the examining finger is enabled to feel the underlying bone. These cephalhæmatomata are not infrequently mistaken for depressed fractures, but no difficulty should be experienced if the existence of the circumferential ridge be appreciated and if the underlying bone can be felt at the centre of the tumour. In cases of doubt the blood should be drawn off by aspiration and the swelling again examined.

For *differential diagnosis*, see p. 57.

Treatment. The less extensive hæmatomata require no active surgical treatment, the absorption of the clot being aided by protection of the part and by cooling lotions.

Similar expectant treatment is generally advised with regard to the extensive subpericranial hæmatomata, but as infection of the clot may take place, and as its resolution invariably requires a considerable period of time—often many weeks—more active measures can be adopted. The region of the hæmatoma is carefully shaved and cleansed, and, under local anæsthesia, a small incision made through the scalp, the clot squeezed out, and firm pressure applied. Under this form of treatment the patient is well within a few days.

Intracranial birth-hæmorrhages. Attention was first drawn to the question of intracranial birth-hæmorrhages by Little, who showed that a history of difficult labour could be obtained in a large percentage of cases in which children in after-life suffered from uni- or bilateral spastic paraplegia; hence the name, 'Little's disease' or birth palsy. Further information was supplied by Sarah MacNutt, and the whole question was fully investigated by Harvey Cushing.

In all cases a history of difficult and protracted labour can be obtained, with considerable post-partum respiratory difficulties, the child being described as 'blue in the face' for some hours after birth.

The stress and strain which the advancing head undergoes, and the consequent moulding and overlapping of the various segments of the skull, exposes the brain to great alterations of pressure, and throws considerable tension on the intracranial veins. It is, in fact, rather surprising that birth-hæmorrhages are not more common.

The hæmorrhages may be wholly within the meshes of the pia-arachnoid system, but, in the great majority of cases, the lesion is more serious, and the extravasation comes to lie within the subdural space.

Occasionally the bleeding takes place beneath the tentorium cerebelli, the blood-clot lying in relation to the pons and medulla. Such hæmorrhages are said to be observed only in vertex presentations. The more common supratentorial hæmorrhages—usually resulting from difficult breech presentations—either remain more or less localized to a certain region of the cortex, or become widely diffused over the surface and base of the brain.

It is probable that Cushing is correct in his observations with respect to the source of these supratentorial hæmorrhages. He states that the blood is derived from one or more radicles of the superior longitudinal sinus, especially from those veins which, in their upward passage in the sulci of the brain, leave their cerebral beds for a short and comparatively unprotected course, immediately previous to their entry into the lacunæ laterales of the superior longitudinal sinus.

In addition, he points to the very important fact that the localized hæmorrhages are commonly situated in relation to the mid-cerebral cortex, close to the sinus, and on one or both sides of the falx cerebri. In addition, therefore, to the symptoms of general cerebral compression, certain definite localizing symptoms are to be observed, these being in direct proportion to the size of the clot.

In an analysis of 74 autopsies on infants still-born or dying within the first few days, Archibald [1] found 'intrameningeal' hæmor-

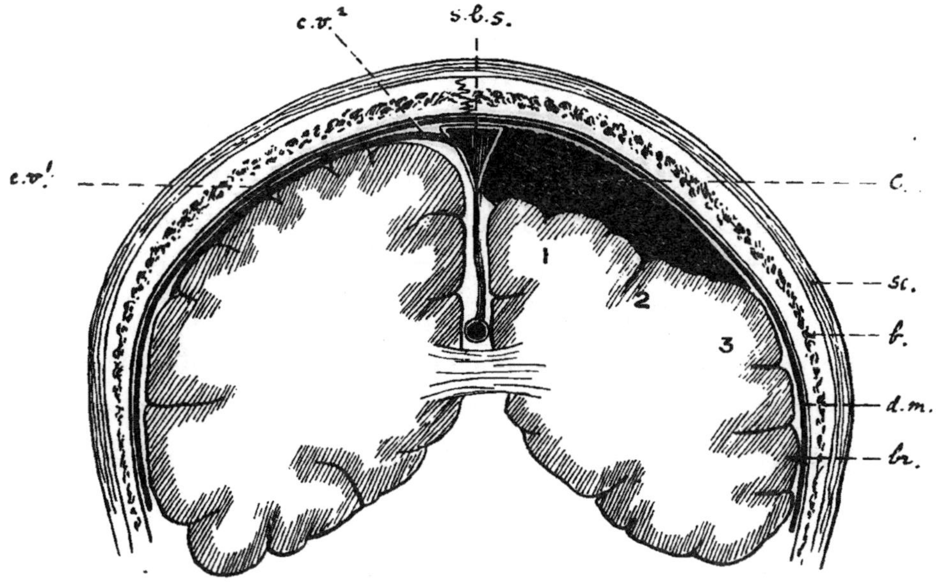

FIG. 25. DIAGRAM TO ILLUSTRATE THE EFFECTS AND POSITION OF A BIRTH-HÆMORRHAGE. *sc.*, Scalp ; *b.*, Bone ; *d.m.*, Dura mater ; *br.*, Brain ; *s.l.s.*, Superior longitudinal sinus ; *c.v.*[1], The protected part of a superficial cerebral vein ; *c.v.*[2], The unprotected part of a superficial cerebral vein ; *c.*, The subdural clot, exercising pressure on (1) the cortical leg arm, (2) the arm area, and (3) the face area.

rhage in 32, in 19 of which it was of considerable extent : and in 5 others there was extra-dural hæmorrhage. In only two or three was effused blood found within the cerebral cortex. The importance of these facts from a surgical point of view cannot be over-estimated.

Symptoms. Besides the history of protracted labour and the 'blue' asphyxiated appearance of the baby, other evidence is to hand with respect to both general and local increase of brain-pressure.

The *general* increase is evidenced first and foremost by the bulging and non-pulsatile anterior fontanelle. The fontanelle may be regarded as an index of intracranial pressure. The margins of the

[1] *American Practice of Surgery.* Bryant and Buck.

fontanelle are outlined with some difficulty, and, owing to the free communication between the intra- and extra-cranial venous systems, the scalp-veins are unduly prominent. The general condition of the child varies according to rise of intracranial pressure. In the more serious cases it may be impossible to arouse the patient: in the slighter hæmorrhages the child may appear but little the worse, with the exception, perhaps, of being rather more irritable than usual.

The effect of the pressure on the medullary centres is shown by respiratory difficulties—irregularities of rhythm, &c.—some retardation in pulse-rate, and increase in blood-pressure. The reflexes are increased and the child is readily thrown into general convulsions.

The effect of the *localized* pressure on the upper Rolandic centres seldom becomes evident till after the lapse of a few days—and often after a longer period—when muscular weakness, twitchings, rigidity, or paralysis—more especially of the contralateral lower extremity—becomes apparent. The mother often draws attention to the fact that the child does not move one of its legs properly.

When the extravasation is extensive, spreading downwards over other motor areas, the upper extremities and even the face may be involved.

When a small hæmorrhage is present, situated on either side of the falx cerebri, both lower extremities suffer and diplegia results.

In some cases, chemosis of the conjunction, œdema of the lids, and proptosis have been observed. In any case an ophthalmoscopic examination should be carried out. Frequently some fullness of the retinal veins and diminution in the calibre of the arteries supply confirmatory evidence.

In the event of doubt in diagnosis, lumbar puncture should be carried out. It should be noted, however, that although the positive evidence of free blood corpuscles points to subdural hæmorrhage, yet that absence of blood in the fluid withdrawn does not exclude the possibility of a localized and more or less encapsulated hæmorrhage. In the event of failure at recognition of the serious lesion present, disastrous results will ensue—monoplegia, diplegia, hemiplegia, epilepsy, and idiocy.

Treatment. The age of the patient must not be allowed to weigh in the balance against operative treatment, for, if due precautions be taken, the new-born child stands operation well. Cushing points out that 'the possibilities of surgical relief are limited to the first week or two after the hæmorrhage has occurred, for old cortical scars can neither be helped by medicine nor by the scalpel'.

The clot can be exposed by craniectomy or by craniotomy. The latter operation results in a more complete exposure, but the shock is undoubtedly more severe. Exposure by craniotomy is advocated by Cushing, and carried out in the following manner: 'An omega-shaped incision just within the outer margin of the parietal bone is carried down to the bone through the scalp and pericranium, and the latter is scraped away so as to expose the thin serrated edge of the parietal bone. Under this a blunt dissector is passed, so that the edge of the bone is tilted up, and then, with a proper cutting instrument (strong blunt-pointed scissors suffice), the bone is incised in a line conforming with the skin incision 1 centimetre or more within the parietal margin. The parietal bone is then broken across at its base. The dura is opened by a curved incision some distance within the bony margin, and the superficial clot broken away or lifted off in fragments, or irrigated away with a gentle stream of warm saline solution. The dura should be accurately sutured, the bone replaced, and the skin closed with suture.'

He reports on 9 cases so treated, with 4 recoveries, apparently complete and permanent. The fatal cases were all associated with extensive extravasation over the entire hemisphere. In 3 cases bilateral exposure was necessitated.

Taking, however, the question into more general consideration, it would appear that equally satisfactory results can be obtained, with a lesser degree of operative danger, by carrying out craniectomy in the manner described in the treatment of 'traumatic subdural hæmorrhage' (see p. 156).

DERMOIDS

Dermoids, in this region of the body, are almost invariably situated in the middle line between nasion and inion, though cases have been described in which congenital tumours, dermoid-like in nature, were situated over the mastoid process and in other regions.

They occur with the greatest frequency over the anterior fontanelle and in the region of the external occipital protuberance. In the latter situation they are specially prone to possess those deep attachments to the dura mater which are further alluded to below. In the great majority of cases careful examination will show that the tumour occupies a depression in the bone, saucer-like in nature, in which the tumour rests. They are seldom freely movable, and are often markedly fixed, being either attached to the pericranium or to deeper structures. They are not attached to the overlying skin. The tumour is irreducible, and pulsation is absent except in those rare cases where, in the presence of a wide gap in the skull, transmitted pulsation may be obtained.

On careful dissection it may be found that the tumour communicates, by means of a small hole in the skull, with the underlying membranes. In more exceptional cases a wide gap in the skull may be found by means of which the dermoid obtains extensive connexion with the dura mater and even with the brain. In rare cases the dermoid may be pedunculated.

Bland Sutton drew attention to this frequent connexion between the dermoid and the membranes of the brain, showing further that the entire tumour may lie on the inner side of the occipital bone.

The following account affords further information as to the nature and origin of cephalic dermoids.

'Morphologically considered, the bony framework of the skull is an additional element to the primitive cranium which is represented by the dura mater, and the term extra-cranial should be applied to all tissues outside the dura mater. Early in embryological life the dura mater and skin are in contact ; gradually the base and portions of the side wall of the membranous cranium chondrify, thus separating the skin from the dura mater. In the vault of the skull, bone developes between the dura mater and its cutaneous cap, but the skin and dura mater remain in contact along the various sutures even for a year or more after birth. This relation persists longest in the region of the anterior fontanelle and the neighbourhood of the inion. Should the skin be imperfectly separated, or a portion remain persistently adherent to the dura mater, it would act precisely as a tumour germ and give rise to a dermoid. Such a tumour may retain its original attachment to the dura mater, and its pedicle become surrounded by bone ; the dermoid would lie outside the bone but be lodged in a depression on the surface, with an aperture transmitting its pedicle. On the other hand, the tumour may become separated from the skin by bone; it would then project on the inner surface or between the layers of the dura mater. If this view of the origin of dermoids be accepted, we must modify our teaching and say that the depressions in which dermoids of the cranium are lodged arise as imperfections in the developmental process, and are not due to absorption induced by pressure; further, the fibrous connexion of such dermoids with the dura mater is primary, not accidental.' [1]

Treatment. When of inconsiderable size, and when intracranial connexions are absent, of doubtful existence, or of slight extent, the sooner the tumour is removed the better. The dura mater should not be opened unless absolutely necessary, in which case it should be carefully sewn up and the scalp-flap replaced without drainage.

When possessing deep and extensive connexions, careful dissection may still allow of the complete removal of the dermoid. It is impossible to foretell with certainty whether it is possible to remove the tumour until its basal portion is exposed. The operation may be a formidable one.

SOME POINTS IN THE DIFFERENTIAL DIAGNOSIS BETWEEN CEPHALOCELES, DERMOIDS, AND CEPHALHÆMATOMATA

Cephaloceles (congenital).	*Dermoids.*	*Cephalhæmatomata.*
Present at birth.	Present at birth.	Usually appears after birth.
In middle line, especially over occiput and base of nose.	In middle line, especially over anterior fontanelle.	Always to one side of the middle line, and usually over the parietal bone.
Firm or fluctuating.	Firm.	Fluctuation over central part only.
Perhaps translucent.	Not translucent.	Not translucent.
Perhaps pulsates.	Does not pulsate.	Does not pulsate.
Perhaps reducible, in whole or in part.	Irreducible.	Very slightly, if at all.
Perhaps swells up on straining.	No alteration.	Very slightly, if at all.
Perhaps associated with cerebral symptoms.	No cerebral symptoms.	No cerebral symptoms.
Gap in skull felt.	Depression in bone common, actual gap comparatively rare.	Deceptive raised margin, no actual central depression.

[1] *Tumours, Innocent and Malignant.* Bland Sutton.

HYDROCEPHALUS

The conditions that lead up to internal hydrocephalus are classified by Parkes Weber [1] in the following manner :—

1. 'Cases secondary to and part of the phenomena of tuberculous or any suppurative meningitis, comparable to pleural effusions due to tuberculous or any septic invasions of the pleura.

2. Cases resulting from the presence of tumours, &c., analagous to the pleuritic effusions accompanying tumours, &c., situated close to or involving the pleura.

3. Ordinary infantile or congenital hydrocephalus, which is, in some cases at least, due to intra-uterine meningitis.

4. Internal hydrocephalus supervening on the epidemic or sporadic type of posterior basic non-suppurative meningitis.

6. Simple idiopathic internal hydrocephalus of adults or older children due to serous ependymitis or ventricular meningitis.

7. Traumatic cases.'

This classification possibly includes all the various grades and degrees of internal hydrocephalus, but for all practical purposes the cases may be grouped into two classes, congenital and acquired, both of which may be either acute or chronic.

Congenital internal hydrocephalus. The condition may be recognized soon after the birth of the child, or the enlargement of the head may only become apparent some weeks or months later. The slow development and the insidious nature of the enlargement, as observed in many cases, may lead to some confusion between the late congenital and the early acquired varieties. However, the absence of any symptoms pointing to meningeal inflammation between the time of the birth of the child and the hydrocephalic development usually allows of correct classification.

It is doubtful whether congenital internal hydrocephalus can be ascribed to malformation of the inter-ventricular channels and occlusion of the passages by means of which the cerebro-spinal fluid escapes into the cerebral subarachnoid space, or whether the development is dependent on hypersecretion from the ependyma and choroid plexuses. Virchow showed that occasionally there was an actual

[1] *Brain*, 1902, p. 140.

formation of small grey-red masses, about the size of a hemp-seed or cherry, in the walls of the ventricles, but other authorities deny the existence of such changes, and consider that the hydrocephalic condition is entirely dependent on congenital malformation.

It would, however, seem more probable that we have to deal with two distinct varieties of congenital internal hydrocephalus, one resulting from intra-uterine ependymal inflammation (? syphilitic), the other dependent on congenital malformations, especially in the region of the fourth ventricle, where the foramina of Majendie, Key, and Retzius are regarded as permitting the outward escape of the fluid secreted from the lining membrane and choroid plexuses of the ventricles.

Acquired hydrocephalus. Acquired hydrocephalus, whether acute or chronic, presents certain antecedents or associations which enable us to have a more clear idea as to the pathological conditions present.

In the majority of cases it is secondary to basic meningitis which, whether tuberculous or not, results in matting of membranes and in the development of adhesions. The normal flow of cerebro-spinal fluid from the ventricular to the cerebral subarachnoid spaces is thus impeded.

Similar interference to the flow of cerebro-spinal fluid may be caused by the growth of a tumour, especially those which originate in the subtentorial region.

Progress of the case. Whether the progress of the case be acute or chronic, the ultimate results are much the same. The fluid in the ventricular spaces may be increased up to 1,000 c.c. or more, pressure effects being exerted on the surrounding parts, with the following results :—

A. The soft cerebral substance is slowly but surely compressed, with the result that the sulci on the surface of the brain are more or less obliterated, distinction between the white and grey matter may be lost, the ventricular spaces are enormously dilated, and, in the most marked cases, a mere shell of brain may intervene between the ventricles and the surface of the brain.

This cerebral compression results in the development of two main groups of symptoms, those referable to the general increase in the intraventricular pressure and those due to regional compression.

The more general results are headache, vomiting, optic neuritis and atrophy, slow pulse-rate, somnolence, and coma. The temperature is variable, more commonly rising during the more acute stages of the disease, and falling to normal or subnormal during the quiescent periods.

Localizing features are to be found in squints, inequality of pupils, retraction of the head and neck, dyspnœa, and dysphagia, whilst compression of the cortical motor centres is evidenced by twitchings, convulsions, and spasticity of the limbs. General convulsions are by no means uncommon. Remissions and intermissions of both local and general symptoms are frequently observed, paralyses, for example, fluctuating in depth and character.

B. The bones comprising the vault of the skull become greatly thinned and widely separated from one another, the fontanelles enlarged, and the sutures unduly prominent. The head becomes enlarged in all directions, and its increased weight renders the child incapable of retaining postural control, the head being top-heavy and falling about in all directions.

The bones of the base share in the deformity. The pressure exerted on the orbital plates of the frontal bone force the globe in the downward direction in such a manner that the infra-corneal sclerotic is obscured by the lower lid, whilst the supra-corneal portion is unduly prominent. The bony eminences in the region of the sella turcica are diminished in size, the middle fossa of the skull flattened from side to side, and the posterior fossa from before backwards. In such cases the skull assumes an almost dolicocephalic appearance. In any case, the disproportion between the enlarged skull and diminutive face is a marked feature.[1]

The scalp becomes stretched, hairs are sparse and brittle, and the veins dilated.

[1] In estimating the size of the head, the following tables—after Bonnifay—will be useful :—

Age.	*Circumference of head* (average).
Birth to fifteenth day . . .	343 millimetres (approximate).
Fifteenth day to 2 months . .	368 ,, ,,
At 3 months	388 ,, ,,
Six months to 1 year . . .	429 ,, ,,
One year to 2 years	459 ,, ,,

Treatment. *Indications for operation.* The results obtained by operation for internal hydrocephalus are not sufficiently encouraging to enable the surgeon to urge immediate operative treatment.[1] Still, it is perfectly clear that he cannot possibly carry out surgical treatment with benefit to the patient if the ventricular distension is allowed to progress to such a degree that marked cortical flattening and degeneration occurs. No fixed probationary period can be laid down as a guide, each case must be judged on its own merits. Special attention should be paid, however, to the disks and lower extremities. Any suggestion of optic neuritis or spasticity should be regarded as urgently demanding operative interference.

Lumbar puncture cannot be expected to confer other than temporary benefit even under the most favourable circumstances, whilst, in the event of interference in the normal communication between the ventricular and cerebro-spinal spaces, no relief can be anticipated. Connal recommends that lumbar puncture should be carried out daily, or twice daily, over extended periods of time. This operation, however, is by no means devoid of danger, and the results obtained by such treatment are not at all satisfactory.

Operation. Operations are carried out (*a*) with the object of withdrawing fluid from the distended ventricular cavities (ventricular puncture), and (*b*) to establish a communication, or short-circuit, between the ventricular space and other spaces (ventricular drainage).

Normal rapidity of growth of the head

During the first 3 months . . .	44 millimetres (approximate).		
During 3 to 6 months . . .	41	,,	,,
From 6 months to 1 year . . .	30	,,	,,
During second year	14	,,	,,

It should be noted that enlargement of the head can only take place during the years previous to synostosis of the skull bones. Leonard Guthrie (Harveian Lecture, March 17, 1910) writes, 'I cannot find from any recorded cases of hydrocephalus acquired in later childhood and adult life that an increase in the size of the head has been any aid to diagnosis, and I believe it is true that internal hydrocephalus acquired after the sutures are set is hardly distinguishable from a non-localizable intracranial new growth giving rise to headache, vomiting, and optic neuritis.'

[1] The treatment for acquired hydrocephalus dependent on tumour formation is discussed elsewhere. This section deals with the congenital variety and with those cases of acquired hydrocephalus not due to obstruction by tumours.

Ventricular puncture. This operation may be carried out through the anterior fontanelle, through the frontal bone, or over the descending cornu of the lateral ventricle.

Through the anterior fontanelle. The region of the fontanelle is shaved and cleansed in the usual manner, after which the surrounding parts are cut off from the field of operation by a large sheet of gauze or lint, in which a hole is cut sufficing to allow of exposure of the site of election for puncture.

The patient should be in the recumbent position, the head well towards the end of the table. The operation is performed without an anæsthetic or under local anæsthesia. A site is chosen at the outer angle of the fontanelle, about 1 inch away from the median antero-posterior line, thus avoiding all possibility of injuring the superior longitudinal venous sinus. The trocar and cannula, of small size, is passed directly inwards, towards the base of the skull, for a distance of not more than 2 inches. The trocar is withdrawn and the fluid allowed to escape slowly. If the cerebro-spinal fluid escapes at high pressure, the flow should be regulated by the finger placed over the mouth of the cannula, and, in any case, it is inadvisable to allow of the withdrawal of more than 50 c.c. (approximately 1½ ounces) at one sitting. The cannula is withdrawn and the site of tapping covered with collodion gauze. Even when adopting all precautions the operation is not without danger, and, added to this, is the fact that few surgeons care about introducing an instrument blindly into the cerebral cortex—the risk of puncturing one of the distended superficial cerebral veins is sufficiently obvious.

Through the frontal bone. Tillmanns, in recommending this procedure, states that 'the needle should be inserted about 2 centimetres from the central line and 3 centimetres from the precentral sulcus. You strike the ventricle at a depth of from 3 to 5 centimetres'. He claims that this method leads to satisfactory results. It is open, however, to all the objections of puncture through the fontanelle.

Over the descending cornu of the lateral ventricle. This operation is strongly recommended by Keen on the ground that excellent drainage is supplied. A point is mapped out on the skull which lies 1¼ inches behind the external auditory meatus and the same distance above Reid's base-line. If the postero-lateral fontanelle be open a small trocar and cannula may be introduced at the upper angle of the space—thus avoiding the lateral sinus—and passed inwards in a direction towards the summit of the opposite ear. If the fontanelle be closed, a scalp-flap is framed and a bone-disk removed with a $\frac{1}{4}$–$\frac{1}{2}$ inch diameter trephine. The dura should not be opened. The evacuating instrument is then introduced through the membrane in the same direction as before. In either case it should not be passed for a greater distance than $1\frac{1}{2}$ inches, and, in all cases, the exploration should be of a progressive nature, that is to say, the trocar should be withdrawn once for each $\frac{1}{2}$ inch of brain substance perforated. The escape of cerebro-spinal fluid must be regulated in the manner previously described.

If trephining has been necessitated, the bone-disk is not replaced, thus allowing of subsequent tappings through the trephine-hole, this gap now taking the place of a patent postero-lateral fontanelle.

Keen's method of ventricular puncture presents many advantages over other methods, though still open to the objection that the actual central puncture is done blindly.

Ventricular-subdural drainage. A point is mapped out on the scalp which corresponds to the surface-marking of the descending horn of the lateral ventricle (see p. 3), and, with this point as a guide, a scalp-flap is framed, the base of which lies immediately below the indicated spot whilst its convexity is situated between $1\frac{1}{2}$ and 2 inches above. This flap should not include the pericranium. The flap is turned down to its base, the pericranium stripped aside and a disk of bone removed, at the upper part of the exposed bone, with a $\frac{1}{4}$ or $\frac{1}{2}$ inch diameter trephine. The bone is usually very thin.

When this disk is removed, the dura is separated from the bone, and, with the aid of a strong pair of scissors, the bone is cut in such a manner as to form a bone-flap, the margins of which lie well within those of the scalp-flap (see Fig. 26). This flap is broken across at its base, turned down, and covered with gauze.

At the lower portion of the exposed dura mater, a crucial incision is made through the dura mater and a blunt-pointed trocar and cannula introduced at the centre of the exposed brain, all visible vessels being avoided. The diagnosis is now confirmed—by the withdrawal of the trocar and the escape of cerebro-spinal fluid.

By the introduction of a bundle of horsehair or catgut, passed through the cannula so as to project into the ventricular cavity, and, after the withdrawal of the cannula, tucked, with respect to the proximal ends, into the subdural, extra-dural, or subaponeurotic spaces, it is obvious that drainage may be established between the

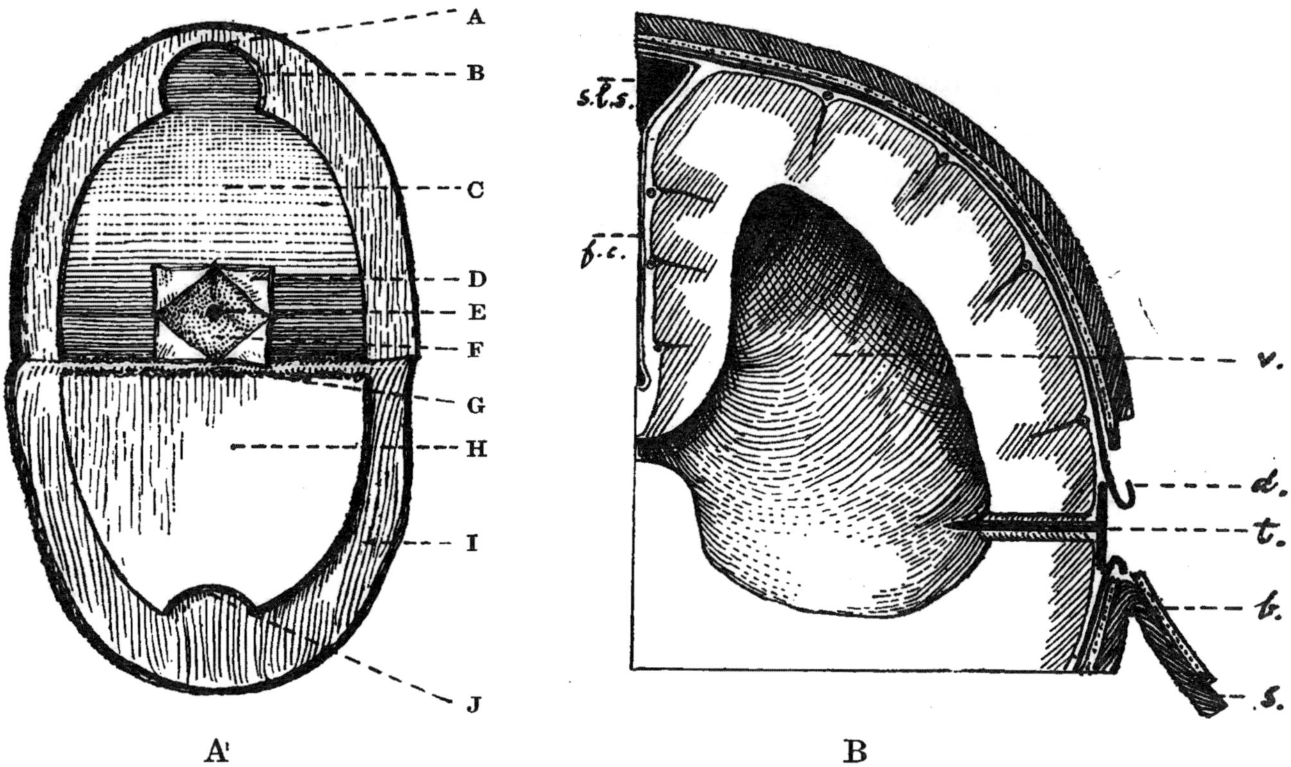

FIG. 26. DIAGRAMMATIC REPRESENTATION OF THE AUTHOR'S OPERATION FOR HYDROCEPHALUS INTERNUS. A. The osteoplastic exposure of the brain (A, The bone; B, Upper two-thirds of trephine hole; C, Dura mater; D, The four dural flaps; E, Site of brain perforation; F, The brain; G, Line of fracture of bone-flap; H, The bone-flap; I, The Scalp; J, Lower third of trephine hole). B. Ventriculo-subdural drainage (*s.*, The scalp; *b.*, The bone; *d.*, The dura mater; *v.*, The lateral ventricle; *t.*, The drainage medium between the ventricular cavity and the subdural space; *s.l.s.*, Superior longitudinal sinus; *f.c.*, Falx cerebri).

ventricles and the other regions. Experience showed, however, that drainage into the subaponeurotic space usually converted the condition of hydrocephalus into one of cephalocele (see Fig. 27), the fluid collecting as a localized fluid tumour over the region of exploration, whilst extra-dural drains did not permit of sufficiently rapid reabsorption of fluid. Subdural drainage gave the best results, the cerebro-spinal fluid being brought into relation with the pia-arachnoid meshwork of vessels. It would, of course, be infinitely preferable if the ventricular fluid could be brought into direct relation with the veins of the *subarachnoid* space, for the cerebro-spinal tension and venous pressure are equal, and all excess of cerebro-spinal fluid would be absorbed as soon as it is formed. This course is, however, impossible to carry out. We have, therefore, to rest content with less

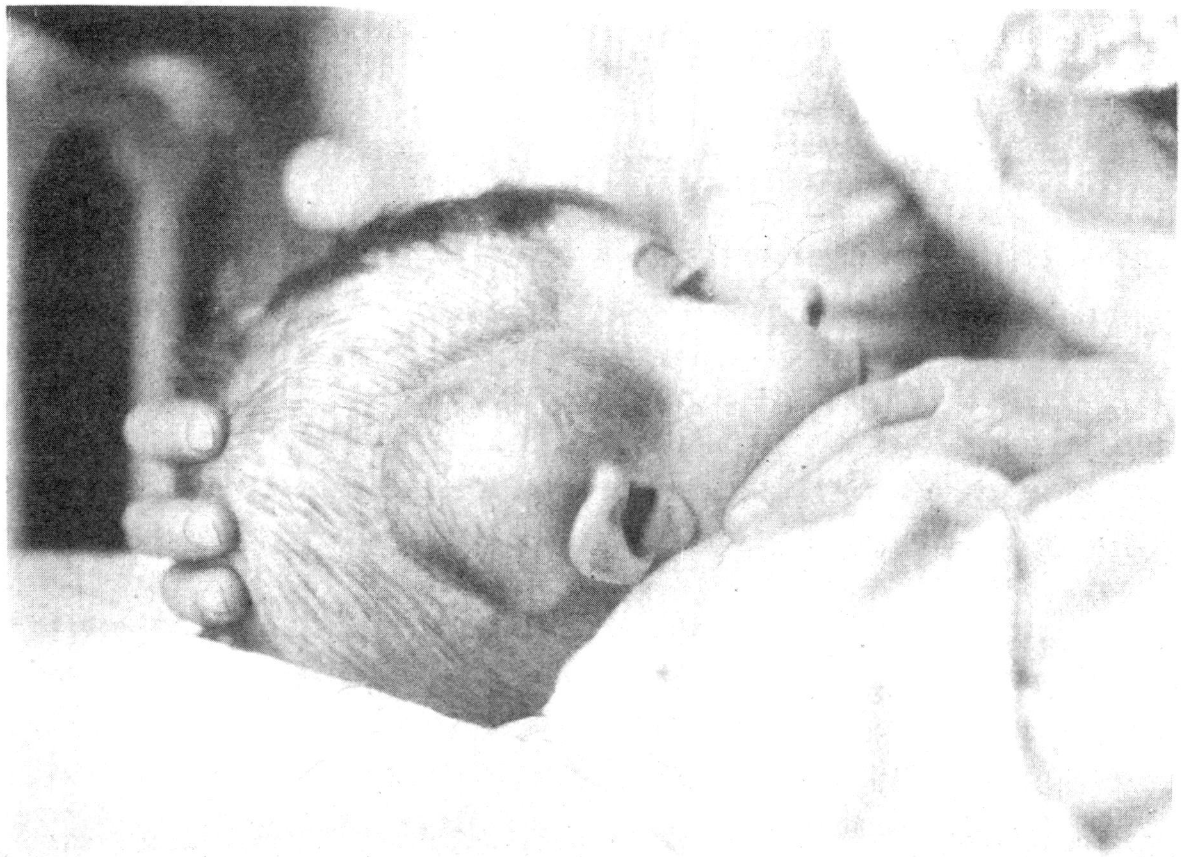

FIG. 27. THE CONVERSION OF HYDROCEPHALUS INTERNUS INTO CEPHALOCELE.

direct contact, drainage into the *subdural* space. This ventricular-subdural drainage, as obtained by horsehair, catgut, and silk, apparently leads to but temporary benefit, probably owing to falling together of the brain substance and obliteration of the adventitious passage.

Silver tubes and bone tubes have been utilized, but the results are sometimes disappointing. In one of my recent cases the two halves of a bone tube were utilized. The tube was cut across in an oblique manner at about its centre, the two parts set at right angles to one another and sewn together with silk. One arm is introduced into the ventricle, the other tucked underneath the dura mater. The child improved considerably, but the method is not altogether satisfactory and by no means easy of application. In another case I utilized strands of silver wire. The depth of brain-tissue necessary to reach the ventricular cavity was measured, and two or three strands of wire introduced so as to project well into that space, then steadied with forceps whilst the proximal ends were bent at right angles to the surface of the brain and tucked underneath the dura mater. The method was unsatisfactory.

Tubular drainage is not essential, for the fluid escapes from the ventricle as much alongside the tube as through its lumen. Still, I believe that tubular drainage is preferable to other methods, and, realizing the difficulty of introducing a right-angled tube—one arm to project into the ventricle, the other to lie beneath the dura mater—Messrs. Arnold & Son are now making for me small and light right-angled silver tubes so constructed that each limb can be inserted independently, after which they can be locked together. This method appears to overcome many of the difficulties previously encountered. The tube is inserted after the formation of the osteoplastic flap, as described above. The four dural flaps are then united, preferably by cross union of their apices, the bone-flap is replaced, and the scalp-flap sewn accurately into position. Collodion gauze, applied to the wound, aids in the prevention of cerebro-spinal escape.

The scalp and bone-flaps are framed, and the dural incision carried out low down, so as to make the opening to the brain as valvular as possible. All these precautions are taken to avoid leakage of cerebro-spinal fluid, a most troublesome complication—adding to the risk of infection and often resulting in an acute eczematous condition of the surrounding skin.

By this method it is hoped that a permanent fistulous communication will be formed between the lateral ventricle and the subdural space.

Ventriculo-abdominal drainage. The following method of drainage has been devised by Cushing: ‘It having been established that the ventricle can be emptied by the lumbar route, and that the withdrawal of fluid is not prejudicial to the child’s well-being, the following procedure is carried out. A laparotomy is performed; the posterior layer of peritoneum to the left of the rectum is split; the body of the fifth lumbar vertebra, just under the bifurcation of the vessels is exposed; the bone is trephined and one-half (the female portion) of a silver cannula, exactly the size of the trephine, is inserted and held in position. The child is then turned on his face and a laminectomy performed; the subarachnoid space is opened, the strands of the cauda separated, and the posterior half (male portion) of the cannula is invaginated, so that it locks into the portion inserted anteriorly. Both wounds are then closed. The fluid for a time finds its way into the peritoneal cavity, but ultimately into the retro-peritoneal space whence it is taken up by the receptaculum chyli, as experimental observations have shown.'

Cushing has carried out this operation in 12 cases with a considerable degree of success.

Recently, another method of treatment has been carried out by Cotterill.[1] A large semilunar flap is made from the occipital region, exposing the bone. Trephine circles are made on either side of the median ridge, and the intermediate part of the bone, together with the posterior part of the foramen magnum, is removed. The dura mater is opened and the occipital sinus ligatured. The lateral lobes of the cerebellum are then held apart, and the thickened arachnoid over the posterior part of these lobes and over the roof of the fourth ventricle exposed. This roof is opened. The wound is then closed.

By this method drainage from the ventricle is said to be re-established. Though without personal experience of this extensive procedure, one cannot avoid expressing considerable doubt as to its advisability.

My own experience would lead me to the following conclusions:—

1. Whilst recognizing that internal hydrocephalus usually demands surgical interference, it is only in some few cases that material benefit results. Some recent successful cases point to the possibility of better results in the future.

2. The operation which promises the best results, combined with the least risk to the patient's life, is that described as ventriculo-subdural drainage.

[1] *Review of Neurology and Psychiatry*, vol. ix, No. 1, p. 1.

CHAPTER IV

FRACTURES OF THE SKULL

General considerations. Fractures of the skull do not form more than one-twentieth part of the fractures admitted annually into the hospitals, but, in spite of this relative infrequency of occurrence, the difficulties attendant on diagnosis, the numerous associated complications, and the all-important question of treatment, invest this subject with a special interest.

The whole question of skull fractures is beset with difficulties, many of which, it is hoped, will be swept away in this and subsequent chapters.

Brief allusion must first be made to some important points in connexion with the anatomical structure of the skull, such as bear relation to fractures and aid in the appreciation of the extent and mechanism of the fracture.

The **vault** varies in density to a remarkable degree, not only in its several parts, but also in different individuals. Cases have now and again been recorded in which a very trivial blow, totally insufficient to produce any definite osseous lesion in the normal individual, has resulted in the production of a vault or basic fracture. Each case, therefore, must be judged on its own merits.

The vault derives its strength from its shape and structure. The two tables are of equal strength, and, for the most part, separated from one another by a variable amount of diploic tissue. This diploe is most abundant in the frontal, parietal, and upper occipital regions. These parts are proportionately strong. Two regions are practically devoid of this inter-tabular buffer—the squamo-temporal and cerebellar (see Figs. 29 and 50). A recognition of this comparative weakness is of great practical importance in view of the fact that both these regions are liable to special lesions—injury to the middle meningeal artery in the first case, and, in the second, cerebello-medullary lesions. Nature's ' mistake ' in providing coverings unsuited to requirements has been compensated for in part by additional protection—the temporal and nuchal muscles.

Further, not only does the skull vary in density in its several parts, but it is also ribbed and strengthened by various bony bars

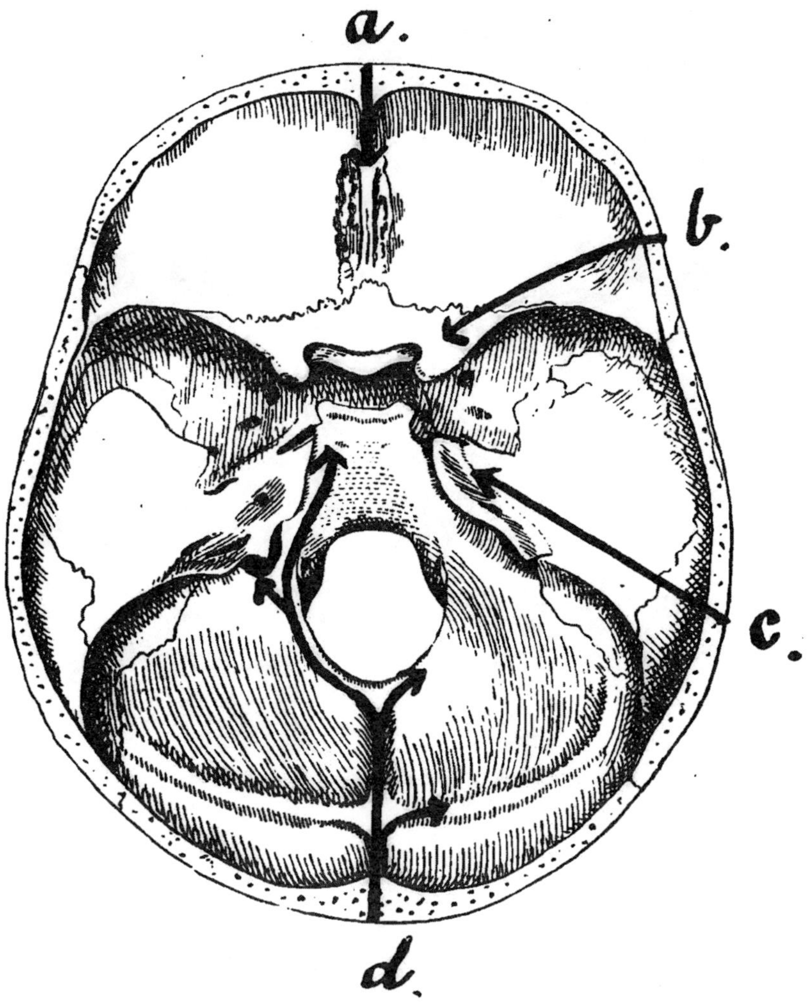

FIG. 28. DIAGRAM ILLUSTRATING THE LINES ALONG WHICH FORCES RECEIVED ON THE VAULT ARE TRANSMITTED TO THE BASE. (For further description, see text.)

and buttresses that pass up from base to vault (see Fig. 28). These 'ribbings' are seen to extend upwards from the crista galli, from the external angular frontal process, from the auditory region, and from the occipital protuberance. Presumably, these 'ribbings' were so constituted for a definite purpose; in any case, it is clear that they play an important part in the reception and conduction of forces to the base of the skull. It is apparent, moreover, that the parts intervening between these 'ribbings' are liable to injury in direct proportion to their general position and strength. The deep groovings of the bone for the reception of the middle meningeal artery

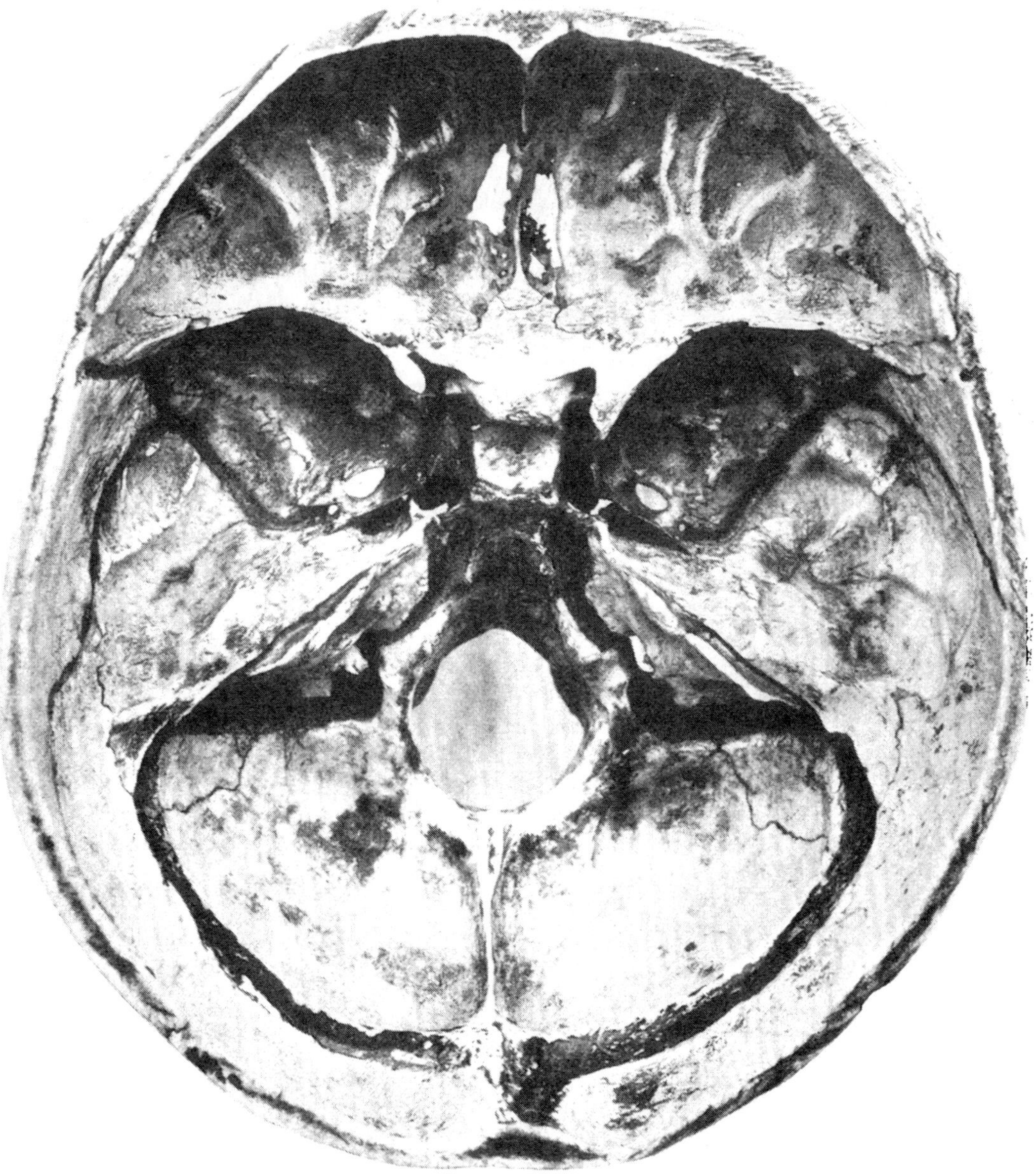

FIG. 29 A. THE BASE OF THE SKULL.

afford an additional source of weakness to the bone in the squamo-temporal region. (See Fig. 50).

Further reference will be made to the relative strengths of the various regions of the skull. Sufficient has been said to show that nature has provided the skull with various paths by means of which forces applied to the vault can be conducted and distributed to the base.

Before, however, proceeding to discuss the effects produced on the base of the skull, it is necessary to add that nature provides other

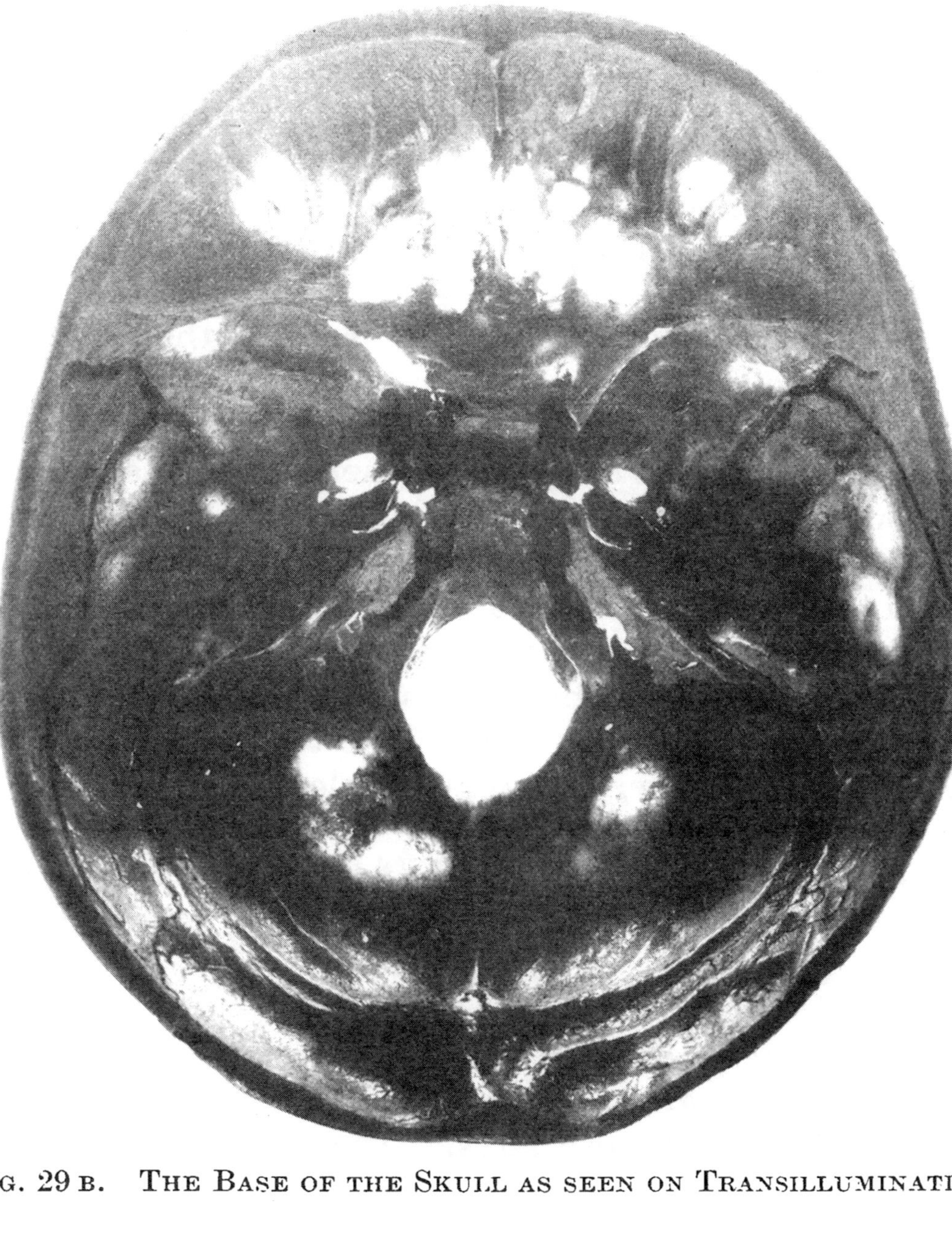

FIG. 29 B. THE BASE OF THE SKULL AS SEEN ON TRANSILLUMINATION.

methods by means of which the intensity of a blow, delivered over the vertex of the skull, is diminished. The forces are broken up and distributed in the following manner :—

1. Though the force tends to travel in the direction of the applied force, yet the convexity of the skull allows of the dissemination of that force over a large superficial area.

2. The intervention of cartilage or fibrous tissue between two or more of the component bones of the vault tends to diminish the intensity of the force, to break it up and to alter its direction.

3. The bony ridges, along which the forces tend to travel, themselves terminate blindly (see Fig. 28). Thus,

(*a*) Forces passing from the frontal region converge, more or less, to the crista galli.

(*b*) Forces from the external angular frontal process pass along the wings of the sphenoid bone to the anterior clinoid process.

(*c*) Forces from the auditory region are projected along the summit of the petrous bone towards the apex of that process and to the posterior clinoid process.

(*d*) Forces applied to the occipital region travel inwards along the internal occipital crest to the strengthened margins of the foramen magnum, or are projected outwards along the lateral sinus ridges. In the former case, the force either passes forwards towards the dorsum ephipii and so again reaches the posterior clinoid process, or is directed more laterally towards the jugular process of the occipital bone, there meeting the fibrous tissue intervening between that process and the corresponding part of the temporal bone.

4. All forces, whether transmitted along the internal occipital crest, the temporal bone, the sphenoidal wings, or the crista galli of the ethmoid, are further transmitted to the dura mater attached to those prominences and ridges. The dura mater undoubtedly plays an important part in the reception and transmission of the forces.

5. The forces all show a tendency to converge towards the pituitary region, the great 'water-cushion' of the brain—a region bounded by the clinoid processes. That these processes receive a considerable part of the forces transmitted is confirmed by the fact that they are frequently torn away from their basic attachments. This is especially the case with respect to the attenuated base of the anterior clinoid process.

It is obvious, therefore, that forces tend to be transmitted from the vault to the base, and yet the base is, in many respects, the weakest part of the skull. It is perforated by numerous foramina, it is hollowed out in places for the formation of air sinuses and for the reception of the integral portions of the auditory apparatus. Furthermore, it presents a more or less plane surface, one differing in all respects from the marked convexity of the vault. Those forces, therefore, which are received by the base of the skull are not subjected to that diffusion which forms so conspicuous a feature in the case of the vault.

All these points tend to show that the base of the skull is more or less unsuited for the reception of severe blows, direct or transmitted, whilst, on the other hand, nature has taken into consideration and provided fairly adequately against the dangers incident to vault injuries.

It is not proposed at this stage to discuss further the relative strength of vault and base. Points, other than those already enumerated, will be brought forward in subsequent sections.

FRACTURES OF THE BASE OF THE SKULL

Fractures of the base of the skull are produced in two ways :—

1. By violence applied *directly* to the base—perforating wounds of the orbit, bullet-wounds through the mouth and base of skull, the driving inwards of the bones of the face, the driving upwards of the condyle of the jaw (the 'knock-out' blow of the pugilist), and, as the result of heavy falls on to the feet or buttocks, the upward driving of the condyles of the occipital bone.

2. By violence applied *indirectly*—blows applied directly to the vault and transmitted to the base. This variety will be considered first as it receives the greatest prominence in surgical textbooks. Various explanatory theories have been advanced, of which the following are the more important :—

(*a*) **Aran's theory of irradiation.** This theory states that 'fractures of the base result as extensions from fractures of the vault, the fracture following the shortest anatomical route to the base'. Although this theory must be accepted as offering a satisfactory explanation for the occurrence of a certain proportion of basic fractures, such, for instance, as result from a blow applied directly to the vertex, it certainly cannot be accepted as accounting for the great majority of basic fractures. The theory was advanced on the hypothesis that basic and vault fractures were necessarily co-existent.

That combined lesions of this nature are frequently in evidence is not to be doubted for one instant. It is, however, 'putting the cart before the horse' to say that the vault fracture is always the primary lesion. Such is by no means the case.

(*b*) **The bursting and compression theories.** The skull is here regarded as an highly elastic sphere, compression of which leads to diminution in the diameter along the axis of greatest pressure, bulging occurring in other diameters. The bulging exceeding the limits of elasticity a fracture occurs, the line of fracture varying according to the different features present. Thus, when the lines of fracture run parallel to the direction of the compressing force the bone bursts open along the convexity (bursting fractures), and when the lines of fracture run at right angles to the direction of the compressing force a fracture by compression is said to result (compression fractures).

These theories are based on experiments carried out on the cadaver, the skull being enclosed in a tight-fitting box and subjected to pressure sufficing to bring about a fracture. Undoubtedly, the head may be compressed between two forces, as, for instance, when a person is knocked down in the street, the vehicle passing over the head, or, as in a case recently under my care, where a boy, hanging by his feet from the side of a barge, was crushed between the barge and the wharf as the vessel swung inwards with the tide. Cases of bilateral compression are, however, of infrequent occurrence, the great majority of basic fractures resulting from blows applied directly at the region of the level of the base of the skull (see p. 76), or from the forward propulsion of the body, the head coming into violent contact with a resisting object, as, for instance, when a person is thrown out from a motor-car, the head striking against a tree, brick wall, &c. In the first case, there can be no question of bilateral compression, and in the second the compression is exerted between the vertex and the occipital condyloid region.

Moreover, the fundamental points on which the bursting and compression theories are grounded are based on erroneous principles. The skull cannot in any sense be regarded as a sphere, nor does it possess the requisite elasticity to bulge and allow of compression in the manner that the theory demands. The skull, in reality, forms rather less than two-thirds of a sphere, the base passing inwards from the lower limits of this partial sphere in a more or less horizontal plane. This can be readily verified by placing the skull on a table so that its base corresponds to the surface of the table. The elastic properties of the skull have also been greatly exaggerated, and far too little attention has been paid to the peculiar anatomical formation of the base.

(*c*) **The contre-coup theories.** Fractures of the base occasionally occur in which evidence is conclusive that the blow was received on the vault, the vault itself remaining uninjured. Such cases have given origin to this theory, one stating that 'from the point struck a wave is transmitted through the semi-fluid brain, producing a fracture at some more distant point'. Helferich, for instance, maintains that isolated fractures of the orbital roof, and more rarely of other parts of the base, are produced by the influence of hydrostatic pressure. There can be no question that waves are transmitted through the brain and cerebro-spinal fluid, but that such waves should be capable of producing a basic fracture is, in my opinion, beyond the bounds of possibility. The theory is opposed to all my experience of basic fractures, and the cases brought forward in support are capable of a much more probable explanation. The base is undoubtedly the weakest part of the skull, and a blow on the vault may fail to produce a local lesion and yet, when the force is transmitted to the weaker base, may there bring about a more definite result. For instance, it is by no means uncommon to find that a blow on the frontal region fails to fracture the vertical plate of that bone and yet suffices to produce a fracture, often comminuted, of the orbital plate of the frontal bone or of the cribriform plate of the ethmoid, two fragile plates, either of which may shatter like a plate of glass from the effect of forces transmitted across them. In further support of this theory, the following case, recently under my care, may be cited. The patient received a heavy blow over the left occipital region. A fracture passed inwards across the left cerebellar fossa towards the posterior border of the foramen magnum, and a second fracture, entirely distinct from the first, passed across the right orbital plate of the frontal bone. In this case, the force conducted across the base, from behind forwards, failed to fracture the strong basi-occiput, but succeeded in producing a more definite lesion on reaching the fragile orbital plate.

Some of the celebrated surgeons of the last century insisted that the course pursued by basic fractures was to be explained on anatomical grounds, but their views have been neglected and theories based on experimental evidence have been accepted in their place. All experiments, such as those previously mentioned, are useless, and definite conclusions can only be gained by carrying out in every case the following method of investigation: (1) by obtaining in the first case an accurate history as to the manner in which the injury was received; (2) by noting all visible and palpable signs of external injury; (3) by careful observation of all the clinical symptoms during the progress of the case; (4) by comparison of such with the lesions found in case of death.

Over 300 cases have been investigated by me after these principles. In about 30 per cent. of the cases sufficient evidence was obtained to show that the basic fracture resulted and extended from a primary fracture of the vault. These cases were to be explained by Aran's theory of irradiation. This theory, however, errs in stating further that the fracture follows the shortest anatomical route to the base. This is not correct, for the line of fracture corresponds to the direction of the applied force and is influenced to a very large extent by the resistance offered, the weaker areas being picked out and the strong buttresses avoided. It is only in the most severe cases that the fracture travels to and traverses across the base in such a direction as to show that, for the time being, all laws are in abeyance.

In about 5 per cent. of cases the fracture resulted from bilateral compression, from falls on to the buttocks, &c., and from blows applied to the angle of the jaw. These cases afforded examples of the bursting and compression theories.

On the other hand, in over 60 per cent. cases, the injury was received over one of the following situations: (1) in front, over the frontal eminence or supra-orbital ridges; (2) in the antero-lateral region, over the external angular frontal process; (3) in the lateral region, over the lower temporal, auricular, and mastoid regions; (4) in the posterior region, over the superior curved line of the occipital bone or over the external occipital protuberance.

In all these cases, therefore, the blow was inflicted at or near the level of the base of the skull, the resultant fracture being a fracture by direct violence, the fracture traversing the base and splitting it much in the same way as a chisel splits a board of wood. The 'grain' of the wood may be regarded as representing the weaker basic lines, and any 'knot' the resistance offered by the strong basic buttresses,

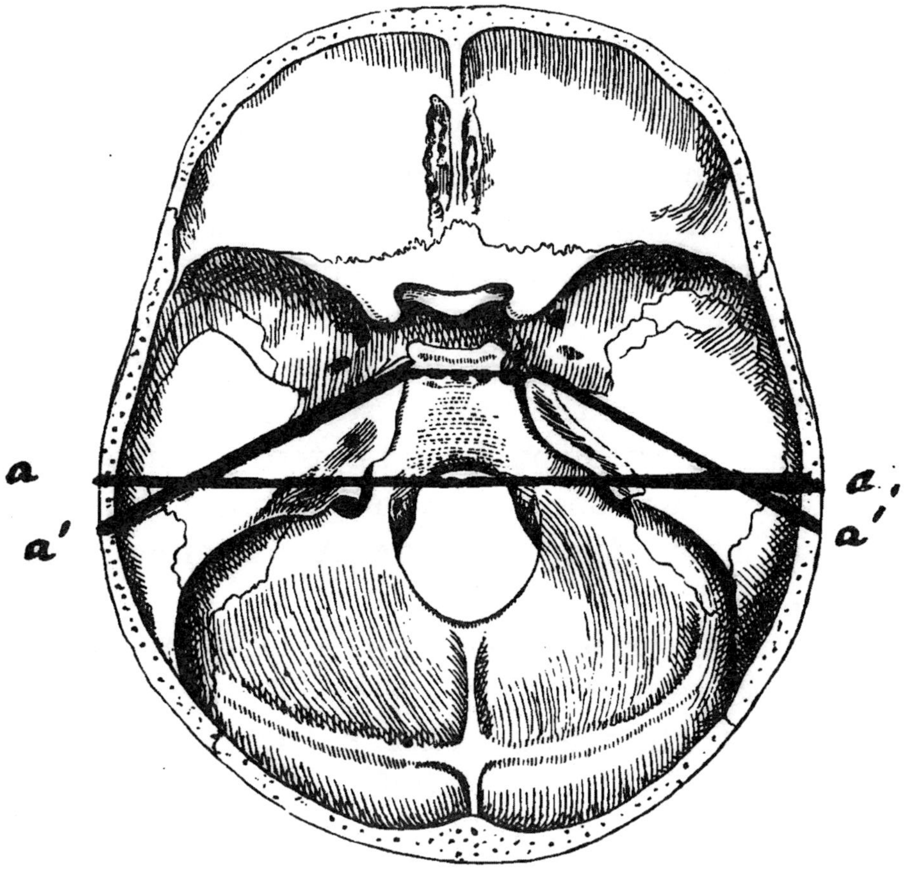

FIG. 30. PLAN OF THE BASE OF THE SKULL. *a*, *a*, The transverse pre-condyloid line ; *a′*, *a′*, The line pursued, in whole or in part, by the 'typical' basic fracture.

the forces being momentarily turned aside, but soon again passing onwards, parallel to the original direction, but not necessarily in the same straight line.

Any blow delivered at or near the basic level tends *primarily to involve the weaker area, the base, passing secondarily upwards on to the vault.* One may go even so far as to say that in most combined vault and basic fractures, the vault fracture is a secondary development, the basic fracture being the primary lesion.

There is, however, still another important anatomical feature bearing on the mechanism of basic fractures, one that must necessarily come into force in the greater number of such fractures. The base of the skull may be said to consist of two parts, one lying anterior to the condyles of the occipital bone, the other posterior to and including the condyles with their vertebral attachment. These two segments are united to one another by a weak chain—represented by a line drawn from one external auditory meatus to the other, with, as a connecting link, the sphenoidal sinus in the middle line.

When the base of the skull is viewed from below, it will be seen that the weak line includes both Glaserian fissures, both petro-sphenoidal sutures, both foramina lacera media, with the sphenoidal sinus again as a connecting link. The two parts of the skull are, to all intents and purposes, merely cemented together by the union of the basi-sphenoid and basi-occiput. Consequently, if a blow be received on the antero-lateral region of the head, the anterior segment tends to be split off from the more fixed posterior part, the fracture following the weak line previously indicated. This weak line occupies so important a position in the mechanism of basic fractures that careful observation will show that the greater number of middle fossa fractures follow that line, wholly or in part. Such a fracture of the middle fossa may be termed 'the typical fracture of the base of the skull' (see Figs. 30, 34 and 39).

Summary of theories. Aran's theory of irradiation, with certain modifications, accounts satisfactorily for about 30 per cent. of basic fractures.

The contre-coup theory may be rejected entirely.

The bursting and compression theories are unsatisfactory, accounting for not more than about 5 per cent fractures.

The majority of cases result from direct violence applied at or near the basic level, the fracture passing across the base in the general direction of the applied force, but not necessarily in the same straight line.

Up to this point certain facts and theories have been discussed, such as bear on the general mechanism of basic fractures. It now remains to consider other factors that exercise influence on the general direction of the fracture.

The influence of sutures on the line of the fracture. Complete maceration of the skull is always essential in endeavouring to estimate in what way the various sutures of the skull influence the extent and direction of a fracture. Sutural separation is generally regarded as of infrequent occurrence. An examination of a large number of macerated skulls has shown, however, that sutural separation is in reality of common occurrence. Certain sutures show a special liability to such changes, especially the masto-occipital, the petro-occipital, and the petro-sphenoidal. Separation of the sutures is more common in the young adult ; in the infant and in the old such conditions are seldom observed.

Allusion has already been made to the fact that forces transmitted from the vault to the base, or vice versa, undergo a marked diminution in intensity when the sutures of the skull are encountered, the 'fracture' showing a marked disposition to follow the line of the suture. When the force is excessive, all rules are temporarily in abeyance, but, under ordinary circumstances, the separation along the line of a suture corresponds fairly accurately with the dentations and serrations of the suture involved. Sutural separation without actual fracture is a possible occurrence, but is decidedly rare. Such isolated fractures are confined, more or less, to the sagittal suture in the vault, and the masto- and petro-occipital sutures in the base.

The influence of air-sinuses, &c., on the line of the fracture. The *sphenoidal sinuses,* two in number, are usually separated from one another by a thin septum. This septum is, however, often deficient, and a single cavity exists. The sinuses make their appearance about the seventh or eighth year ; they vary greatly in size but, when fully developed, occupy the greater part of the so-called body of the sphenoid, extending backwards almost as far as the junction of the basi-sphenoid and basi-occiput, and spreading outwards into the wings of the sphenoid and over the roof of the orbit.

The sinus is bounded on all sides by a thin lamella of bone ; its roof forms part of the middle fossa of the skull, the sides are separated by a thin bony wall from the cavernous venous sinus, and the floor aids in the formation of the roof of the naso-pharynx. There exists, therefore, in the very centre of the base of the skull—in the region of the so-called buttress of connexion between the posterior and anterior segments of the skull—an exceedingly weak area, one which must be implicated in the great majority of basic fractures. The 'weak line' of the base of the skull—previously referred to—is now still more accentuated.

The sphenoidal sinus is involved in at least 40–50 per cent. of basic fractures, comminution of the sinus wall being often so excessive that a probe can be passed with the greatest ease from the middle fossa into the naso-pharynx. Blood is thus allowed to escape readily into the naso-pharynx, and a source is opened up for the possible development of meningeal infection.

Reference to the various illustrations of fractures of the base will supply further evidence as to the special liability of the sinus region to injury. It will be seen that nearly all fractures that pass one middle fossa to the other, or from one middle fossa to the opposite anterior fossa, traverse this region.

The *frontal sinuses*, also two in number, are separated from one another by a thin osseous septum. Up to the age of puberty these sinuses are either absent or represented by a small cell. Subsequently, they develop rapidly, often extending into the orbital roof. The upper and inner boundary—usually very fragile—assists in the formation of the anterior fossa of the skull. The outer boundary—the perpendicular plate of the frontal bone—is much more dense, and, consequently, a fracture of the outer wall is almost necessarily associated with a fracture involving the inner or orbital boundary, that is to say with a fracture of the anterior fossa.

The ethmoid cells. The ethmoid bone consists of a collection of cells which communicate with the nasal cavity (middle and superior meati), and which are merely separated from the anterior fossa of the skull by the thin cribriform plate. This plate of bone is of so fragile a nature that splintering occurs in the great majority of anterior fossa fractures. The special dangers that arise from the possibility of meningeal infection are obvious.

The auditory region. That part of the petrous bone which encloses the auditory apparatus, and which transmits the seventh and eighth pair of nerves, is proportionately weakened and correspondingly liable to fracture. The special details of these fractures are dealt with on p. 102.

The influence of basic foramina. It has often been stated that a basic fracture is arrested on meeting one of the larger foramina of the skull. With this view I am not in agreement, for not only are the larger foramina frequently involved, such as the foramen lacerum

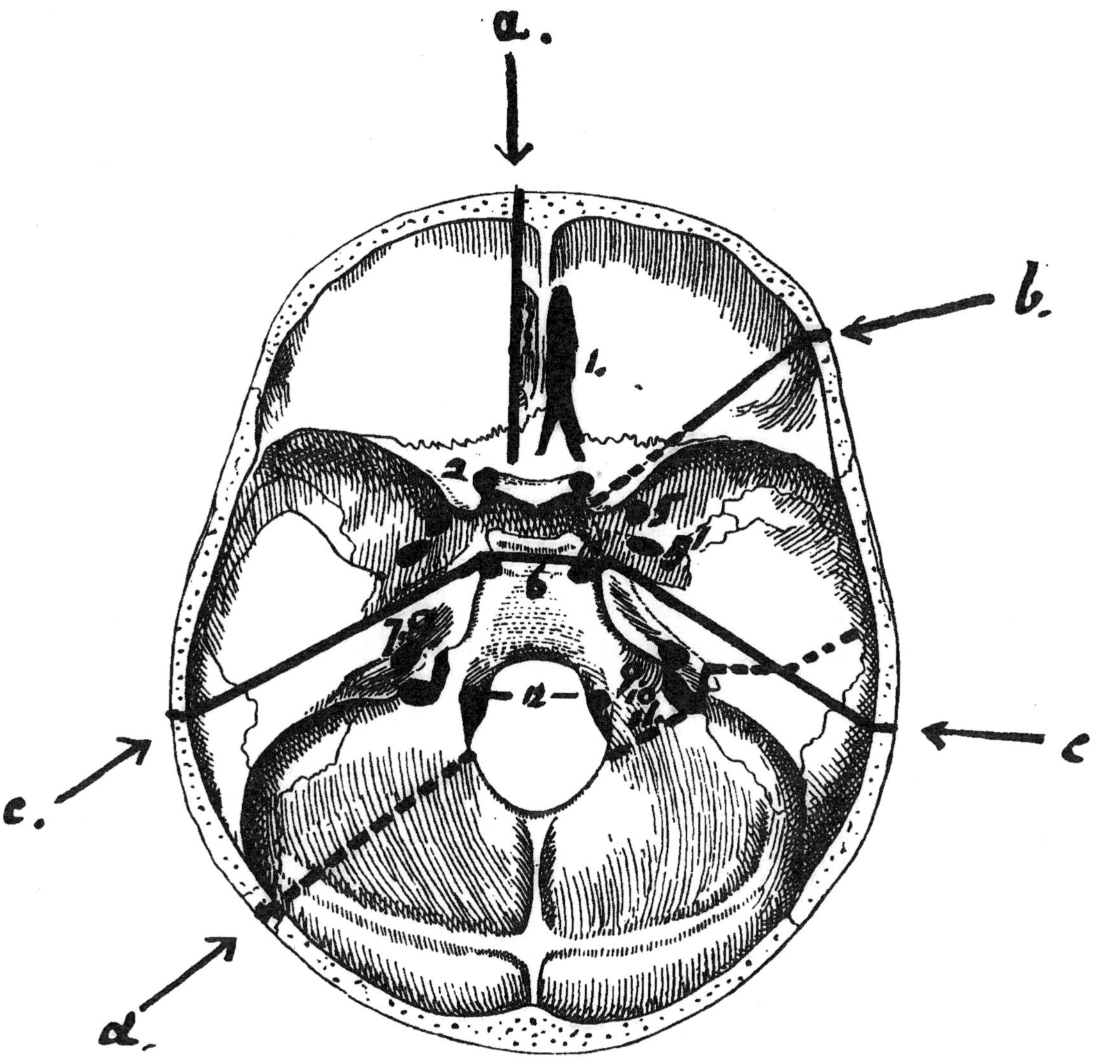

FIG. 31. TO ILLUSTRATE THE RELATION OF BASIC FRACTURES TO CRANIAL NERVES.

posterium and medium, but the largest foramen of all, the foramen magnum, is often implicated. It will be granted that certain foramina are but rarely involved, but this is due to the fact that they are aside of the chosen and definite paths of basic fracture. Thus, the foramen ovale and the foramen spinosum are only exceptionally involved because they lie immediately anterior to the petro-sphenoidal suture, whilst the anterior condyloid foramen—transmitting the hypoglossal nerve—is rarely implicated because it lies internal to the usual posterior fossa fracture. On the other hand, the foramen lacerum medium is involved in nearly every fracture that passes from one middle fossa to the other.

The probable line of basic fracture in any given case. When the various weaker lines and areas are taken into consideration, and when the direction and site of the applied force are known, one is generally enabled to foretell with considerable accuracy the probable transbasic course of the fracture. After investigating over 300 cases, I was enabled to frame the following rules with respect to the probable line of transbasic fracture.

Direction, &c., of the applied force.	*Probable resultant basic fracture.*
1. Force applied to the median frontal region.	The fracture passes backwards from the perpendicular plate of the frontal bone to the cribriform plate of the ethmoid, thence between the optic foramina to the body of the sphenoid, the thin sinus roof being usually comminuted. From there the fracture diverges to the opposite side, and tearing off the posterior clinoid process, passes along the petro-occipital suture to the jugular foramen, being then continued on the other side of that foramen along the masto-occipital suture, and so again to the vault.
2. Force applied to the lateral frontal region, in the situation of the external angular frontal process.	The fracture passes across the anterior fossa towards the sphenoidal fissure, tearing away the anterior clinoid process, and again comminutes the roof of the sphenoidal sinus. Progressing onwards, with or without fracturing the posterior clinoid process, the fracture passes either along the anterior part of the petrous bone at its junction with the greater wing of the sphenoid towards the opposite middle and external ears, or along the petro-occipital suture to the jugular foramen, and continued along the masto-occipital suture as in the previous case.

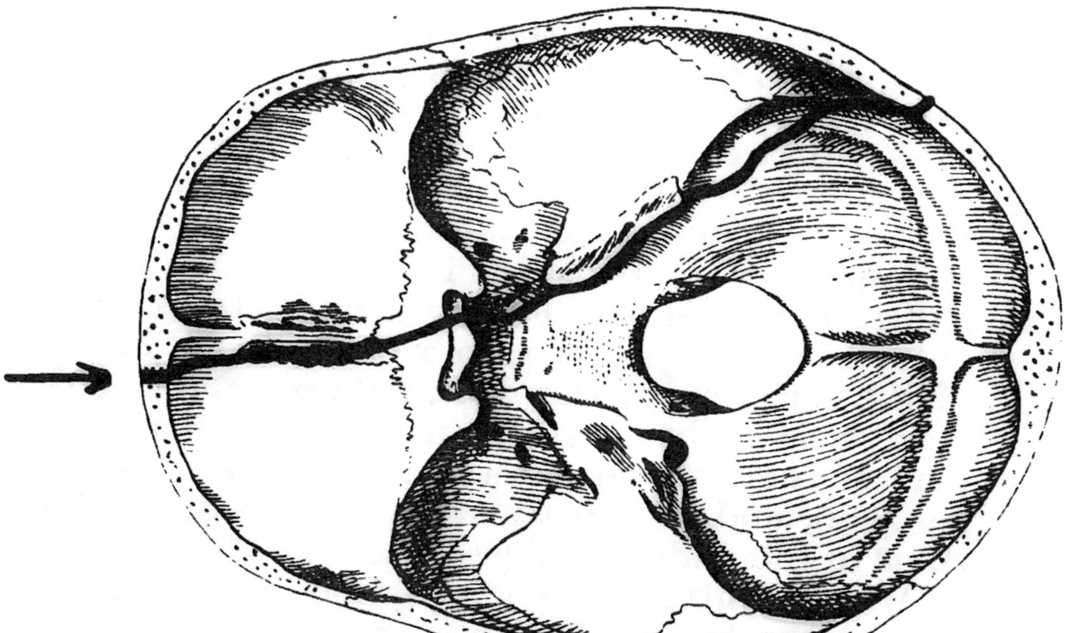

FIG. 32. DIAGRAM OF LINES PURSUED BY BASIC FRACTURES. Force applied to the median frontal region.

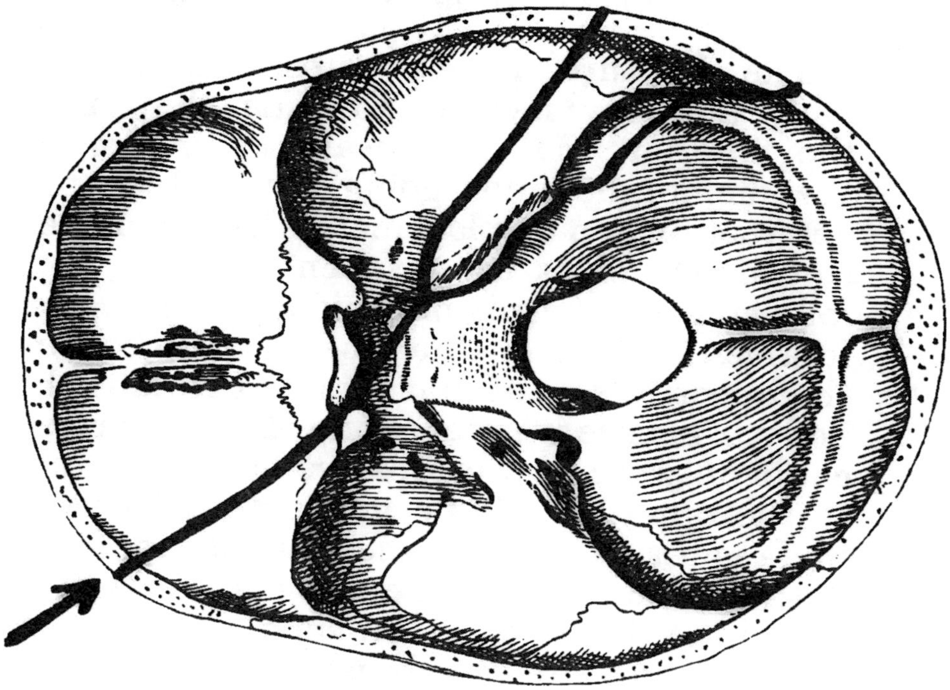

FIG. 33. DIAGRAM OF LINES PURSUED BY BASIC FRACTURES. Force applied to the lateral frontal region in the situation of the external angular frontal process.

Direction, &c., of the applied force.	*Probable resultant basic fracture.*
3. Force applied to the region of the external ear.	The fracture passes across the roof of the bony auditory meatus towards the junction of the anterior and inner walls of the middle ear, the membrane undergoing a variable amount of destruction and displacement. The fracture is then continued across the tegmen tympani, and after following the petro-sphenoidal suture reaches the foramen lacerum medium, being again continued on the opposite side of that foramen to the sphenoidal body. Thence it pursues one of two courses. Most commonly the fracture passes backwards obliquely to the opposite middle and external ears, following a course similar to that already indicated.

In such cases the fracture may extend on each side up on to the vault in such a manner that the two segments are merely united by the soft parts; whether the fracture be so complete or not, a more minute examination of the line of separation will evidence many interesting points. An inspection of the anterior aspect of the posterior fragment shows that the fracture passes just in front of the geniculate ganglion of the facial nerve, the ganglion being laid bare, whilst its petrosal branches are usually torn. The fracture also passes anterior to the Eustachian tube and the horizontal part of the internal carotid artery. On examining this posterior fragment the following structures will be seen, passing from without inwards: the posterior half of the external auditory meatus, the mastoid antrum, the lacerated membrane and the ossicles of the middle ear, the geniculate ganglion of the facial nerve, the Eustachian tube, the horizontal part of the internal carotid artery, the Gasserian ganglion, and the posterior half of the sphenoidal sinus in the middle line (see also Fig. 39).

After reaching the sphenoidal body, the alternative course for the fracture to pursue is to pass towards the opposite sphenoidal fissure and, tearing off the anterior clinoid process, to be directed across the anterior fossa, parallel to the original direction but not in the same straight line.

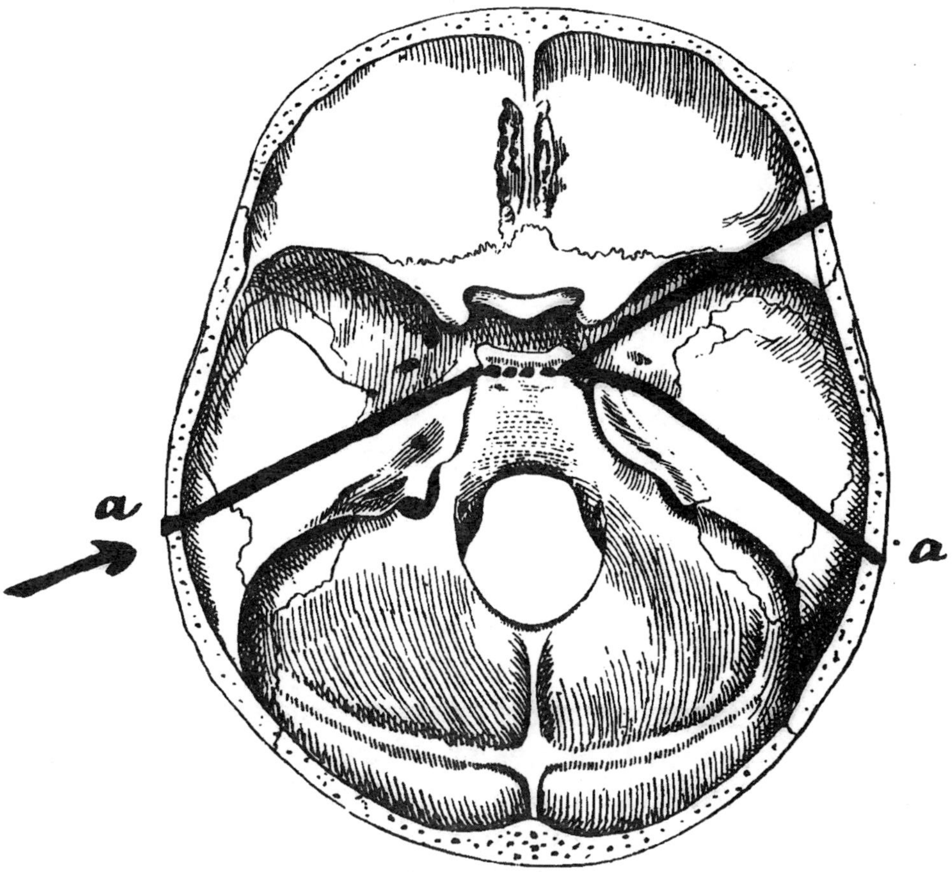

FIG. 34. DIAGRAM OF LINES PURSUED BY BASIC FRACTURES. Force applied to the region of the external ear. *a . . . a*, The 'typical' basic fracture (see also Fig. 30).

Direction, &c., of the applied force.	*Probable resultant basic fracture.*
4. Force applied to the mastoid region.	The fracture follows the occipito-mastoid suture to the jugular foramen, and is again continued on the opposite side of that foramen along the petro-occipital suture towards the apex of the petrous bone. It then passes across the sphenoidal body to the sphenoidal fissure of the opposite side, and so across the anterior fossa. It is especially common in this particular variety of fracture to find fissures diverging from the region of the sphenoidal sinus forwards towards the cribriform plate of the ethmoid, these fissures usually passing between the optic foramina. This fracture is also peculiar in so much that, when the degree of separation along the occipito-mastoid suture is excessive, there is special liability to a tearing of the lateral sinus wall as the sinus begins to turn downwards and inwards.
5. Force applied to the lateral occipital region.	The fracture passes across the thin cerebellar fossa and strikes the foramen magnum immediately behind the condyle. Starting again from a similar point on the opposite side of the foramen, the fracture passes outwards to the jugular foramen. Again, two courses are now available, the fracture either cutting outwards across the body of the petrous, 'external' to the internal auditory meatus and cutting across the facial nerve in the region of the geniculate ganglion, and finally terminating in the roof of the middle ear, or else passing along the petro-occipital suture and so to the foramen lacerum medium, the sphenoidal fissure, and the anterior fossa as in the previous case.

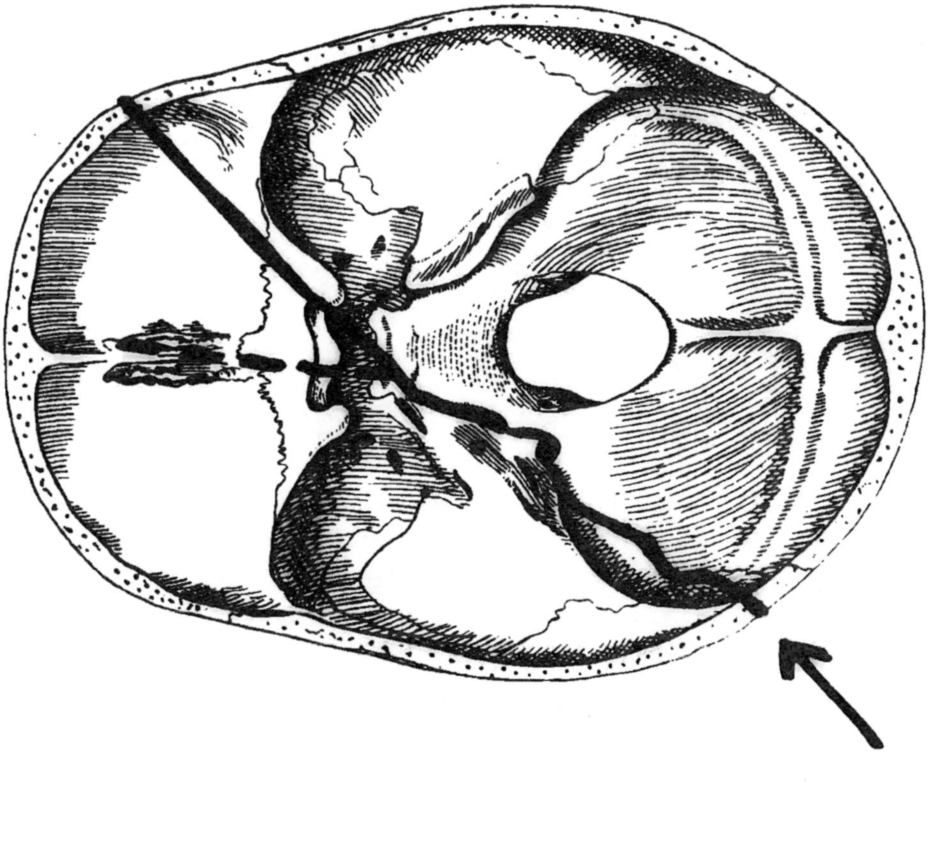

Fig. 35. Diagram of Lines pursued by Basic Fractures. Force applied to the mastoid region.

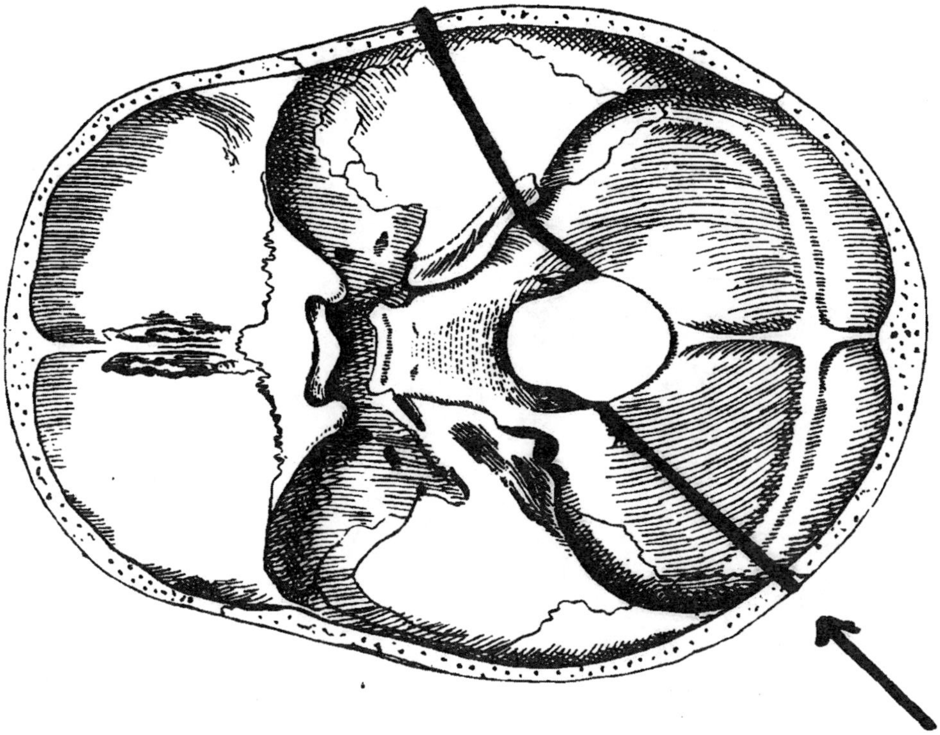

Fig. 36. Diagram of Lines pursued by Basic Fractures. Force applied to the lateral occipital region.

Direction, &c., of the applied force.

Probable resultant basic fracture.

6. Force applied to the posterior occipital region.

The resultant fracture varies according to the direction of the applied force. A force which is applied to the posterior occipital region at right angles to the transverse axis of the skull results in a fracture which, on reaching the posterior margin

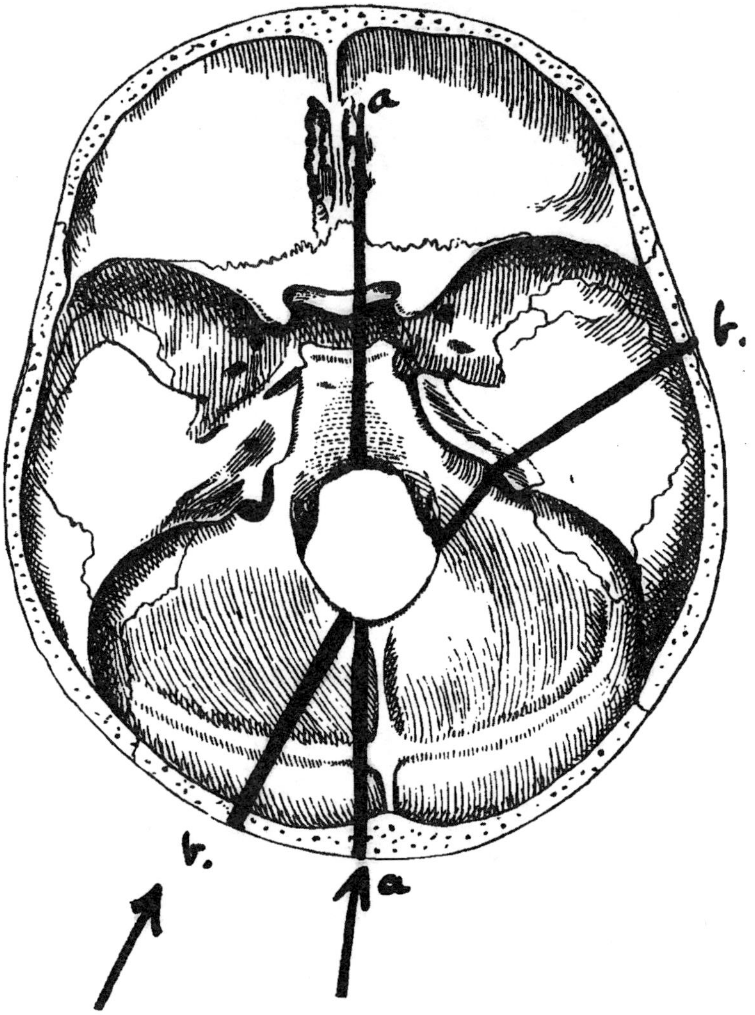

FIG. 37.
DIAGRAM OF LINES PURSUED BY BASIC FRACTURES. Force applied to the posterior occipital region, the fracture following the course *a. a.* or *b. b.*, according to the direction of the applied force.

of the foramen magnum, is continued again on the opposite side of the foramen along the dorsum ephipii. When the force is more oblique in direction (as is usually the case) the fracture traverses the thin cerebellar fossa to the outer margin of the jugular foramen, and then follows one of the two courses indicated in the previous case.

More commonly the fracture cuts across the petrous bone.

Summary. Basic fractures tend to follow certain definite paths, this transbasic course varying according to the direction of the force applied and the site of application of the same. Whether the fracture completely traverses the base depends on the character of the force and the resistance offered, for bases, as well as vaults, vary greatly in strength. To every rule there must be exceptions, and cases are at hand in which the fracture appears to have obeyed no law, or in which the force applied was of so forcible a nature that the fracture traversed the base, regardless of all the ordinary rules.

The principles enumerated above were formulated by me some four years ago, and, in spite of certain adverse criticisms, I am more than ever convinced that the rules are correct, and that time and research are alone required to add to the strength of my assertions.

SYMPTOMS RESULTING FROM FRACTURE OF THE BASE OF THE SKULL

The symptoms resulting from a fracture of the base of the skull vary according to the particular fossa fractured. From a general point of view, the following symptoms require consideration :—

Hæmorrhages.
Escape of cerebro-spinal fluid.
Escape of brain-matter.
Escape of air from the air-sinuses into the surrounding tissues.
Involvement of certain cranial nerves.

Symptoms pointing to fracture of the Anterior Fossa.

Hæmorrhages : (*a*) *Subconjunctival hæmorrhage* usually makes its appearance at the outer canthus of the eye, progressing inwards towards the corneo-scleral margin, and, in the most severe cases, completely surrounding the cornea, bulging the conjunctiva forwards in such a manner as to constrict the field of vision. The extravasated blood is usually bright red in colour, makes its appearance within a few hours of the accident, and reaches its maximum within thirty-six to forty-eight hours.

In some cases a condition of subconjunctival œdema (chemosis) is observed. This also usually originates at the outer canthus.

Taken by themselves, neither hæmorrhage nor œdema are of any great diagnostic value. Both conditions, however, aid materially in confirming the diagnosis.

The blood is almost invariably completely absorbed, and no ill effects remain.

(*b*) *Palpebral and peri-palpebral hæmorrhage* is seen in most cases of fracture of the anterior fossa. This form of hæmorrhage differs from the one mentioned above in that it usually commences at the inner canthus of the eye, thence progressing in the outward direction. The extravasated blood may be wholly anterior to the suspensory ligaments of the lid, in which case it may be surmised that the fracture only involves the perpendicular plate of the frontal bone. More commonly, however, the cribriform plate of the ethmoid shares in the lesion, in which case palpebral, peri-palpebral, and subconjunctival hæmorrhage are all present.

(*c*) *Orbital hæmorrhages* may be so extensive that marked forward protrusion of the globe exists. The time at which proptosis makes its appearance, and the degree to which it progresses, vary according to the nature of the lesion. Thus :—

Proptosis severe, appearing almost at once,	implies	a fracture associated with injury to the cavernous sinus or internal carotid artery.
Proptosis moderate, and appearing after a few hours,	,,	a fracture involving the walls of the orbit, the blood being derived from lacerated ethmoidal and other small vessels.
Proptosis appearing days or weeks after the accident, usually progressive,	,,	a fracture involving the region of the sphenoidal body and complicated by the formation of a fistulous communication between the cavernous sinus and the carotid artery (see Traumatic orbital aneurysm).

(*d*) *Retinal hæmorrhages.* Fleming, in 1902, reported 12 cases of fracture of the skull, all except one being fractures of the base, in which retinal hæmorrhages were present. All cases were associated with hæmorrhage into the subarachnoid space, and when this hæmorrhage was of a unilateral nature the retinal changes were likewise one-sided. It was also found that in 4 cases of cerebral hæmorrhage without osseous lesion retinal hæmorrhages were present in three, these three being all associated with considerable effusion into the subarachnoid space.

These observations are not only of value in the general diagnosis of intracranial lesions, but are also of considerable importance in the differential diagnosis between extra- and intradural hæmorrhages.

(*e*) *Hæmorrhage from the nose and mouth* is almost invariably present in fractures of the anterior fossa, with the inference that the fracture involves the cribriform plate. The blood—derived mainly from lacerated ethmoidal vessels—escapes from the anterior nares or, passing back into the naso-pharynx, escapes by the mouth or is swallowed, to be vomited up later.

Escape of cerebro-spinal fluid. Blandin, of the Hôtel-Dieu, drew attention to this condition in the year 1840. The fracture involves the cribriform plate of the ethmoid, and is associated with laceration of the overlying dura mater and arachnoid, and of the prolongations of those membranes along the olfactory nerves.

The escape of cerebro-spinal fluid from the nose may be regarded as diagnostic of a fracture of the anterior fossa, in spite of the fact that Goucard, Malgaigne, and others describe cases in which, as the result of a severe fracture of the petrous bone (middle fossa) without laceration of the membrana tympani, the fluid escaped along the Eustachian tube to be expelled by mouth and nose.

At this stage, it will be necessary to allude more fully to the general question of cerebro-spinal discharge from the nose, mouth, and ear. The symptom is an important one, though undoubtedly of far less frequent occurrence than stated in text-books. This was proved by Crandon and Wilson, who reported 27 cases in which there was a cerebro-spinal discharge out of a total number of 530 cases examined. Phelps mentions 13 in a series of 286 cases of fractured base. My experience coincides with these statements.

The escape of a slightly blood-stained fluid from the ear and nose does not necessarily imply that the fluid is cerebro-spinal in nature, for it has been proved on numerous occasions that fluid may escape in considerable quantities without the existence of a basic fracture. In such cases the fluid is derived either from the membranous labyrinth (the liquor cotunnii) or from the mucous membrane lining the ear and nose, the result of great vaso-motor dilatation of aural and nasal vessels.

If the fluid be cerebro-spinal in nature, the natural inference is that the subarachnoid space is opened up to the exterior, either directly or indirectly along the course of a cranial nerve. A chemical analysis of the fluid will determine the nature thereof, provided that the fluid be collected EARLY.

Thus, cerebro-spinal fluid is rich in chlorides, contains little or no albumen, but shows a trace of a reducing substance, allied to pyro-catechin,	whilst	fluid derived from other sources contains chlorides, a fair amount of albumen, and no sugar.

Certain factors, however, must be taken into consideration which diminish the value of these chemical tests, for, though the fluid be cerebro-spinal in nature, the admixture of blood at once interferes with the delicacy of the test. Furthermore, even in the event of a profuse discharge of cerebro-spinal fluid, the first part collected alone contains sugar, the discharge soon becoming nothing more or less than a serous exudation.

The fluid is almost certainly cerebro-spinal if the discharge begins within twenty-four hours of the accident, if it be practically colourless, fairly profuse, and continuing for two or three days, perhaps longer.

Though the discharge usually originates early, cases are recorded in which the flow commenced some weeks after the accident. The discharge may continue for hours or for weeks. Sir W. Savory recorded a case in which fluid escaped for one month from both ears. The quantity also varies greatly, usually a few ounces, but sometimes many pints. Sir W. MacCormac recorded a case in which 10 pints escaped within five hours. A profuse discharge is due to the fact that, as the original cerebro-spinal fluid drains away, its place in the subarachnoid space is taken by a serous exudation from the cerebral venous system. This exudation occurs as soon as the subarachnoid pressure is sufficiently reduced, the serous exudation progressing till the venous and cerebro-spinal pressures are again equal.

As regards the *prognosis*, it is interesting to note that the escape of cerebro-spinal fluid implies of necessity that the subarachnoid space is opened up to the exterior, with all attendant dangers of meningeal infection, yet that the prognosis is generally favourable. One might even go further and state that the prognosis in such cases is rather more favourable than under more ordinary circumstances. Thus, Battle records 36 cases with a mortality of 25 per cent., the general mortality of fractured base being about 44 per cent. My own experience tallies with these statistics. The more favourable result hinges no doubt on the fact that the prolonged outflow tends to wash away organisms existent in the aural and nasal passages.

With regard to any special points in treatment, it is obvious that syringing of ear or nose is absolutely contra-indicated. The cavities should be *lightly* plugged with gauze, the dressings to be renewed as soon as they are soaked. The patient must also be prevented from interfering with the dressings.

With regard to the routine use of urotropin to guard against the advent of meningitis, see p. 116.

Escape of brain-matter from the nose. This diagnostic symptom is of very rare occurrence. For its development the following factors are requisite :—

Great comminution and destruction of the anterior fossa.

Severe local laceration of the brain (frontal lobes).

A copious discharge of blood and cerebro-spinal fluid.

A general increase in the intracranial pressure.

One case only of this nature has come under my own observation, that of a man whose right nostril was blocked with brain substance. He died shortly after admission into the hospital, and at the post-mortem examination the above conditions were found.

Escape of air from the air-sinuses into the surrounding regions. When the fracture involves the frontal, ethmoidal, and mastoid sinuses, any sudden increase of the intrasinus air-pressure, such as is caused by sneezing, blowing of the nose, &c., may force air into the surrounding tissues. A distinction must be made between those cases in which the pericranium overlying the seat of fracture is torn and those in which it remains intact. In the former case, the escaping air may spread widely into the neighbouring loose tissues, leading to a condition of 'surgical emphysema'. In the second case, the air remains confined to a smaller area, giving rise to a soft, more or less rounded swelling. Gentle palpation of this swelling imparts to the fingers that crackling sensation peculiar to the condition. Firm pressure results in diminution in the size of the tumour, the contained air being forced back into the sinus cavity. Such localized collections of air are known as 'pneumatoceles'.

As regards the special *treatment* of these conditions, the patient must, in the first case, be warned against straining of all sorts. Pneumatoceles require no other treatment. The condition soon disappears if the patient recovers. In widespread surgical emphysema, an incision should be made over the injured sinus, thus allowing of the direct escape of the air expelled from that sinus.

The involvement of nerves. The following nerves may be involved in anterior fossa fractures :—

(*a*) *The olfactory nerve.* The great majority of anterior fossa fractures traverse the cribriform plate, necessarily injuring the fine branches of the olfactory bulb. The bulb itself may be lacerated, with or without injury to the under surface of the frontal lobes. Sir Prescott Hewitt considered that anosmia, or loss of smell, resulted most frequently from blows applied to the back of the head, the frontal region being injured by contre-coup. From my own experience it would appear, however, that anosmia, whether uni- or bilateral, whether transient or permanent, generally results from direct injuries of the cribriform plate with associated lacerations of the olfactory nerves. It is difficult to estimate the presence or degree of immediate loss of smell on account of the general condition of the patient and because the nostrils are usually more or less filled with blood coagulum. Experience shows, however, that early loss of smell is the rule and total and permanent anosmia the exception. Anosmia is usually associated with some degree of loss of taste.

(*b*) *The optic nerve.* Many cases have been recorded in which visual defects resulted from blows applied to the head. The blindness may be partial or complete, immediate in onset or developing at some future date. In the latter case, the loss of vision is due to retinal changes or results from post-neuritic atrophy.

The occurrence of complete or partial blindness as the immediate result of the injury is, at first sight, difficult to explain, for the vast majority of anterior fossa fractures avoid the immediate vicinity of the optic foramina, passing by preference between the two foramina or diverging towards the sphenoidal fissures. Small fissured fractures not infrequently radiate through the optic foramina, usually, however, of so slight a nature as to be incapable of leading to any gross lesion of the optic nerves. Hæmorrhage into the sheath of the nerve is probably responsible for a certain proportion of cases, more especially those in which there is a peripheral concentric loss of vision, the more central fibres escaping. It is possible, also, that cases evidencing temporal or nasal blindness may be due, as J. J. Evans[1] thinks, to a contre-coup contusion of the nerve through it being forcibly driven against the bony boundaries of the foramen. Taking into consideration, however, the very frequent presence of a fracture through the anterior clinoid process (see p. 82), and the usual displacement of that process, it would appear probable that immediate and more or less complete loss of vision results from the compression and crushing of the optic nerve by reason of the pressure exercised by a displaced clinoid process.

The following statistics add confirmation to this view. Thus, Callen collected 17 cases in which the optic nerve was compressed by osseous fragments in the region of the optic foramen, whilst Holder observed injury to the bones entering into the formation of the foramen in 53 out of 86 cases of fracture involving this region.

The prognosis varies according to the cause of the blindness. When resulting from concussion of the nerve trunk or from hæmorrhage into its sheath, certain fibres may regain their function. In the majority of cases, however, that have come under my own observation, blindness of the affected eye was immediate and permanent.

(c) *The nerves passing through the sphenoidal fissure.* The ophthalmic division of the fifth nerve is rarely injured to such a degree as to cause anæsthesia of all the regions supplied. Blood extravasation into the surrounding regions, or direct involvement of one of the branches of the nerve, often results in areas of anæsthesia, and some few cases have been recorded in which there was complete anæsthesia of both cornea and conjunctiva, with subsequent ulceration and sloughing. The nasal nerve may be implicated as the result of a fracture involving the cribriform plate, whilst the supra-orbital and supra-trochlear branches may be damaged by fractures of the vertical plate of the frontal bone.

The third nerve is similarly liable to injury, in any part of its orbital course. It is quite exceptional, however, for the whole trunk to be affected, some of the branches being taken, others left. The fourth nerve is also occasionally involved, generally in association with other orbital nerves.

[1] *Brit. Med. Journ.*, September 11, 1909, p. 645.

When anæsthesia or paralysis of muscles results from pressure exercised on the nerves by extravasated blood, the ultimate prognosis is not unfavourable. When due to direct implication, in the line of the fracture, the prognosis is much more uncertain, partial or complete loss of function resulting.

SYMPTOMS POINTING TO FRACTURE OF THE MIDDLE FOSSA

External hæmorrhages. (*a*) *Hæmorrhage into the temporal region.* The extravasated blood may either be confined to the temporal region—temporal hæmatoma—or diffused throughout the subaponeurotic space. A temporal hæmatoma is always highly suggestive of a fracture involving the temporal fossa, especially in the event of marked outward bulging, with stretching and discoloration of the overlying tissues. In many cases also the hæmatoma pulsates, in which case it can be presumed that the fracture of the temporal fossa is associated with hæmorrhage from a lacerated middle meningeal artery (see Fig. 38). In such cases the application of pressure to the hæmatoma may lead to the development of fits on the contra-lateral side, originating in the face or arm regions and spreading to the higher cortical motor area.

(*b*) *Hæmorrhage from the ear and mouth.* The great majority of middle fossa fractures involve the external auditory meatus, passing inwards across the roof and floor of the middle ear towards the body of the sphenoid. Examination will show that the fracture passes inwards towards the junction of the inner and anterior walls of the middle ear, that is to say, towards the tympanic orifice of the Eustachian tube. The membrana tympani undergoes a variable degree of destruction. In the lesser cases the membrane is torn in its upper and front part only—in the region of the membrane of Shrapnell—whilst in the more serious cases it may be completely destroyed. The blood that escapes from the ear is derived from those vessels that supply the lining cuticle of the external and middle ears, from the numerous tympanic vessels, from the lateral sinus, and from the middle meningeal artery. The amount of blood which escapes varies according to the source of the hæmorrhage. When hæmorrhage occurs from the smaller vessels, the blood either clots in the external meatus or trickles from the ear. In the most severe cases the hæmorrhage is profuse and long-continued. Some years ago a case came under my observation that threw light on the probable source of such severe hæmorrhages.

A man was admitted into the hospital, suffering from profuse hæmorrhage from the ear as the result of a fall down an area. The bleeding continued for fourteen hours, soaking the dressings and continuing so long as the man lived. At the post-mortem examination

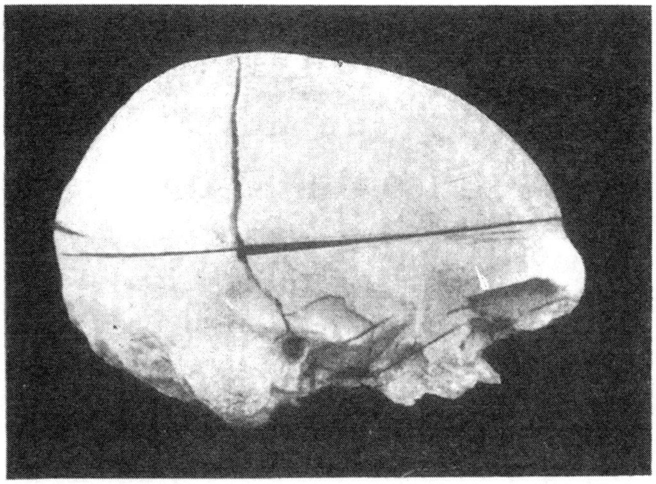

A

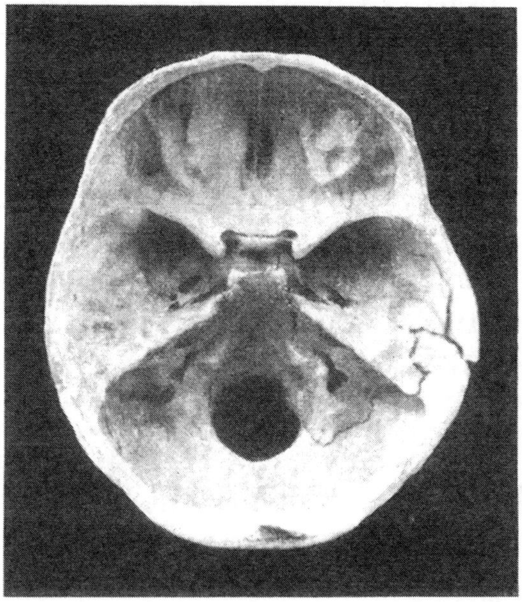

B

FIG. 38. TO ILLUSTRATE THE PROBABLE SOURCE OF PROFUSE HÆMORRHAGE FROM THE EAR. A, The fracture involves the roof of the external auditory meatus. B, Comminution of the tegmen tympani, the fracture involving the groove for the posterior branch of the middle meningeal artery.

an extensive comminution of the tegmen tympani was discovered, the fracture being associated with great extra-dural extravasation of blood from a lacerated middle meningeal artery. The extra-dural hæmorrhage was enabled to escape through the tegmen tympani into the middle ear, and thence by means of the lacerated membrana tympani (see Fig. 38).

Profuse and long-continued hæmorrhage from the ear should always arouse suspicion as to the possibility of injury to the middle meningeal artery. Since meeting the case recounted above, many similar cases have come under my care, and, in several instances, guided by this symptom alone, operative measures have been carried out successfully.

The two following cases show, however, that the extra-dural extravasation may be derived not only from the middle meningeal artery but also from the lateral sinus.

'A man fell down an area and suffered from continuous hæmorrhage from the ear. He remained in bed for a few days, and then, becoming tired of confinement, got up, walked some distance on a cold and frosty day, and visited a *sage femme*. On returning home he complained of feeling ill, the hæmorrhage from the ear ceased, and shortly afterwards he became unconscious and died. The autopsy showed an extensive fracture of the petrous bone with extensive extra-dural hæmorrhage from a torn lateral sinus and from a lacerated meningeal artery.' [1]

The man had remained fairly well so long as the extra-dural blood was permitted a free means of escape through the tegmen tympani and external auditory meatus, but, so soon as clotting occurred, compression symptoms developed and the man died in that condition.

'A man, 50 years of age, fell down, striking his head against the kerb. On admission it was seen that blood was trickling freely through a torn membrana tympani. He rapidly became unconscious and died. The post-mortem examination revealed a fracture involving the middle ear and external auditory meatus, passing backwards across the lateral sinus, in which region there was a large extra-dural extravasation of blood.' [2]

The above statements are confirmed by Dwight,[3] who, in 146 autopsies, found that, in 69 per cent. cases of fracture of the middle fossa of the skull, there was bleeding from the ear, and that in 29 per cent. cases the fracture was associated with laceration of branches of the middle meningeal artery.

Although hæmorrhage from the external auditory meatus may be regarded as almost diagnostic of a middle fossa fracture, especially of that variety previously described as the 'typical basic fracture', yet the blood may be derived from a torn membrana tympani or from laceration of the lining cuticle of the external meatus. Aural

1 Chassaignac, *Plans de la Tête*, 1842.

2 Milligan, *Trans. of the Otolog. Soc.*, vol. viii, p. 69.

3 *Boston City Hosp. Reports*, 1894.

examination will soon prove whether the blood is coming *through* a rent in the membrane, in which case the diagnosis is clear. Sometimes bleeding takes place from both ears, a symptom practically diagnostic of the transverse middle fossa fracture known as the 'typical basic fracture'.

The following statistics will supply further information as to the relative frequency with which hæmorrhage occurs from ears, nose, and mouth, and the proportionate mortality. The cases were collected and tabulated by Crandon and Wilson.

	Cases.	*Lived.*	*Died.*	*Mortality.*
Hæmorrhage from the ear	281	170	111	39 per cent.
Hæmorrhage from both ears	47	16	31	66 per cent.
Hæmorrhage from the nose	44	17	27	61 per cent.
Hæmorrhage from the mouth	168	73	93	33 per cent.

Special points in prognosis and treatment. It is not possible to formulate any very definite prognosis when the hæmorrhage takes place from one ear only, though the mortality is about 40 per cent. When bleeding takes place from both ears the outlook is more grave, the mortality being about 66 per cent.

With regard to special treatment, two points are obvious: (1) that syringing of the ear is absolutely contra-indicated, on the ground that such treatment carries with it a considerable risk of bringing about meningeal infection; and (2) that plugging the external meatus with strips of gauze is an unsurgical form of treatment, insomuch as the escape of blood from the ear is an important factor in preventing compression of the brain, more especially in those cases where hæmorrhage is profuse. Under the last named conditions, operative measures—exploration for a torn meningeal artery or lacerated venous sinus—are to be carried out.

Hæmorrhage from the mouth may be slight or copious, according to the source from which the blood is derived. In the former case, the bleeding takes place from sphenoidal and pharyngeal vessels, in the latter from the cavernous sinus or from the internal carotid artery (see p. 148), the bone being shattered in the region of the sphenoidal body, with comminution of the walls of the contained air-sinus.

Escape of cerebro-spinal fluid. This condition was first investigated by Van der Wiel in 1727, and more completely by Langier in 1839. The majority of those middle fossa fractures which involve the petrous portion of the temporal bone pass immediately anterior to the genu of the facial nerve (see p. 102), and it follows, therefore, that the fracture cannot so involve the dural and arachnoid prolongations of that nerve in such a manner as to allow of the escape of cerebro-spinal fluid. This fact probably explains another fact, namely, that aural cerebro-spinal discharge is an infrequent symptom in middle fossa fractures. On the other hand, as a result of blows applied to the occipital region, a fracture originating in the posterior fossa may cut across the petrous bone, almost at right angles, in such a manner as to sever the seventh nerve in the region of the genu (see Fig. 41). This is the usual nature of a basic fracture associated with the escape of cerebro-spinal fluid from the external auditory meatus. More rarely, this particular class of fracture is unaccompanied by any injury to the tympanic membrane, in which case the fluid may escape along the Eustachian tube into the nose and naso-pharynx (see p. 91). Cerebro-spinal fluid may also escape from the nose and mouth in middle fossa fractures in the event of extensive injury to the basi-sphenoid with involvement of the overlying cisterna basalis. The following case exemplifies that condition :—

A man suffered from a severe fracture of the middle fossa. Three weeks later there was a sudden and profuse discharge of cerebro-spinal fluid from the nose. Meningitis developed and the patient died. The basi-sphenoid was extensively comminuted, the overlying membranes torn, whilst a probe could be passed readily from the cranial cavity into the naso-pharynx.

Special points in prognosis and treatment. The question of cerebro-spinal discharges has been discussed previously (see p. 91). It is therefore merely necessary to lay further stress on the fact that syringing of the ear is absolutely contra-indicated, for reasons already stated. The ear should be cleaned out with wool and gauze and *lightly* packed with strips of gauze, these to be renewed when soaked with fluid. When the cerebro-spinal discharge is long continued, acute eczema of the side of the neck may develop as a result of the irritating effect of the fluid. Under these circumstances it is advisable to adopt precautionary measures, painting the skin with ‘ new skin ’ or collodion. Ointments are of but little use. The eczema will clear up so soon as the discharge ceases.

Escape of brain-matter. The conditions needful for the discharge of brain-matter from ear or nose have been enumerated previously (see p. 93). There are but few cases recorded in literature, and one case only has come under my own observation :—

A lad, 11 years of age, fell some distance out of window on to his head. He was admitted under the care of my colleague, Mr. Lockwood. On admission he was unconscious, and was bleeding freely from the right ear and nose. Shortly afterwards it was noticed that brain-matter was issuing from the right external auditory meatus, sufficient brain-matter being obtained to fill a teaspoon. The extensive nature of the brain-injury was confirmed by the fact that the left arm and leg were paralysed for some days. On the fourth day the boy regained consciousness and recognized his relations. From this period onwards he made an uuinterrupted recovery. I have seen the lad on various occasions, the last time one year after the accident. At that time he was an exceedingly bright and intellectual boy.

Special points in treatment and prognosis. The brain-matter should be gently wiped away from the ear, and the meatus cleansed and lightly plugged with gauze. Operative measures are required in the event of the development of symptoms pointing to brain compression. The prognosis must necessarily be unfavourable, but, as the conditions are almost entirely confined to the young, the most astonishing recoveries are reported.

Involvement of nerves. The second and third divisions of the fifth nerve pass respectively through the foramen ovale and the foramen rotundum, two foramina which lie anterior to the petro-sphenoidal suture, a suture traversed by the majority of middle fossa fractures. These two nerves are therefore seldom involved.

In all the cases of fractured base which have come under my observation I have never seen the foramen rotundum implicated, and in one case only was the foramen ovale involved.

In certain rare instances, a fracture, passing in the antero-posterior direction, may cut across the apex of the petrous bone in close relation to the cavum Meckelii—the bed of the Gasserian ganglion —in which case all three terminal divisions of the fifth nerve may suffer. Thus, a case was reported by Lee in 1853 in which, seven weeks after the accident, the following symptoms were present:—anæsthesia of the left face and forehead, anterior two-thirds of tongue, and left nostril, together with weakness of the left masticating muscles, and an opaque left cornea.

The sixth nerve. The sixth nerve may be involved either by itself or in conjunction with other cranial nerves. In the latter case the paresis is due to blood extravasated in the sphenoidal fissure or in the orbital cavity. In the former case the nerve is injured where it grooves the lateral aspect of the dorsum ephipii, a process frequently fractured in lesions of the middle fossa. Fractures tend to pass obliquely across this process, one nerve usually escaping. The prognosis as to functional recovery is very problematical.

The seventh and eighth nerves. There can be no doubt that the seventh nerve, on account of its complicated intrapetrous course, is more frequently involved than any other cranial nerve. Köhler records 22 cases in 48 middle fossa fractures. My own experience coincides closely with Köhler's, facial paresis or paralysis being noted in nearly 50 per cent. cases of middle fossa fracture.

The question of facial nerve implication is so intimately associated with involvement of the eighth nerve that the two subjects must be considered together. Thus, cases may be classified as follows:—

1. Cases of paresis of the facial nerve with a variable degree of deafness.

2. Cases of complete facial paralysis with complete deafness.

The greater number of middle fossa fractures involve the middle and external ears, as is evidenced, amongst other symptoms, by hæmorrhage from the ear. Some degree of facial paralysis is frequently existent, not always evident at first sight, but requiring careful examination and comparison between the two sides of the face. The fracture involves both roof and floor of the external ear and passes inwards towards the junction of anterior and inner walls of the middle ear, the membrana tympani undergoing a variable degree of destruction whilst the ossicles may also be injured. Thence, the fracture passes inwards towards the petro-sphenoidal suture in such a manner that the geniculate ganglion of the facial nerve is exposed and laid bare on the anterior aspect of the posterior portion of the skull.

The facial nerve, therefore, escapes direct injury except in so far that the ganglion may be compressed by blood-clot or fragments

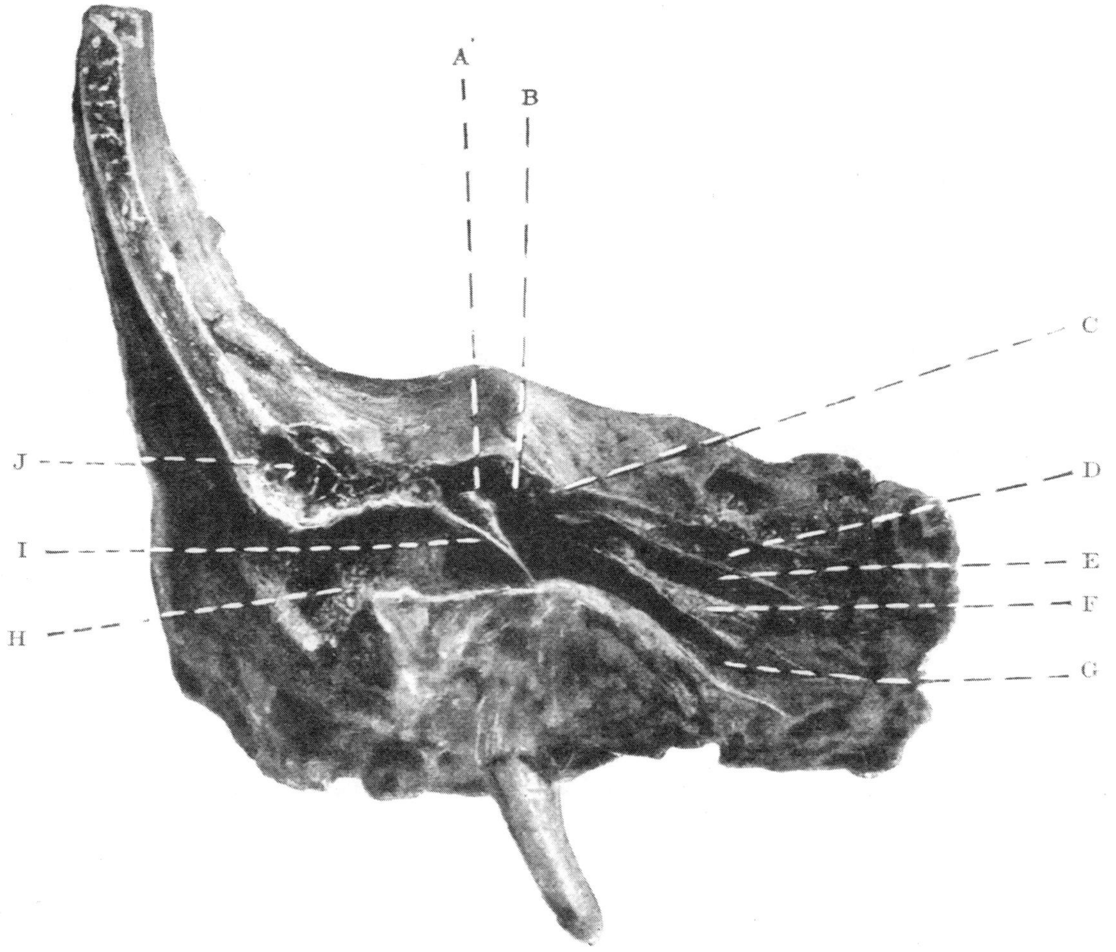

FIG. 39. TO SHOW THE RELATION OF A TYPICAL BASIC FRACTURE TO THE MIDDLE EAR AND ITS ADJUNCTS. A, Malleus ; B, Middle ear and aditus ; C, Geniculate ganglion (facial nerve) ; D, Groove for great superficial petrosal nerve ; E, Canal for tensor tympani muscle ; F, Processus cochleariformis ; G, Eustachian tube ; H, External auditory meatus ; I, Membrana tympani ; J, Mastoid cells.

of bone. Partial loss of function results. In most cases the blood is absorbed and a complete recovery may be anticipated. The degree of deafness is directly proportionate to the damage incurred by the membrana tympani and ossicles.

In the second group of cases a different picture is obtained. Usually the result of blows applied to the occipital region, the fracture traverses the thin cerebellar fossa towards the outer angle of the jugular foramen, thence cutting across the petrous bone, external to the internal auditory meatus, and terminating, usually by comminution, in the tegmen tympani. It is in the transpetrous part of the fracture that the damage is done, for, not only is the facial nerve cut across in the region of the ganglion, but the auditory apparatus

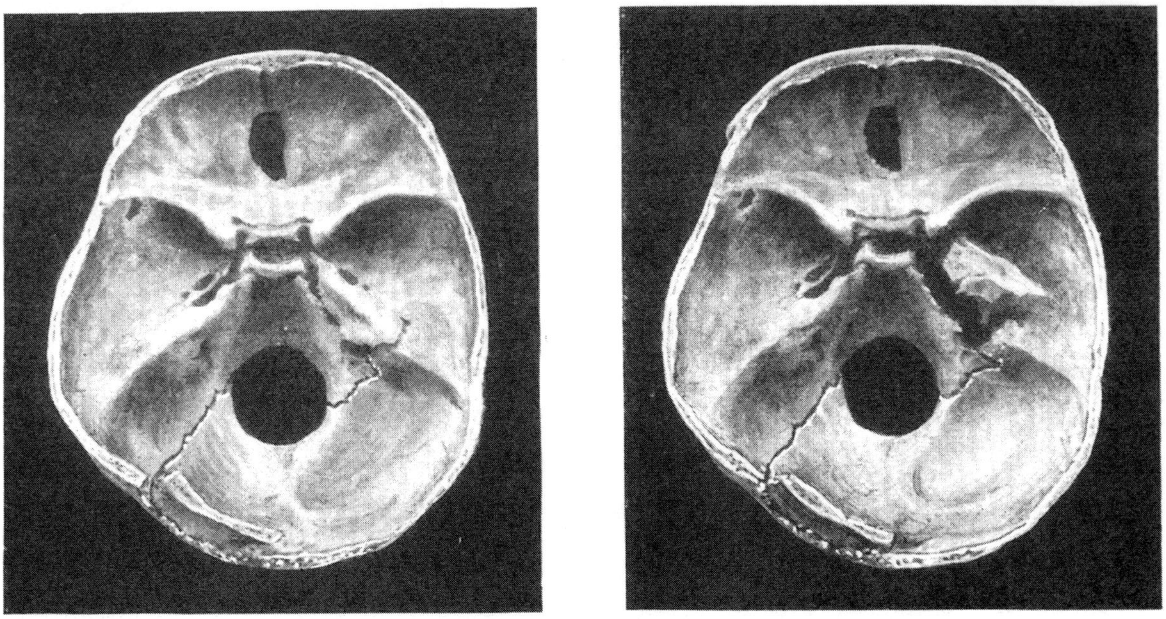

A B

FIG. 40. TO SHOW THE RELATION OF BASIC FRACTURES TO THE PETROUS BONE. A, The basic fracture, resulting from a force applied to the left occipital region. follows the course depicted in Fig. 36. B, The inner half of the petrous bone, being loose, is thrown forward so as to show the relation of the fracture to the integral parts of the petrous bone.

is also severed into two parts. The exact line of the fracture is shown in Figs. 40 and 41.

In this class of fracture, though facial paralysis and deafness are both immediate in onset and permanent in duration, there is, in many cases, no bleeding from the ear as the membrana tympani may be uninjured.

The facial nerve may also be implicated in that rare type of basic fracture which was described by Lèon Boullet in 1878, under the title of 'Fracture of the Mastoid portion of the Temporal bone'. This fracture is fully described on p. 108. It will suffice to mention that the mastoid process may be torn away from the base of the skull, the facial nerve being lacerated as it descends the aqueductus Fallopii.

Bilateral facial paralysis is exceedingly rare. Two cases were described by the late Professor von Bergmann. Its occurrence is pathognomonic of the typical basic fracture (see p. 84).

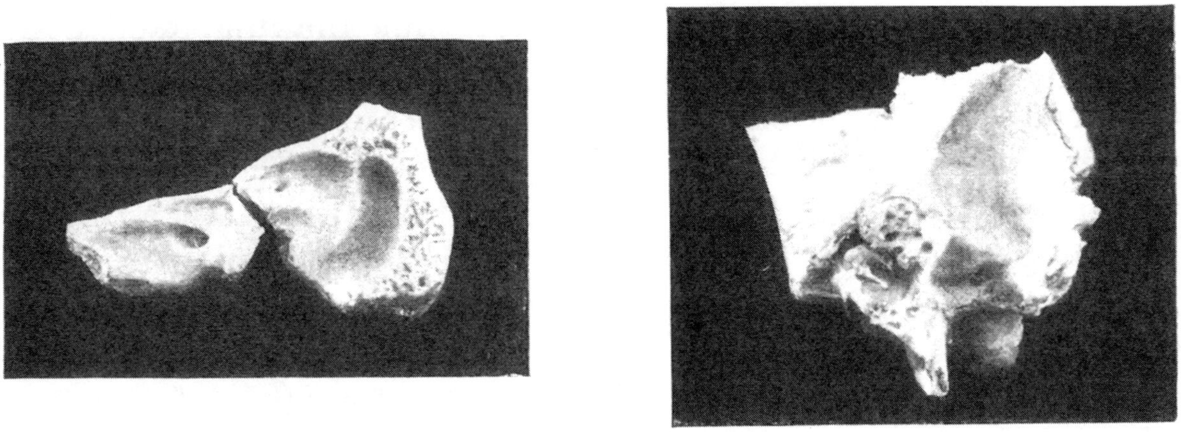

A B

FIG. 41. TO SHOW THE RELATION OF BASIC FRACTURES TO THE PETROUS BONE. A shows the course pursued by an antero-posterior fracture of the petrous bone. Note that it lies external to the internal auditory meatus. B shows—enlarged—the inner aspect of the outer fragment. Note the relation of the fracture to the semicircular canals, and that the membrana tympani and ossicles are quite uninjured.

Complete facial paralysis may be associated with the following symptoms :—

Epiphora, conjunctivitis, and keratitis (from paralysis of the orbicularis palpebrarum).

Loss of taste (from involvement of the chorda tympani).

Impaired nasal air-entry (from paralysis of dilator alæ muscle).

Impaired acoustic sensibility (from paralysis of the stapedius).

Impaired mastication (from involvement of the buccinator muscle).

Impaired secretion of saliva (from the cutting off of the secretory and vaso-dilator fibres of the chorda tympani).

Lastly, it is necessary to add that facial paralysis developing some days or weeks after the accident, though sometimes dependent on degeneration of nerve-fibres as the result of pressure in the region of the geniculate ganglion, may also arise from an ascending neuritis or from meningeal infection.

SYMPTOMS POINTING TO FRACTURE OF THE POSTERIOR FOSSA

External hæmorrhages. In fractures of the posterior fossa, blood effused into the deeper tissues of the scalp has considerable difficulty in coming to the surface and thus making itself evident. Furthermore, the resistance offered by the nuchal muscles tends to confine the blood to the subtentorial region, thus adding to the already grave prognosis of fractures in this region. On careful palpation, however, it will be noted that the nuchal tissues present a doughy or boggy condition, whilst ecchymosis becomes evident after twenty-four to thirty-six hours. A peculiar ecchymotic patch is occasionally observed, appearing in front of the mastoid process and travelling upwards in a curved direction, concavity forwards, following the outline of the ear. It is said to result from the tracking of blood along the course of the posterior auricular artery. Whether this is the case or not, the hæmorrhage usually implies a separation along the line of the masto-occipital suture.

Escape of cerebro-spinal fluid.
Escape of brain-matter. } Neither of these symptoms are present.

Involvement of nerves. When dealing with fractures of the middle fossa, allusion was made to the implication of the seventh and eighth pair of nerves as the result of a fracture traversing the posterior fossa of the skull towards the outer angle of the jugular foramen and cutting across the petrous bone (see p. 104).

The ninth, tenth, and eleventh cranial nerves may be injured in the same variety of fracture. These three nerves are, however, so protected by their dural sheaths that they generally escape injury.[1]

In the following cases the nerves were involved :—

The patient was admitted suffering from a fracture resulting from a blow on the posterior parietal region. During the next four days no special symptoms developed. On the fifth day, during a sudden attack of dyspnœa and dysphagia, death occurred. A fissured

[1] Delfau and Günther narrate a case in which death occurred from pressure on the tenth nerve. (*Deutsche Klinik*, Berlin, 1853.)

fracture was found which extended into the jugular foramen, a region occupied by blood-clot.

A man committed suicide by means of a pistol-bullet fired through the mouth. The bullet lodged against the under surface of the petrous bone, tearing the jugular vein and lacerating the nerves passing through that foramen.

In another case the patient was admitted with a fractured base. He progressed favourably until the tenth day when, on sitting up suddenly in bed, he was seized with rigors, dyspnœa, and dysphagia, dying shortly afterwards. A basic fracture was found, practically dividing the skull into two parts and involving the jugular foramen. Displacement had occurred with consequent compression of the ninth, tenth, and eleventh nerves.

The twelfth nerve. The anterior condyloid foramen is most favourably situated with respect to the course pursued by posterior fossa fractures. No instance of its involvement has come under my own observation.

Stierlein records a case in which the tenth and twelfth nerves were injured, with inability to speak or swallow, paralysis of the right half of the tongue, soft palate, vocal cords and pharyngeal constrictions. Death resulted in seven weeks.

The late Professor von Bergmann [1] mentions a case of hypoglossal paralysis together with paralysis of the sterno-mastoid and trapezius muscles (eleventh nerve).

For *treatment* of basic fractures, see p. 116.

FRACTURE OF THE BASE OF THE SKULL: SUMMARY OF SYMPTOMS

Anterior Fossa.	*Middle Fossa.*	*Posterior Fossa.*
Hæmorrhages. Subconjunctival. Palpebral. Peripalpebral. Orbital. Retinal. From the nose. From the mouth.	*Hæmorrhages.* Into the temporal region. From the mouth. From the nose. From the ear.	*Hæmorrhages.* Into the nuchal region. Into the occipital region. Into the post-auricular region.
Cerebro-spinal fluid. From the nose. From the mouth.	*Cerebro-spinal fluid.* From the nose. From the mouth. From the ear.	*Cerebro-spinal fluid.* None.

[1] *System of Surgery*, vol. i, p. 93.

Anterior Fossa.	*Middle Fossa.*	*Posterior Fossa.*
Brain-matter. From the nose.	*Brain-matter.* From the ear.	*Brain-matter.* None.
Air-escape. From the frontal sinus. From the ethmoidal cells.	*Air-escape.* From the mastoid antrum.	*Air-escape.* From the mastoid antrum.
Nerve-involvement. Olfactory. Optic. Third. Fourth. Fifth (first division). Sixth.	*Nerve-involvement.* Fifth (second and third divisions). Sixth. Seventh. Eighth.	*Nerve-involvement.* Seventh. Eighth. Ninth. Tenth. Eleventh. Twelfth (?).

FRACTURE OF THE MASTOID PORTION OF THE TEMPORAL BONE

Fractures limited to this region are of rare occurrence. Our knowledge of the condition is obtained from the researches of Lèon Boullét, who first described the fracture in 1876, reporting at the same time 26 cases.

The fracture usually results from sharp blows delivered along the posterior border of the mastoid process, the force acting obliquely from above downwards and forwards. More rarely, the process is detached as the result of a blow delivered immediately above the ear, that organ sharing in the displacement. In either case the detachment is usually of an incomplete nature, mainly on account of the muscular and pericranial attachments in the region involved.

According to Boullet, the following symptoms result :—

Surgical emphysema and pneumatocele. Air escapes from the mastoid cells and antrum into the overlying tissues, either spreading widely through the subaponeurotic space of the scalp and cellular tissues of the neck (surgical emphysema), or remaining localized and forming a tumour of inconsiderable size (pneumatocele). In either case palpation reveals that peculiar crepitation which is pathognomonic of tumours of this nature.

Bleeding from the ear. Hæmorrhage takes place into the middle ear, and, as the tympanic membrane is usually lacerated, the blood escapes from the external ear. In the event of the tympanic membrane being uninjured, the blood may escape along the Eustachian tube into the naso-pharynx.

Boullet also pointed out that certain complications may be associated with the mastoid lesion. These are as follows :—

Immediate.	*Remote.*
Wound of the lateral sinus.	Deafness.
Laceration of dura and brain.	Otitis media.
Injury to the aqueductus Fallopii and paralysis of the seventh nerve.	Caries and necrosis of the petrous bone.

Treatment. The displacement of the mastoid process is of so incomplete a nature that the question of replacement by open operation seldom arises. In the event, however, of intracranial complications, operative treatment must be carried out. Under ordinary circumstances the treatment consists mainly in the prevention of suppuration. When suppuration occurs, frequent cleansing of the ear must be carried out in order to prevent accumulation of pus in middle ear and antrum. This object is to be attained, *not* by syringing, but by gentle irrigation and light packing. Later on it may become necessary to carry out the complete mastoid operation.

FRACTURES OF THE VAULT OF THE SKULL

Fractures of the vault of the skull may be restricted to the vault or associated with a basic fracture. Evidence has been brought forward previously to show that many vault fractures may be regarded as mere upward extension from a primary basic lesion. The limitation of a fracture to the vault depends on the nature of the productive force, the degree of violence used, the site of application, and the direction of the force. Thus, the smaller the weapon, the greater the violence, the nearer the site of application to the vertex, the more direct the blow, the greater is the tendency to vault limitation. Again, compound fractures are much more liable to vault limitation than simple fractures, as is proved, for instance, by the reports of Sir Prescott Hewitt—20 compound fractures in which the fracture was restricted to the vault of the skull, and 56 simple fractures in which the base was involved in all but one.

Fractures of the vault may involve :—

(*a*) the external table only;
(*b*) the internal table alone;
(*c*) the whole thickness of the skull.

Fractures of the external table alone. These fractures are excessively rare. Their existence was even doubted till the recent South African War, when Makins [1] saw one case of this nature. They appear to be due to the impact of a glancing bullet (see p. 297). A 'gutter-shaped' depression results, the comminuted fragments of the external table being carried away or distributed in the region of the lacerated scalp (see Chapter IX).

Fractures of the internal table alone. Ambrose Paré drew attention to this class of fracture in 1652, but it remained for Teevan to investigate more fully the condition in 1865. Previous to Teevan's investigations, it had been considered that the internal table of the skull was the more brittle, and that fractures confined to the internal table were to be explained on that hypothesis. Teevan, however, demonstrated the incorrectness of such a theory, for, on firing bullets through the skull, from without inwards and from within outwards, it was found that on all occasions the more distal table suffered the more severely. This was explained in the following manner:—the fracture of the proximal table was produced by the bullet, whilst that of the distal table resulted, not from the passage of the bullet alone, but also from various fragments of bone driven along with the bullet.

Teevan's experiments also proved that a fracture of the internal table alone could be produced mechanically, this being in obedience to the law that 'when a pressure is applied to a body the fracture commences on the line of extension, not that of compression'.

Fractures of the internal table are undoubtedly more common in those situations where diploic tissue is prevalent, e.g. in the frontal, parietal, and upper occipital regions. In the squamo-temporal and cerebellar regions fractures of the internal table are almost unknown.

Teevan also stated that 'but little force is required to produce

[1] *Surgical Experiences in South Africa.*

such a fracture, and that they are produced usually by some small body, such as a stone '.

Fractures involving the whole thickness of the skull. Fractures which involve the whole thickness of the skull may be :—

(*a*) Simple or compound.

(*b*) With or without depression.

When depressed, the fragments of bone may be either loose or interlocked, forming in the latter case the so-called pond and gutter fractures.

(*c*) Elevated, usually from sabre-cuts.

(*d*) Fissured, stellate, comminuted, punctured, &c.

(*e*) Explosive.

Symptoms associated with fracture of the vault. A diagnosis of fracture of the vault is made :—

On the evidence obtained by local examination.

On the evidence supplied by symptoms dependent on injury to the intracranial contents.

The various intracranial lesions are discussed elsewhere (see Chapters III and IV).

Evidence supplied by local examination. A compound fracture will be most readily determined by digital examination, previous to which the scalp-wound must be carefully cleansed. Digital examination is greatly preferable to investigation with the aid of the probe. In any case care must be taken to avoid mistaking one of the sutures of the skull for a fissured fracture.

In simple fractures the diagnosis is frequently obscured by an extensive subaponeurotic or subpericranial hæmatoma. Irregularities of surface are more or less diagnostic of a solution in the surface of the bone, and a linear hæmatoma is of corresponding clinical value. In any case, the presence of an extensive hæmatoma must be regarded as of so suggestive a nature that exploration is called for, more especially when prolonged concussion or compression are co-existent. Such treatment is imperative when the hæmatoma —whether diffuse, localized, or linear—pulsates, such a condition implying a breach in the surface of both bone and dura with communication between the extra-cranial and some intra-cranial hæmorrhage.

Pringle [1] lays stress on the value of percussion as an aid to diagnosis.

'The patient's head must be supported beneath the occiput, the mouth either open or shut—it matters not, so long as it is the same throughout the examination—and the skull is struck sharply with the finger. When a fracture is present, two changes in note may

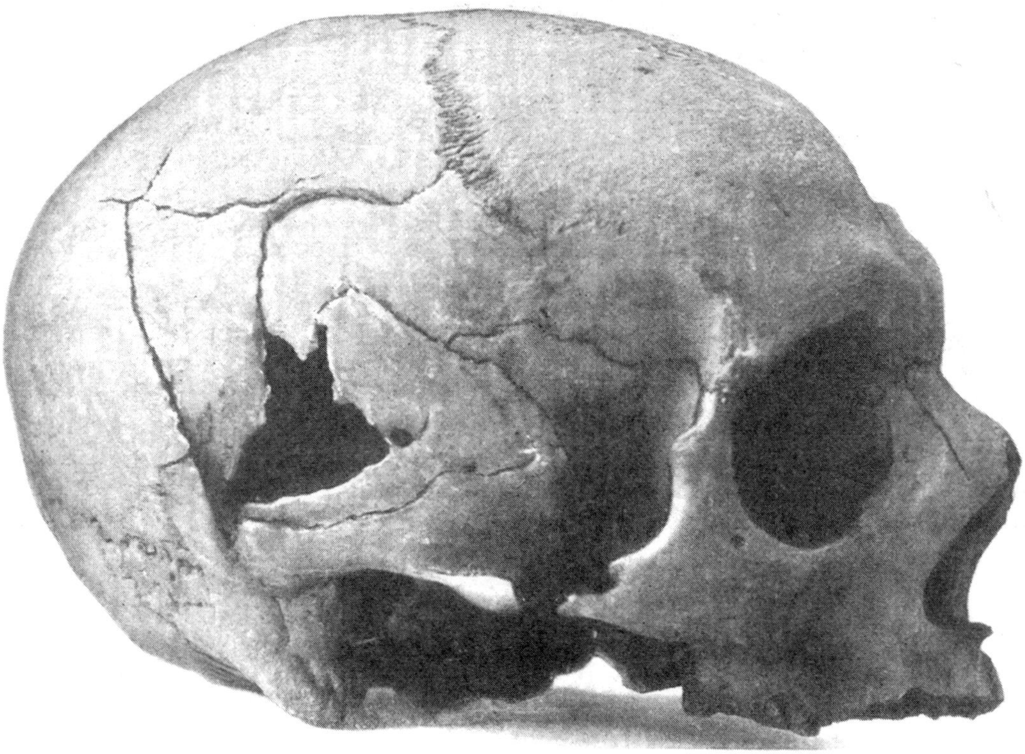

FIG. 42. A COMMINUTED FRACTURE OF THE SKULL.

be elicited. Either a note lowered in pitch over the fracture zone, or, in addition, a definite crack-pot sound. The note elicited is most typical when comminution is present, and some fragments loose. A fracture of a T or L or V-shape gives the best crack-pot sound, and the crack quality is always most pronounced when the percussing finger comes over the angular portion of the bone. Hæmorrhage into the subaponeurotic region blurs the note.'

If time and occasion permit, an X-ray photograph will clinch the matter.

When the fracture involves the internal table alone, the symp-

[1] *Edin. Med. Journ.*, 1909, p. 526.

toms are less definite. Teevan stated that this class of fracture does not lead to the development of any symptoms unless :—

The middle meningeal artery be injured.

The dura mater and brain be irritated.

The brain be compressed.

He also adds that the existence of the following features suggests the nature of the injury :—

The history of a slight blow, probably with a small body.
The blow situated over the parietal region.

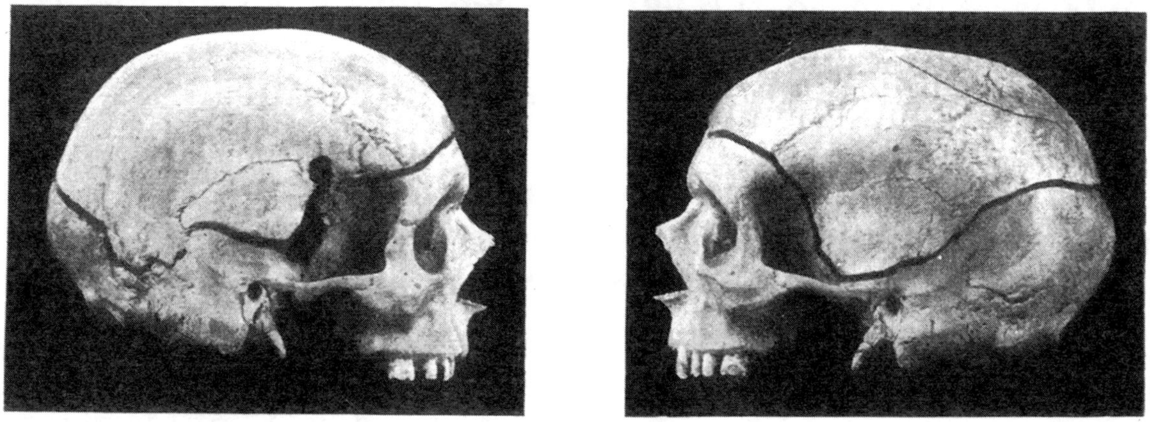

A B

FIG. 43. AN EXPLOSIVE FRACTURE OF THE VAULT OF THE SKULL. A shows the right side of the skull and the site of entry of the bullet. B shows the extension of the fracture round the left half of the skull. In the left upper parietal region (Fig. B) a fissured fracture is seen where the bullet failed to perforate the skull.

Chronic fixed pain, some days or weeks afterwards, with symptoms of brain-irritation or encephalitis, and even suppuration, suggesting irritation of the meninges and brain by spicules of bone.

Compression and paralysis on the opposite side of the body some hours afterwards, as the result of injury to the middle meningeal artery.

Symptoms of compression early and slight, combined with partial paralysis of the opposite side of the body.

'The less definite the symptoms of compression, the greater the reason to believe that they are caused by the internal table only.'

Before entering into the question of *treatment* of fractures of the skull, it is essential that allusion should be made to the *temperature in its relation to head-injuries.* The great importance of temperature changes in the consideration of operative treatment will be manifest when discussing the treatment of fractures of the base.

The temperature in its relation to head-injuries. The various temperature changes observed in cases of head-injury have afforded a subject prolific in discussion. Broca, Battle, Guyon, Walsham, and others have endeavoured to deduce facts from the examination of head cases, but the results have been rather indefinite. In over 300 cases that have come under my observation, accurate records of the temperature charts were obtained, the patients were watched throughout their illness, and in the case of death, the autopsies were attended.

The following deductions were made :—

1. That, for a variable period of time after the injury, the temperature is always subnormal—sometimes so low that it cannot be registered. This is the period of shock.

2. That the patient may die in this state of shock, but that, if he lives, reaction takes place and the temperature rises.

3. That this rise in temperature is, in fatal cases, rapid and progressive. In one case the temperature rose 6° in seven hours, in another 8° in four hours. Death occurs when the temperature is at its highest—anything up to 106°, and even more when registered in the rectum.

4. That the temperature may rise to a moderate height, and there 'mark time'. This is the 'crisis' of the case. A subsequent fall in temperature generally indicates recovery, a further rise usually points to a fatal termination.

5. That the rise of temperature is independent of any special osseous lesion, since similar changes are observed in fractures of the vault and in fractures of the base.

6. That laceration of the brain is present in the majority of cases in which marked temperature changes are observed, but that the changes in temperature are totally independent of any special regional brain-injury.

Richet arrives at the conclusion that two hypotheses present themselves, accounting for temperature changes in general : (1) that there are certain temperature regulators in the encephalon which, when excited, become stimulated in function; (2) that the cortical injury acts in a sort of reflex manner on the regulatory centres situated in the pons or bulb.

Attention was also drawn to the experiments of Lorin and van Benedin, who, after excising the two cerebral hemispheres of a pigeon, showed that the heat regulatory centre was preserved intact, proving that the corpus striatum is not necessarily the head-office for heat-regulation in general.

Till, therefore, more evidence comes to hand with respect to heat-regulation in general, one cannot go beyond the broad statement that, in severe head-injuries, definite temperature changes occur, that the changes are independent of any special lesion of bone or brain, that they are generally associated with some brain-injury, and that they are probably due to the influence exerted by the lesion on the heat-regulating centres in the region of the pons and bulb.

With regard to the value of the temperature, both with respect to prognosis and treatment, a very much more definite statement can be made.

First with respect to the **prognosis**. All cases of head-injury may be grouped into four classes, according to the changes of temperature present.

Group 1. The temperature, at first subnormal, undergoes a rapid and progressive rise. Prognosis most unfavourable.

Group 2. The temperature, at first subnormal, rises gradually to 101° or 102° and there 'marks time'. This hesitancy marks the crisis of the case, further elevation indicating a fatal result, whilst a fall offers every hope of recovery.

Group 3. The temperature, at first subnormal, rises to normal and remains at that level. Prognosis very favourable.

Group 4. The temperature, at first subnormal, remains subnormal. The condition of shock persists, and the prognosis is most unfavourable.

Practically all cases of head-injury fall readily into one or other of these four groups, and the temperature chart presents so clear a picture that it must be regarded as of the greatest possible value in estimating the prognosis in any given case. In other words, the temperature chart affords an almost infallible guide both to prognosis and treatment.

With respect to alteration in temperature on the two sides of the body, the clinical value of such changes must, from my own observations, be regarded as of a very indefinite nature.

It now remains to discuss the value of temperature changes with respect to treatment.

Treatment of Fracture of the Base of the Skull. In the earlier paragraphs of this chapter the special treatment of aural and nasal hæmorrhages and cerebro-spinal discharge was discussed, and some allusion was made to the necessity of exploring the middle fossa in cases of profuse arterial or venous aural bleeding. The general treatment of basic fractures now requires description, previous to which, however, space must be made for a short account of the routine treatment by Urotropin—as advised by Crowe and Cushing—as a prophylactic against the development of meningeal infection. The following is a summary of Crowe's paper[1] on the 'excretion of Urotropin in the cerebro-spinal fluid and its therapeutic value in meningitis'.

1. Urotropin, when given by the mouth, invariably appears in the cerebro-spinal fluid.

2. The largest amount of Urotropin is present in the cerebro-spinal fluid from thirty minutes to an hour after the ingestion of the drug.

3. After doses of Urotropin, within therapeutic limits, a sufficient amount of the drug appears in the cerebro-spinal fluid to exercise a decided inhibitory effect on the growth of organisms inoculated into this fluid after its removal from the body.

4. Following a subdural inoculation of dogs and rabbits with streptococcus, 60–80 grains of Urotropin a day, given under conditions which insure absorption, will markedly defer, and in some cases prevent, the onset of a fatal meningitis.

5. In view of these observations, the prompt administration of Urotropin is advised in all clinical cases in which meningitis is a possible or threatened complication, or even when meningeal infection has actually occurred.

[1] *Johns Hopkins Hospital Bulletin*, April, 1909.

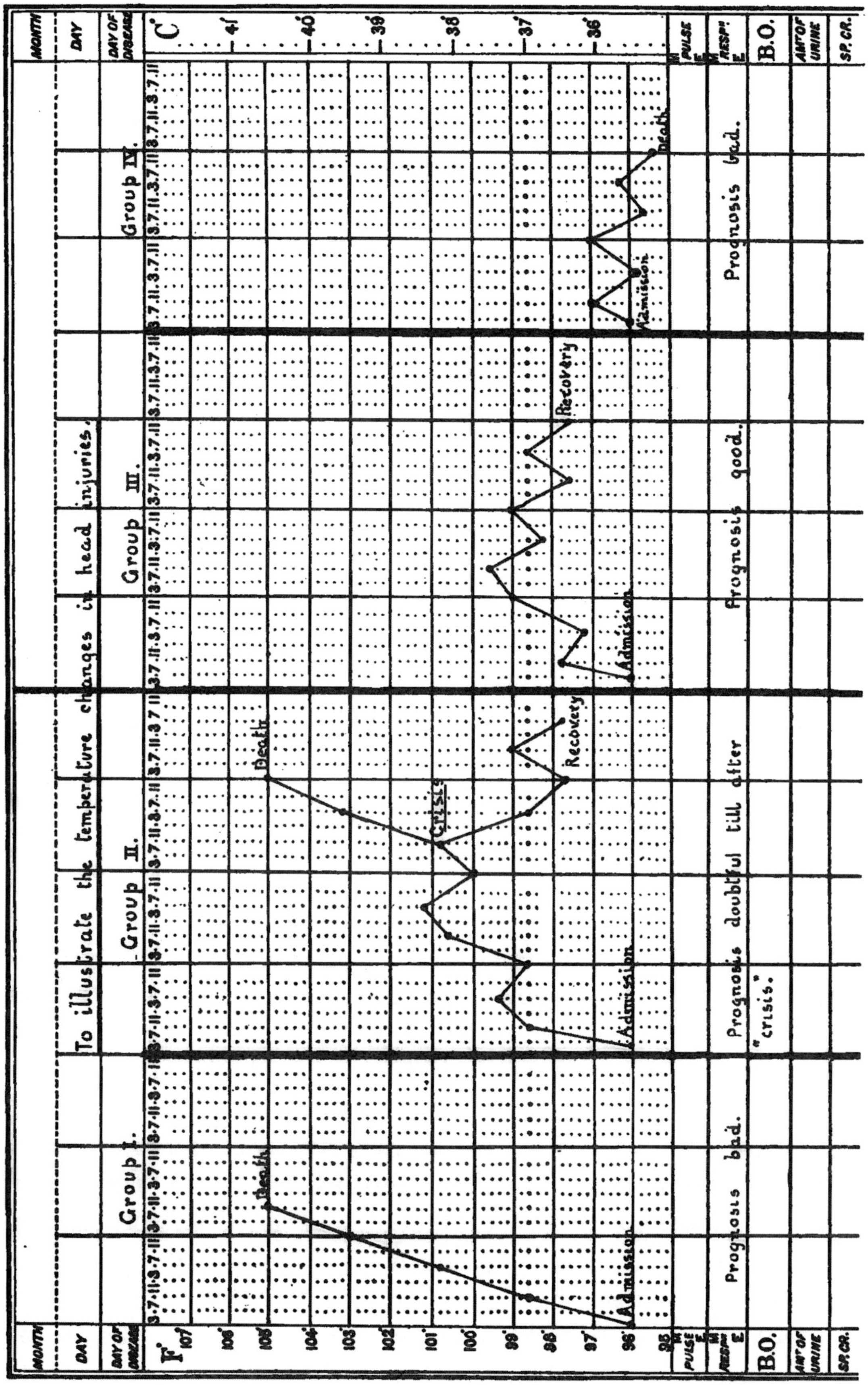

FIG. 44. A TEMPERATURE CHART ILLUSTRATING THE CHANGES IN TEMPERATURE OBSERVED IN HEAD-INJURIES. (For description, see text.)

Acting on these suggestions, I am accustomed to treat all head cases with this drug, 10–20 grains three times a day by mouth. It may be given per rectum, though probably with less satisfactory results. Traumatic cases are treated as soon as possible, other cases receive their dose for two or three days previous to the operation, the drug being continued till all fear of possible meningeal infection has vanished.

In discussing the general treatment of basic fractures, it must be accepted that the basic fracture in itself requires no treatment. Danger or death is dependent on intracranial complications, and an uncomplicated basic fracture demands no active surgical treatment. The special treatment applicable to cases complicated by hæmorrhages, both external to and beneath the dura mater, is discussed in the next chapter. It is therefore only necessary to enter into those cases of fractured base which are associated with concussion, irritation, and compression of the brain—in other words, the *average* case of fracture of the base of the skull.

The surgeon must always be guided by the general condition of the patient—the blood-pressure, character of pulse, state of respiration, depth of unconsciousness, &c.—but, in my opinion, the temperature chart affords perhaps the most valuable basis on which rules can be formulated guiding the surgeon in his general line of treatment.

Thus (1) **when the temperature remains subnormal** the patient is in a condition of severe cerebral shock, due, in the majority of cases, to contusion or laceration of the brain, the grosser lesion being most commonly situated either at the apex of the temporo-sphenoidal lobe or at the anterior inferior part of the frontal lobe. The patient is, however, suffering from shock, and the treatment advocated for that condition in general is equally applicable to these cases in particular. The patient should be placed in the so-called head-down position, and the extremities firmly bandaged from below upwards. The vaso-motor depression should be combated by the administration of rectal or intra-venous infusions of saline solution, to each pint of which is added 1 drachm of a 1 in 1,000 solution of Adrenalin Chloride. It is at once obvious that, whilst combating the condition of shock, this mode of treatment may tend at the same time to encourage fresh bleeding if the brain should have been lacerated, or if intracranial vessels should have been torn. For this reason I regard rectal infusion as the more safe of the two methods, in spite of the fact that intra-venous infusion brings about a more rapid improvement in the patient's condition. The effect of the infusion must be carefully observed, and as soon as the blood-pressure rises and the temperature shows a tendency to rise—say from the subnormal to the normal—the infusion process must be stopped, and the further progress of the case observed.

The risks attendant on this mode of treatment are obvious, but in their consideration, it must also be borne in mind that if the patient remains in the collapse stage, without evidencing any sign of reaction, he will inevitably die. If the treatment advocated should tide the patient over this stage and induce a definite reaction, as exemplified by rise of blood-pressure and elevation of temperature, the further treatment of the case can be considered under the next group.

(2) **When the temperature rises progressively** the patient evidences symptoms pointing to compression of the brain—coma, slow pulse, noisy and stertorous respiration, hot skin and turgid face. Later on, as a result of the increasing pressure, the medullary centres begin to show signs of exhaustion, the pulse-rate increasing, and the respiration becoming Cheyne-Stokes in character.

Whether these symptoms result primarily from the nature of the lesion, or secondarily after the adoption of those measures advocated for the collapse stage, it matters not. Our indications with respect to treatment are clear. The increasing intracranial pressure must be reduced. This desideratum is preferably carried out by the ligature of a bleeding meningeal artery, or by the occlusion of a torn venous sinus, but unfortunately, such a course is frequently out of the question. We have, therefore, to deal with an increased and increasing intracranial pressure, without definite localizing features. For this condition we have at our disposal the following measures: venesection, lumbar puncture, and 'decompression' operations.

Venesection. I regard venesection as a valuable means of reducing the intracranial pressure. It is mainly of use in those cases that hover between slight compression and the fully-developed condition. Venesection may therefore be regarded as of special advantage in those cases that show elevation of temperature to about 101° and there 'mark time'. The 'bleeding' should be carried out after exposure of the median basilic, external jugular, or internal saphenous veins, preferably from the first-named site. The amount of blood to be withdrawn varies according to the individual circumstances of the case, but, in general, the escape of blood should be encouraged till the pulse becomes soft, frequent and compressible. On an average, the quantity of blood withdrawn varies from 10–20 ounces. The operation not infrequently turns the scale in favour of the patient. Venesection may also be carried out in combination with 'decompression' operations.

When applied to suitable cases and carried out with discrimination, venesection often tides the patient over the stage of 'crisis'. The most careful observation is needed in estimating the quantity of blood to be withdrawn, the pulse, blood-pressure, respiration, and temperature affording an adequate guide.

Lumbar puncture. In spite of the apparent advantages of this method, it must, I think, be acknowledged that lumbar puncture is of but little use in reducing the general intracranial pressure. Consequently, in spite of the fact that this procedure has been strongly recommended, experience shows that it is of little practical use. This statement, based on personal experience, is at variance with the opinion of some other surgeons. For instance, de Quènu reports 7 cases of fractured skull which were 'cured' by this treatment, one of them requiring to be punctured eight times. Lumbar puncture assists the diagnosis, but I am doubtful whether it improves the prognosis.

'Decompression' operations. 'Decompression' operations may be carried out over the cerebellar fossa or over the temporal region of the skull. In **cerebellar decompression** a suitable scalp-flap is turned down and the trephine applied over the centre of the exposed occipital bone. After the removal of the disk the wall of the cerebellar fossa is cut away with the craniectomy forceps, up to the line of the lateral sinus above, to the mastoid process in front, to the vicinity of the foramen magnum below, and almost up to the middle line on the inner side. The bulging dura mater is incised in a crucial manner, right up to the margins of the osseous gap, all

meningeal vessels that cross the line proposed for dural section being under-run with a fully-curved needle threaded with catgut. A small drainage-tube is inserted between the dura and the cerebellum and brought out through the most dependent part of the scalp-flap. The flap is then sutured in position. The drainage-tube should be stitched to the skin and withdrawn twenty-four to forty-eight hours later, according to the progress of the case.

I have carried out this operation on several occasions, but in spite of some immediate improvement in the condition of the patient, the remote results have been so unsatisfactory that I have abandoned the operation entirely. The effect of this cerebellar decompression is too radical, the medullary centres strongly object to such heroic attempts at pressure relief.

Temporal decompression, more correctly known as the **inter-musculo-temporal decompression** operation of Harvey Cushing, leads to very different results. Previous to dealing with the technique of the operation, it will be convenient to enumerate the advantages claimed for this method in general.

(1) The frequency with which the bony lesion occurs in the middle fossa of the skull.

(2) The fact that cerebral contusions are especially liable to involve the tip of the temporo-sphenoidal lobe.

(3) The exposure of the meningeal territory and the ease of determining the presence of an extra-dural hæmorrhage.

(4) The possibility of draining through a split muscle rather than directly through the scalp.

(5) The subsequent protective action of the muscle in case a hernia tends to form in consequence of traumatic œdema.

(6) The subsequent absence of any deformities, the skin incision being carried out for the most part through the hairy portion of the scalp.

The operation. The hair is shaved over the temporal region, with a wide margin to the field of operation. In other respects, those preliminary details should be adopted which are enumerated in Chapter II. The skin incision commences well above and behind the external angular frontal process, is directed along the line of, but below the temporal crest, and curves downwards to terminate

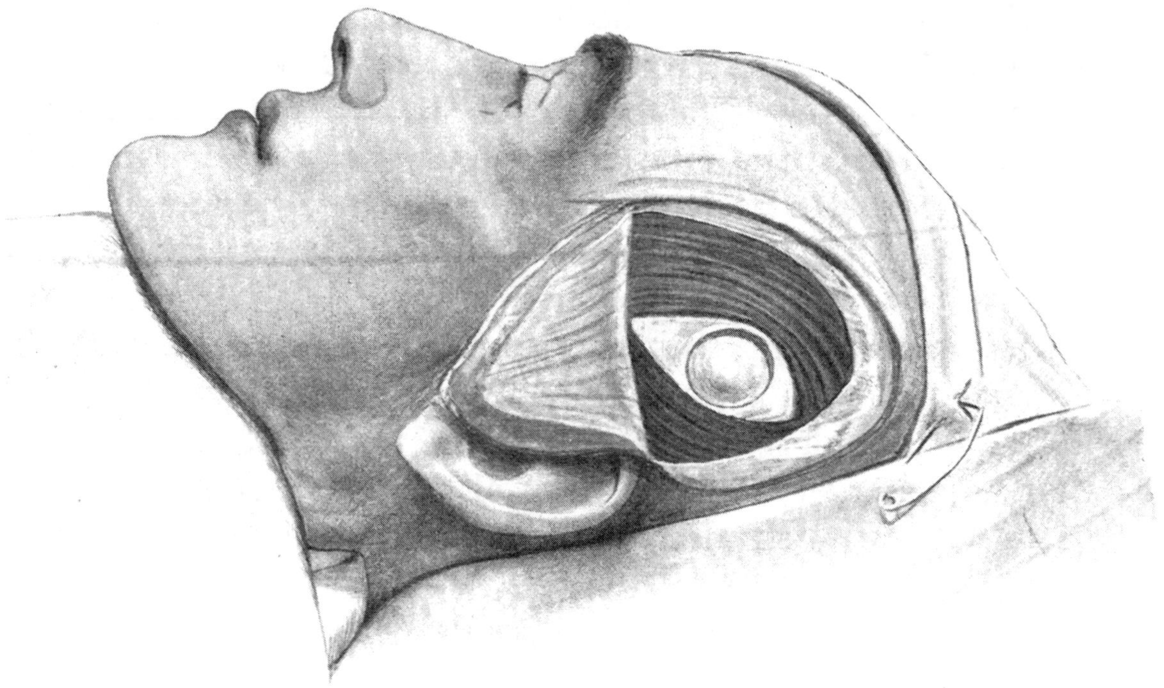

FIG. 45. INTERMUSCULO-TEMPORAL CEREBRAL DECOMPRESSION. *First stage.* The scalp and temporal fascia have been turned down as separate flaps. The temporal muscle is divided in the direction of its fibres, and the exposed bone trephined.

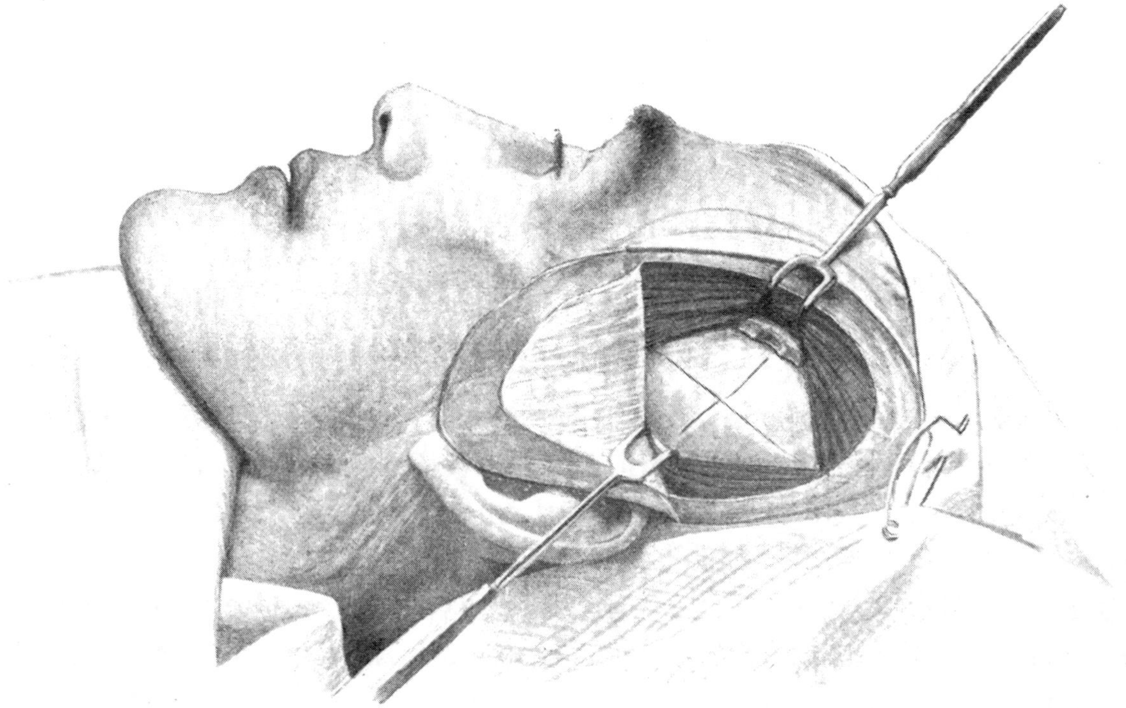

FIG. 46. INTERMUSCULO-TEMPORAL CEREBRAL DECOMPRESSION. *Second Stage.* The temporal muscle is retracted on either side, the bone has been freely cut away, and the bulging dura mater crucially incised.

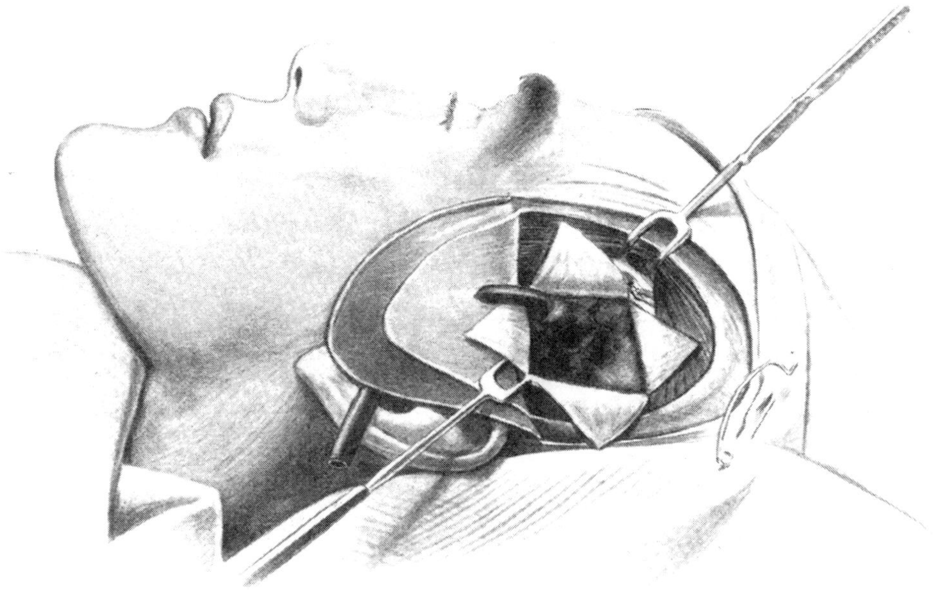

FIG. 47. INTERMUSCULO-TEMPORAL CEREBRAL DECOMPRESSION. *Third Stage.* The dural flaps are turned aside, exposing the lacerated temporo-sphenoidal lobe. A rubber drainage-tube has been inserted beneath the lacerated brain, lying on the floor of the middle fossa of the skull and brought to the surface through the scalp-flap.

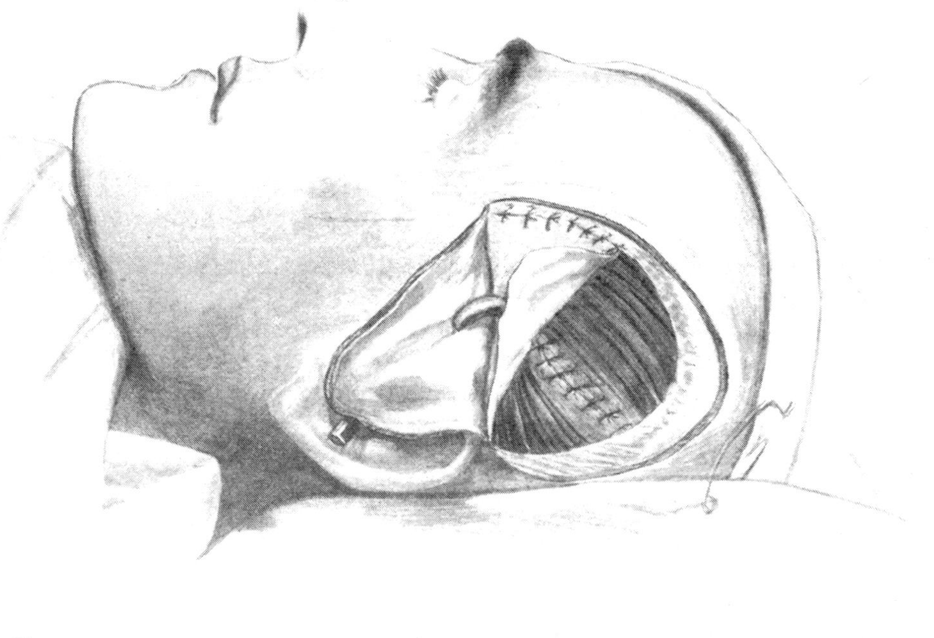

FIG. 48. INTERMUSCULO-TEMPORAL CEREBRAL DECOMPRESSION. *Fourth Stage.* The temporal muscle-fibres have been approximated, and the temporal fascia reunited in part. The drainage tube is seen to emerge through fascia and scalp.

just anterior to the tragus of the ear. Pressure is applied during the formation of the incision so as to control bleeding from temporal arteries. The flap, comprising skin, subcutaneous tissue, and superficial temporal artery, is turned down to a zygomatic base, care being taken to avoid injury to the temporal vessels at the base of the flap. The temporal fascia is then incised, parallel to but immediately below the line of the skin incision, and the fascia also turned down towards the zygoma. The temporal muscle is split in the direction of its fibres, from the temporal crest above to the zygoma below, stripped away from the bone and well retracted in both forward and backward directions. In this procedure care must be taken to avoid detachment of the muscle-fibres from the temporal crest. The area of bone exposed, however, should be as extensive as circumstances permit.

The trephine is applied to the bone, the surgeon aiming at the angle between the anterior and posterior branches of the middle meningeal artery. The disk is removed, the dura separated from the bone, and the craniectomy forceps called into requisition, the bone entering into the formation of the temporal fossa being freely cut away, more especially in the *downward*, forward, and backward directions—in other words, in the general line of the temporo-sphenoidal lobe. In the upward direction the surgeon must be more guarded, more especially when the operation is being conducted on the left side of the head. Broca's area of motor speech must be avoided, for fear of its inclusion in any hernial protrusion that may ensue.

The bulging and probably discoloured dura mater is freely incised, preferably in a crucial manner, though the exact line of such incision is of little importance so long as it is free in character. Needless to say, all meningeal vessels that cross the lines proposed for dural section must first be ligatured (by underrunning with a fully curved needle) on either side of those lines. The four dural flaps are turned aside and the antero-external aspect of the temporo-sphenoidal pole exposed. A small drainage—or drain of rubber tissue—can now be inserted along the floor of the middle fossa skull in the immediate vicinity of any lacerated brain or blood-clot, the drain lying between the dura and the brain, and anchored to the dura mater or muscle by a fine catgut suture.

The four dural flaps are allowed to remain loose over the surface of the brain, whilst the temporal muscle is sewn across from side to side with a few catgut sutures, room being allowed at the lower angle for the emergence of the drain.

The temporal fascia is replaced and carefully united to its upper cut margin, the drain being brought out through the fascia and through a puncture hole made at the most convenient part of the scalp-flap. The scalp-flap is approximated with numerous interrupted silk or salmon-gut sutures.

The tube is allowed to remain for thirty-six hours or more, according to the condition of the patient.

The operation may be carried out on one or on both sides of the skull ; if on the one side only, on that side at which laceration of the brain is probably existent. In connexion with this it is necessary to state that laceration by contre-coup is more common than direct brain-injury. Thus, if the blow be inflicted on the right parieto-occipital region, the operation should be conducted in the left temporal region.

In the absence of all localizing features the decompression should be carried out on the *right* side of the head, in order to avoid all possibility of including, in the hernial protrusion that may result, the motor speech area of Broca.

In cases of severe head-injury the surgeon must be prepared for many disappointments, but, from my own experience, it would appear that Cushing's operation frequently brings about the most satisfactory results.

It should, however, be clearly understood that indiscriminate decompression operations only bring discredit on the method in general. They should only be carried out in suitable cases.

TREATMENT OF FRACTURES OF THE VAULT OF THE SKULL

Indications for operation. It is the general custom to divide fractures of the vault into two groups—those demanding operative treatment and those in which an expectant attitude is advised—and between these two groups a sharp line of demarcation is drawn. There is, however, no such line of demarcation. In the event of the general condition of the patient being compatible with operative interference, such treatment is urgently called for under the following conditions :—

All cases of punctured fracture.

All cases of depressed fracture, whether diagnosed by palpation or by inference, whether simple or compound, whether complicated or not.

All cases of fracture complicated by extra-dural or localized sub-dural extravasation of blood.

All elevated fractures.

All compound fractures.

In all these instances, from the presence of depressed fragments of bone, from associated injury to the intracranial contents, or from other causes, no mere expectant policy should be pursued. The surgeon has to look into the future, to bear in mind the possibility of meningeal infection, and the more remote results of head-injuries in general (see Chapter VI). In other words, early and active surgical interference is imperatively demanded, for not only is it necessary to strain every endeavour to save the patient's life, but the surgeon should also adopt those procedures which guard most effectually against the more remote possibilities of the case.

With regard to *simple* fractures, if it can be determined that the fracture, whether fissured, stellate, or comminuted, is simple and uncomplicated by any serious intracranial lesion, no active surgical treatment is required. The determination of such conditions is, however, quite another matter, always difficult and sometimes, from the presence of overlying hæmatomata, quite impossible.

In the general estimation of these cases it should be borne in mind that simple uncomplicated vault fractures are decidedly rare. For instance, Dwight, in 145 cases of fractured skull that came to autopsy, only found six that evidenced a fissured fracture localized to the vault. It may, of course, be urged that these statistics are fallacious, insomuch as simple uncomplicated vault fractures would probably not come to the post-mortem table. Clinical evidence, however, coincides with Dwight's statistics, and clinical evidence shows, furthermore, that a blow sufficing to fracture the vault of the skull almost invariably results in further injury.

In these doubtful cases the surgeon is greatly aided in his decision by a general review of the patient's condition, more especially by those symptoms which are regarded as exemplifying the clinical conditions of concussion, irritation, and compression.

When the fracture is associated with mild concussion it may be inferred that the brain is practically uninjured, and that operative treatment is not required.

When the fracture is associated with severe concussion it may be inferred that the brain is damaged, to a degree proportionate to the depth and duration of the stage of unconsciousness. The question of operation depends to a very large extent on the general condition of the patient, and more especially on the temperature and temperature changes (see p. 114). With a persistent subnormal temperature it may be inferred that the brain-injury is of a very severe nature, and that operative measures are, for the time being, contra-indicated. In the event of the temperature rising it may be accepted that the patient is passing from the state of shock to that of reaction, operative measures again hinging on the further progress of the case. If the temperature rises progressively, the patient passing from the stage of reaction to that of compression, operative measures are indicated. Under other circumstances an expectant attitude can be adopted.

When the fracture is associated with general cerebral irritation it may be inferred that the brain is contused or slightly lacerated. Under these circumstances operation is, for the time being, not required, and an expectant attitude should be adopted.

When the fracture is associated with compression it may be inferred that the condition is dependent on depressed fragments of bone, or on extra- or intra-dural bleeding. Operative measures are now urgently indicated.

When the fracture is confined to the internal table a diagnosis is only possible when symptoms of localized irritation ensue, either due to pressure exercised on the cortex by spicules of bone or resulting from injury to some intracranial vessel, e. g. the middle meningeal artery. In such cases operation is indicated. Under other circumstances the surgeon must await the developments of the case.

Treatment. *When the fracture is associated with mild concussion.* During the stage of concussion no active treatment is required, beyond putting the patient to bed—with the head low—enveloping him in hot blankets, and applying hot bottles to the extremities. These bottles are wrapped up in flannel: they should never be placed in contact with the patient's skin. As soon as the reaction stage *commences*, the bottles and blankets should be removed, the patient covered with light clothing only, and an ice-bag applied to the head, over the region at which the injury was inflicted. Calomel, in suitable doses, should be given by mouth, and a copious enema administered per rectum. Perhaps the most essential point in the general consideration of the case is the after-treatment. The patient should be kept in hospital or home for at least one month, and for the next three months or more, according to the urgency of the case, he should abstain from all mental and bodily work. At the end of that period of time he may return to work, though still kept under observation.

When the fracture is associated with severe concussion. In the event of persistence of concussion symptoms of a severe type the prognosis is decidedly unfavourable. This prolongation of cerebral shock is undoubtedly dependent in its persistence on severe vaso-motor depression, and in the majority of cases ending unfavourably it will be found that the brain is generally œdematous and regionally contused or lacerated. In cases of this nature the surgeon should confine his attention, for the time being, to an endeavour at terminating this vaso-motor depression, raising the blood-pressure and inducing a definite reaction; the patient being treated after the manner indicated on p. 118.

When the fracture is associated with general cerebral irritation. The patient should be put to bed in a quiet and darkened room, under the continuous attention of a trained nurse. An ice-bag or Leiter's tubes may be applied to the head, though the patient seldom tolerates such attentions. I regard morphia as of the greatest service in this class of cases. It should be given freely, subcutaneously, either by itself or in combination with atropin. I generally order $\frac{1}{4}$ gr. morphia with $\frac{1}{100}$ gr. atropin every six hours, till the irritative symptoms subside.

Insomuch as all evidence tends to prove that general cerebral irritation, as resulting from injury, implies a condition of contusion or superficial laceration, a prolonged period of bodily and mental rest is essential before the patient is discharged from treatment and allowed to return to work—a period of not less than six months.

The operative treatment of fractures of the vault. The usual preparatory treatment is carried out, the scalp-tourniquet applied, a suitable scalp-flap framed and turned down, advantage being taken of all existent scalp lacerations.

The subsequent details vary according to the circumstances of the case :—

Fissured fractures. If, after thorough exposure of the parts, the operator is satisfied that he has to deal with an uncomplicated fissured fracture, the scalp-flap is accurately sewn into position (see p. 16). On the other hand, if the symptoms point to the presence of an extra-dural hæmorrhage, the bone is trephined where the fracture crosses the line of the suspected vessel and the conditions treated as described under middle meningeal hæmorrhage. In subdural extravasation the trephine is applied over that part of the brain, in the immediate vicinity of the fracture, from which the symptoms appear to emanate, and the conditions treated as described under subdural hæmorrhage.

In a certain proportion of cases the symptoms point to a marked increase of intracranial pressure without definite localizing features, a condition pointing to diffuse subdural hæmorrhage, with or without brain laceration. Under such circumstances much may be done to relieve the increased intracranial pressure by carrying out the operation of 'cerebral decompression' (see p. 121).

Depressed fractures. The operative details vary according to the nature of the osseous lesion :—

(*a*) If the depressed fragments of bone are so interlocked that elevation is impossible (e. g. pond and gutter fractures), it will be necessary to trephine in the immediate vicinity of the depression, in order to lessen the mutual attachment of the fragments one to another, so obtaining sufficient purchase for their elevation or removal.

The pericranium is stripped away from the region of the depression (see Fig. 49), and a small trephine applied in such a manner that the trephine circle includes the outer part of the depressed area. Care must be taken to avoid more pressure over the depressed fragments than is absolutely necessary, for fear of causing further damage to the underlying structures. This advice is all the more important when it is realized that the fracture of the internal table is almost invariably more extensive than that which involves the visible external table of the skull.

The disk of bone is removed and the conditions investigated with the dural separator. When the degree of depression and the splintering of the internal table are not excessive, the parts may be elevated into position. In most cases, however, the uncertainty that exists with regard to possible dural injury renders it necessary that the depressed fragments should be elevated and removed, or so raised as to allow of adequate inspection of the dura itself. For this purpose the craniectomy forceps may be required. The dura can now be examined. If torn, the opening may require enlargement, in order to determine whether any osseous fragments have been driven into the brain-substance; all such fragments are carefully removed. Hæmorrhage is arrested, the dura sewn up, and the scalp-flap carefully sutured. Drainage should always be avoided, the risk of infection is too great. As a prophylactic against the development of meningeal infection, the patient should undergo the routine treatment with urotropin (see p. 116).

(*b*) When the depression is of such a nature that the elevation of the fragments can be carried out without preliminary trephining, the fragments are raised with the periosteal separator, and the membranes and brain examined as described above.

In **simple comminuted fractures** the larger fragments of bone are to be replaced in the anticipation that they will live entire, in part, or will act as scaffolding media for the formation of dense fibrous tissue. After removal from the wound, and during the completion of the operation, the vitality of all loose fragments may be preserved by immersion in hot saline solution. All minute fragments of bone should be discarded.

With respect to **compound** fractures, it is necessary that the bone lesion should be fully exposed, all pockets of scalp-tissue being slit up to their termination. Previous to any attempt at examination of the injured bone, further precautions must be taken to avoid subsequent infection, by reason of the bruised and soiled scalp. Such tags of scalp-tissue as appear injured beyond repair should be cut away with the scissors, and in order to avoid or diminish subsequent wound infection, I have been accustomed to swab over the most

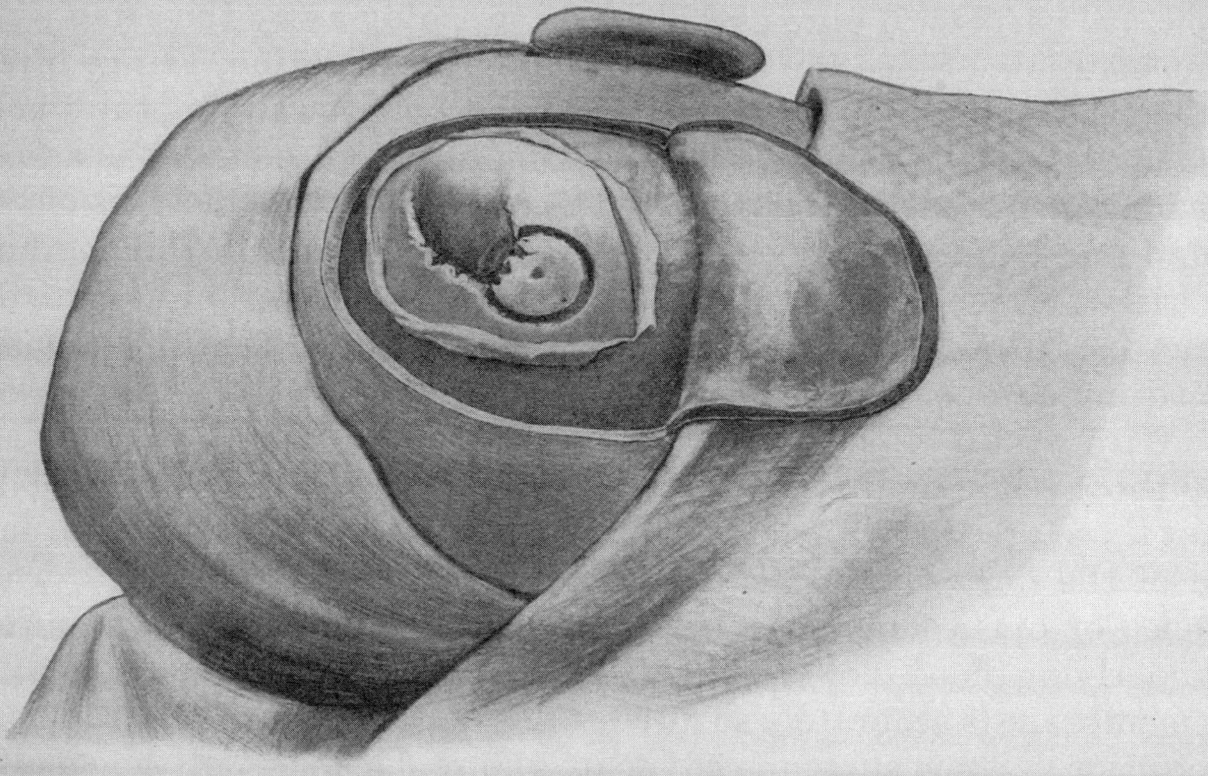

FIG. 49 A. THE ELEVATION OF A DEPRESSED FRACTURE. *First stage.* The trephine circle includes the outer portion of the depressed area.

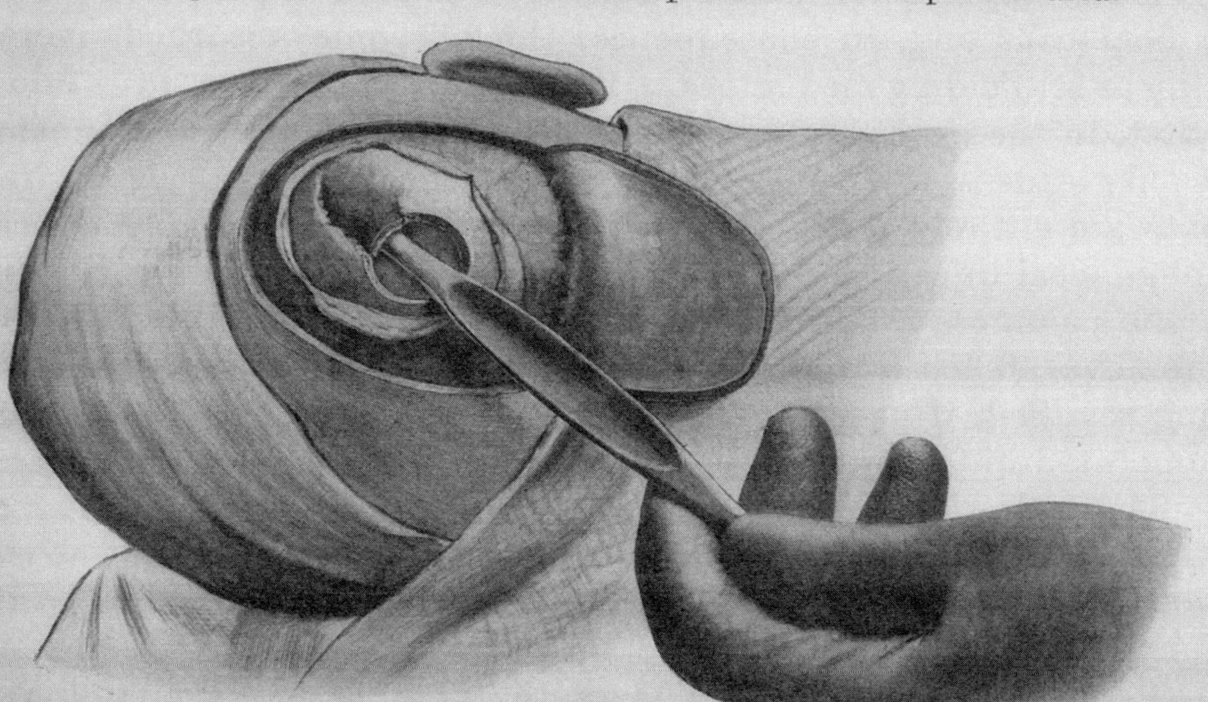

FIG. 49 B. THE ELEVATION OF A DEPRESSED FRACTURE. *Second stage.* The trephine disk has been removed and the elevator is in position.

suspicious parts with pure carbolic acid, washing away the same with saline solution. Since the advent of iodine sterilization, I have often utilized that solution in preference to the carbolic, swabbing the whole surface exposed. I think a combination of the two methods is advisable in more serious cases, utilizing the carbolic for the margins of the wound and iodine for the general surface. By means of this method the risk of meningeal infection and scalp suppuration is greatly reduced. To aid in the prophylaxis, the patient should again be placed under a course of treatment by urotropin (see p. 116).

With regard to the bone, all loose fragments should be removed, only those being preserved which retain their pericranial connexions. Even these are thrown back so as to permit of the maximum inspection of the dura mater. This membrane, if torn, is either sewn up at once or opened up more freely in the investigation and removal of underlying blood-clot or bone-débris. After removing such troubles the membrane is accurately sutured. The bone-flaps are now replaced in position. Some surgeons advocate the replacement of the smaller fragments of bone which have previously been removed. These fragments may be sterilized by boiling, but such a process destroys the bone-cells and, in consequence, they become absorbed, merely acting as scaffolding media for the formation of fibrous tissue. Added to that, in the event of suppuration, the presence of such fragments not only leads to the persistence of a purulent discharge, till the fragments are entirely removed, but also increases considerably the risk of meningeal infection.

As a summary, therefore, it may be laid down that it is necessary to remove all loose fragments of bone, the deficiency in the vault being rectified, if necessary, at a later date by one of the methods enumerated in Chapter VI.

The scalp-flap is accurately sewn up with interrupted salmon-gut sutures, a gauze or cigarette drain being inserted at the most convenient and dependent point, to be removed at the end of forty-eight hours or more according to the progress of the case.

Punctured fractures. Here there is a special liability to dural laceration and in-driving of comminuted fragments of bone. A full exposure of the parts is therefore absolutely essential. The trephine can be applied in the immediate vicinity of the puncture, or, as is often advisable, in such a manner that the punctured area is included in the trephine circle: this latter method may necessitate that the trephining should be carried out without the aid of the guiding fixation-pin, for which process some experience is needed.

After removal of the bone, the craniectomy forceps may be required, to allow of adequate dural inspection. The dura mater is opened up with blunt-pointed scissors, and the brain examined for in-driven fragments of bone. These, when found, are removed. Deeply situated fragments of bone and foreign bodies may be previously diagnosed by means of an X-ray picture.

If possible, both membrane and scalp should be sutured without drainage, but in the event of possible sepsis, a small cigarette drainage-tube should be inserted so as to lie beneath the dura mater on the one hand and emerge through the scalp wound at the other.

Fractures limited to the external table. For this class of fracture the reader is referred to the section dealing with bullet-wounds of the skull (see p. 296).

Fractures limited to the internal table. As previously indicated, the diagnosis of this condition is only practicable when the depression of the osseous fragments, or the hæmorrhage resulting from an injured meningeal vessel, so irritate the dura mater and brain that localizing symptoms ensue. For instance, epileptic fits of a Jacksonian type may develop shortly after the accident, this condition demanding a full exposure of the affected region. The operations required in the treatment of traumatic epilepsy and intracranial hæmorrhages are discussed in subsequent chapters.

THE MORTALITY FROM FRACTURE OF THE SKULL

Whatever the nature of the osseous lesion, the mortality is almost entirely dependent on the question of associated injury to the intracranial contents, more especially the brain.

In the case of fractures purely or mainly basic, of the cases that have come under my care or observation, 116 recovered and 89 died—a mortality of 44 per cent.

Battle, from an examination of 168 cases, puts the mortality at the low figure of 32 per cent., whilst Crandon and Wilson, from an exhaustive series of 530 cases, estimates it at 44 per cent.

The mortality varies according to the *age* of the patient, the death-rate being at its maximum at the two extremes of life—between 50 and 60 per cent. under the age of 5 years and over 60 per cent. after the age of 70.

The mortality varies also according to the *fossa* implicated. Thus, to each fossa there are certain peculiar dangers—to the *anterior* fossa, meningeal infection from the nose, frontal and ethmoidal sinuses; to the *middle* fossa, meningeal infection from the naso-pharynx and ear, and hæmorrhage from the middle meningeal and internal carotid arteries, and from the cavernous venous sinus; and to the *posterior* fossa, laceration of the lateral and sigmoid venous sinuses.

After such consideration of local complications, it would appear that the middle fossa of the skull presents the greatest dangers. Another factor must, however, be taken into consideration—injury to the brain—the commonest cause of death in all head injuries. The main vital centres are grouped in the region of the fourth ventricle, and Leonard Hill has proved that any increase in the intra-cranial pressure exerts its influence most rapidly and most effectually when the lesion is situated beneath the tentorium cerebelli.

One may assume, therefore, that fractures of the posterior fossa are the most dangerous, and that those involving the anterior fossa hold out the best prognosis.

In the case of pure or primary vault fractures the mortality may be estimated by reference to the following table. It is composed from 88 cases admitted into St. Bartholomew's Hospital between the years 1900 and 1906.

Age	Lived	Died	Mortality
Under the age of 5 . . .	8 lived and	2 died.	Mortality, 20 per cent.
,, ,, 10 . . .	2 ,,	,, 3 ,,	,, 60 ,,
,, ,, 15 . . .	6 ,,	,, 0 ,,	,, 0 ,,
,, ,, 20 . . .	10 ,,	,, 3 ,,	,, 23 ,,
,, ,, 30 . . .	9 ,,	,, 1 ,,	,, 10 ,,
,, ,, 40 . . .	16 ,,	,, 9 ,,	,, 36 ,,
,, ,, 50 . . .	3 ,,	,, 7 ,,	,, 70 ,,
,, ,, 60 . . .	2 ,,	,, 1 ,,	,, 33 ,,
Over the age of 60 . . .	3 ,,	,, 3 ,,	,, 50 ,,
	59 lived and	29 died.	Mortality, 37 per cent.

For the remote effects of skull fractures, see Chapter VI.

CHAPTER V

INTRACRANIAL INJURIES : EXTRA- AND SUB-DURAL HÆMORRHAGES. INJURY TO THE BRAIN

HÆMORRHAGES

I. Extra-dural hæmorrhage.

EXTRA-DURAL hæmorrhage may be arterial or venous in origin. In the former case the blood is derived almost exclusively from the middle meningeal artery. When of venous origin the source is usually to be found in a laceration of one of the sinuses of the brain. When blood is poured out from a torn sinus it tends to occupy, and be widely diffused in, the subdural space. A venous extra-dural extravasation is relatively of infrequent occurrence, and the pressure exercised on the brain seldom suffices to permit of the development of local or general symptoms of cerebral compression. On these grounds extra-dural hæmorrhage may be regarded as almost necessarily of arterial origin, and as derived from a torn middle meningeal artery.

Middle meningeal hæmorrhage.

General considerations. The middle meningeal artery enters the middle fossa of the skull through the foramen spinosum, and divides, after a short intracranial course, into two main terminal divisions, anterior and posterior. The *anterior* branch passes forwards towards the anterior inferior angle of the parietal bone, then changing direction and turning upwards and backwards towards the vertex of the skull. The *posterior* branch passes horizontally backwards—grooving the squamous portion of the temporal bone—towards the posterior inferior angle of the parietal bone.

Throughout their intracranial course the main trunk and its terminal branches are embedded in the outer wall of the dura mater, except in the spheno-parietal region, where the anterior branch of the artery usually occupies a channel in the bone—one between ½ and 1 inch in extent.

The anterior branch overlies the pre-Rolandic motor area, whilst the posterior division is related to the temporo-sphenoidal and lower parietal regions—' silent ' areas of the brain.

Middle meningeal hæmorrhage occurs most commonly in connexion with a fissured or comminuted fracture of the temporal region—the result of direct violence. A fracture, however, is not necessarily present, the hæmorrhage may take place on the side opposite to that at which the injury was received (laceration by contrecoup), and both vessels may be involved. Crisp English narrates three cases in which bilateral extravasation resulted. These more rare examples of middle meningeal hæmorrhage are more or less confined to patients suffering from marked arterial degeneration.

Middle meningeal hæmorrhage, uncomplicated by brain injury, is of infrequent occurrence, the associated injuries to bone and brain confusing the diagnosis. Moreover, the special pressure effects are dependent not only on the absence of serious brain lesion, but also on the non-existence of a safety-valve, such, for instance, as is afforded by a comminuted fracture of the bones entering into the formation of the temporal fossa, or of the roof of the middle and external ears. In the former case, blood will force its way into the temporal region, there forming a temporal hæmatoma—one that may pulsate—whilst, in the latter case, the blood escapes freely from the external auditory meatus. It should be noted, however, that pressure applied to the temporal hæmatoma may lead to the development of irritative or paralytic symptoms confined to the muscles of the opposite side of the body, whilst the restriction of aural bleeding, by means of plugs inserted into the ear, will lead to the early development of compression symptoms.

The amount of blood extravasated varies—according to the calibre of the vessel involved—from a drachm to several ounces. The largest coagulum that has come under my observation was 4½ inches in the long diameter and 1 inch in thickness. Krönlein narrates a case in which the clot weighed 9 ounces.

In shape the clot is elliptical; in consistency it is either fluid or jelly-like. During the early stages of its formation it can be readily

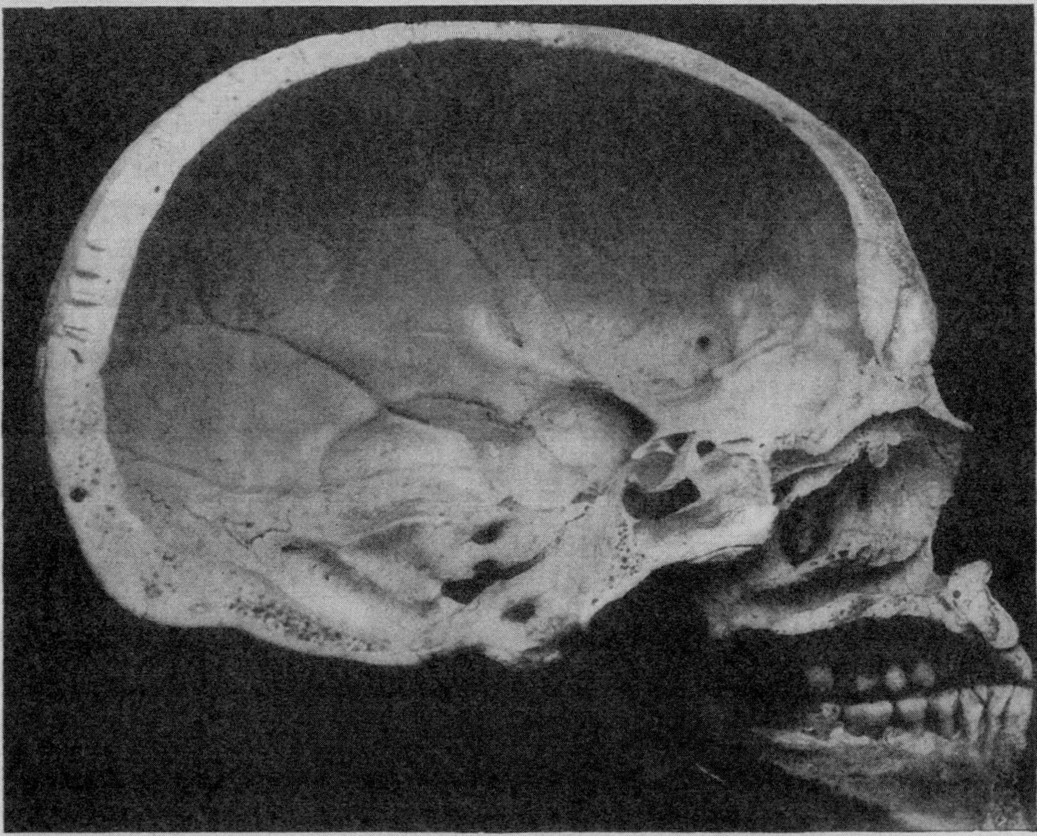

FIG. 50 A. THE INNER ASPECT OF THE SKULL.

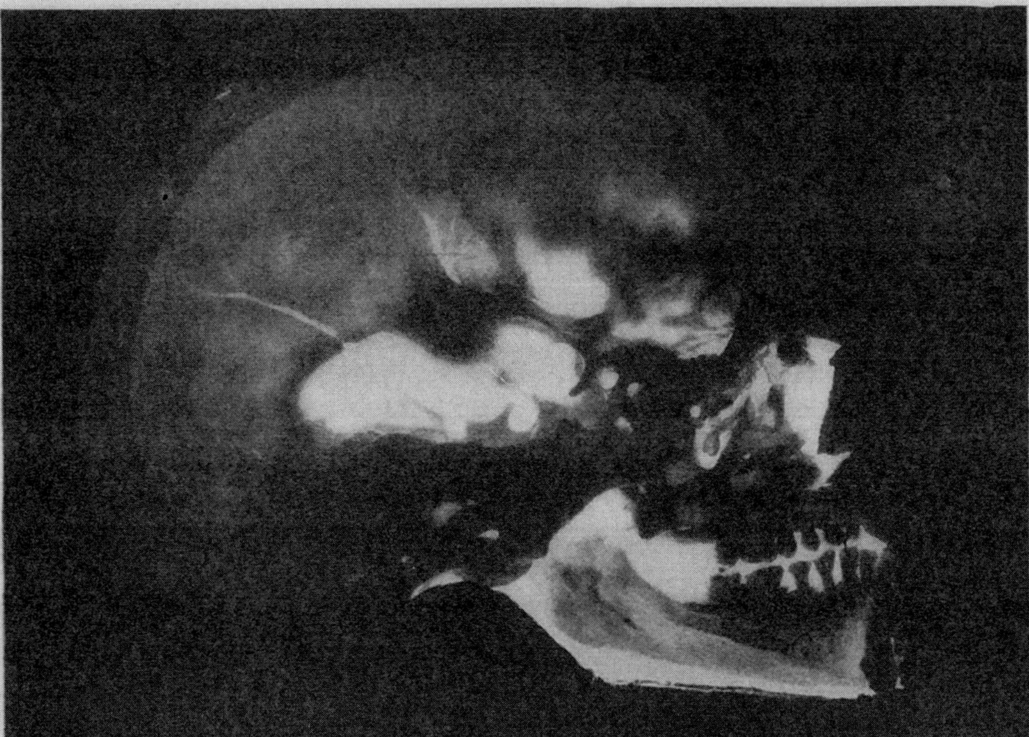

FIG. 50 B. THE INNER ASPECT OF THE SKULL SEEN ON TRANSILLUMINATION.

removed. Later on, it adheres to the dura mater, and, when removed, leaves that membrane rough and discoloured.

Some uncertainty exists as to the relative frequency with which the trunk and the two terminal branches are exposed to injury. There can be no doubt that the majority of cases in which typical clinical symptoms are present are such as evidence injury to the anterior terminal division ; this is due to the anatomical relation of the clot to the motor cortex. Injury to the main trunk is of the rarest occurrence, for the foramen spinosum lies immediately anterior to the petro-sphenoidal suture, the course pursued by typical middle fossa fractures. I have seen one case only, and have read the accounts of two others, in which the foramen spinosum was directly implicated.

The attachment of the dura mater to the sides and base of the skull exercises a most important influence on the direction in which the blood spreads. Firmly adherent to the lesser wing of the sphenoid in front and to the summit of the petrous bone behind, the membrane intervening between these two regions is but loosely attached to, and readily stripped away from, the floor of the middle fossa. As the clot increases in size it exerts considerable mechanical pressure and tends to separate still further the dura from the bone. The anterior and posterior limitations compel the blood to extend first in the outward direction and then upwards towards the vertex of the skull.

Krönlein divides middle meningeal extravasations, according to their regional distribution, into three main groups :—

Temporo-parietal (the most common variety).

Parieto-occipital (rare).

Parieto-frontal (very rare).

Middle meningeal hæmorrhages yielding typical clinical symptoms are of infrequent occurrence, yet such extravasations are very commonly present in severe lesions of the skull. This is evidenced by the fact that middle meningeal hæmorrhage—of a greater or lesser degree—was found in 20 per cent. of all cases of fractured skull, and in 45 per cent. of those in which the middle fossa was involved. My experience is confirmed by Dwight and Nichols. For example, Dwight, in 149 autopsies, notes that middle meningeal hæmorrhage was existent in 49 cases (29 per cent.). He maintains further that the artery is injured in nearly every case in which the fracture, extending from vault to base or vice versa, involves the middle fossa of the skull. Nichols reports 11 cases in 32 autopsies (34 per cent.).

Symptomatology. As the direct result of the blow the patient is 'concussed', remaining in that condition for a variable period of time, a matter of seconds, minutes, or hours, according to the nature of the associated damage to the bone and brain. In the most typical cases, the patient, on regaining consciousness, should recover—again for a variable period of time—complete control over mind and body, returning to work, walking home or visiting hospital or doctor. More usually, however, he remains slightly dazed, though recognizing his surroundings and capable of answering questions. In any case—unless the hæmorrhage is accompanied by grave cerebral lesion—there should be some attempt at recovery, some return to consciousness. The importance of this 'lucid interval' cannot be over-estimated. It should be noted, however, that this interval of consciousness is not of itself absolutely diagnostic of middle meningeal hæmorrhage—it ought to be associated with definite localizing symptoms of brain compression (see below). I have encountered several cases in which this lucid interval was present, and in which operative procedures were carried out in the anticipation of finding an extra-dural extravasation, only to find a subdural hæmorrhage. Such subdural hæmorrhages are not infrequently associated with a similar return to the conscious state, but are rarely—if ever—accompanied by the early development of symptoms of localized brain compression. In the event of doubt as to whether the surgeon has to deal with an extra or subdural extravasation lumbar puncture will probably clear up the diagnosis.

The duration of this 'lucid' interval is exceedingly variable. It is usually a matter of minutes or hours, though both König and Wiesman narrate cases in which eight days elapsed before the onset of definite localized compression symptoms. I also have recollections of a case in which the patient walked some miles across the moor to see his doctor, and finding him away from home, walked home again, then becoming unconscious and dying shortly afterwards.

All depends on the calibre of the vessel injured and on the existence of a safety-valve, by means of which some of the extravasated blood can escape externally (see p. 97).

No rule can be laid down as to the duration of this 'lucid' interval, but all authorities are agreed as to its existence, even though it may be of exceeding short duration. Its importance, from a clinical point of view, cannot be overestimated. It was present in 43 out of 63 cases reported by Jacobson, well marked in 32 (50 per cent.), less marked in 11 (18 per cent.). It was observed in 60 per cent. of cases that came under my care.

During this period the blood is occupied in stripping away the dura from the bone—the larger the vessel the easier the task and the shorter the 'lucid' interval.

The further progress of the case may be considered according to the *general and local effects* of the hæmorrhage.

General effects. As soon as the clot beomes of sufficient size as to exert general pressure on the brain, symptoms of compression become evident, the patient first entering on the stage of 'slow cerebration'. He is dull and apathetic, showing marked delay in responding to questions. As the pressure increases, he gradually passes into a state of unconsciousness.

The pulse becomes full and slow, the blood-pressure rises progressively (to 200 or more mms. of Hg.), respiration is laboured and stertorous, and the temperature raised (rising progressively). The skin is hot, the face turgid and cyanosed. If the pressure is unrelieved, stimulation of the medullary centres gives place to exhaustion, the pulse becoming irregular and rapid, blood-pressure falls rapidly, and respiration is of irregular rhythm and finally Cheyne-Stokes in character. Finally, the patient becomes completely comatose, the pupils are widely dilated, and the cornea insensitive. Both urine and fæces may be passed (through paralysis of the sphincters), the extremities exhibit flaccid paralysis and the reflexes are abolished. Death occurs primarily through paralysis of the respiratory centre.

Local effects. In many cases considerable help to diagnosis may be obtained by external examination—bruising and ecchymosis, or definite hæmatomata, in the temporal or parietal regions. In some cases the hæmatoma may pulsate, and in others the application of pressure to the hæmatoma will lead to the development of fits involving the face and extremities on the contra-lateral side. Copious hæmorrhage from the ear should always arouse suspicion as to the probability of an extra-dural hæmorrhage (see p. 97).

The *anterior* branch of the artery, as it passes upwards towards the vertex, overlies the pre-Rolandic or motor area. The pressure exercised on that region of the brain leads—according to the site

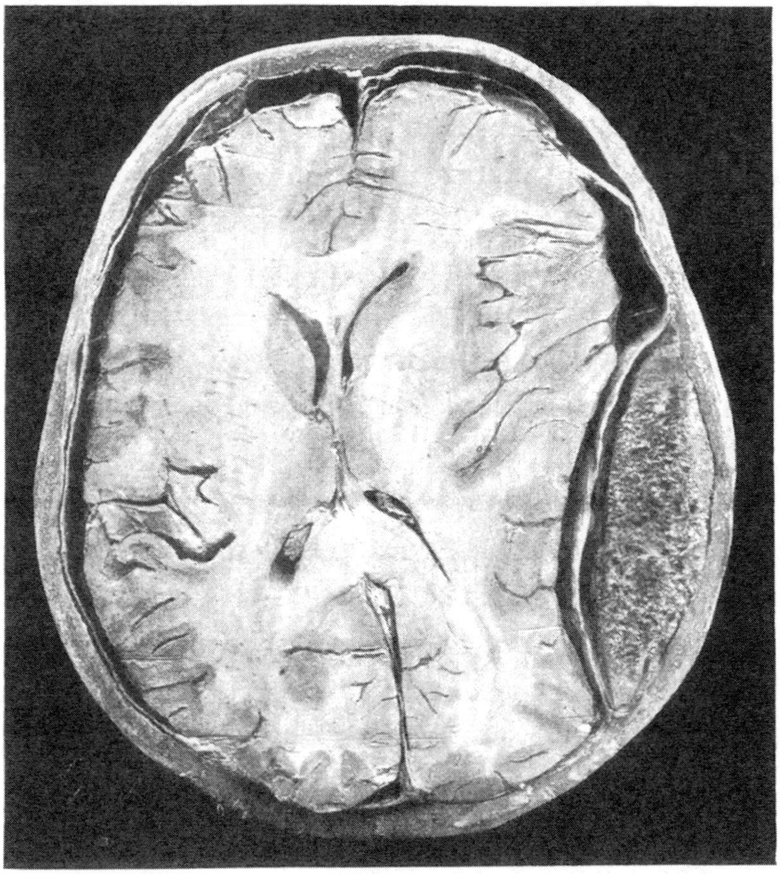

FIG. 51. TO ILLUSTRATE COMPRESSION OF THE BRAIN. As produced by an extra-dural hæmorrhage from the posterior branch of the middle meningeal artery.

of extravasation and the degree of pressure exercised—to the development of twitchings, convulsions, spasticity, or paralysis of the muscles of the face, upper and lower extremities on the contra-lateral side of the body.

The late Professor von Bergmann[1] pointed out that the arm area is most commonly affected, and that the leg area is never alone implicated. Wiesmann[2] states 'that isolated paralysis of the leg area

[1] *Syst. of Pract. Surg.*, vol. ii.

[2] *Deutsche Zeit. für Chir.*, Bd. 4, vols. i and iii.

is never seen, but only paresis when the arm is paralysed, or both may be similarly affected at once; convulsions may precede the affection'.

In discussing the frequency of local compression effects, Wiesmann points out that some abnormal condition of the opposite extremities was only absent in 16 out of a total of 257 cases. In 37 cases reported by Jacobson,[1] hemiplegia, of a greater or lesser extent, was present in 19 (50 per cent.). The same authority explains that 'with regard to the onset of convulsions, if there be restlessness, spasmodic twitchings, or movements of the limbs, it is only too probable that in addition to middle meningeal hæmorrhage, contusion or laceration of the brain-substance will be found at more places than one'.

In cases that have come under my observation twitchings of the muscles of the face and upper extremities were observed in 37 per cent. of cases, and paralysis in the same number. Some alteration in the condition of the muscles on the contra-lateral side was present therefore in 74 per cent. of cases.

If the hæmorrhage be situated on the left side of the brain, both motor and sensory cortical speech areas may be involved, especially the former.

With respect to *reflexes*, it has previously been stated that the reflexes are abolished. This is true with respect to the later stages of fully-developed compression. In the earlier state the reflexes on the contra-lateral side may be increased, the difference between the two sides affording some help in the differential diagnosis.

Pupillary changes are variable. According to Jonathan Hutchinson, the pupil on the affected side becomes dilated, the blood extending inwards towards the cavernous sinus and exercising direct compression of the third nerve. The frequency with which a dilated pupil occurs in cases of middle meningeal hæmorrhage, and the causation thereof, are, however, matters of dispute. Phelps writes as follows: 'Reference to cases cited show that the so-called Hutchinson pupil may be observed as well in hæmorrhages occurring in other situations than the middle fossa, and in some cases of cerebral lesion without injury at all. There is no reason to doubt that it is the result of cerebral contusion, but in what relation they stand to specific cerebral injuries is undetermined.'

[1] *Guy's Hosp. Reports*, 1885–6.

Walton states that ‘ doubtless various factors play an important part in producing the dilated pupil, but if disorders of any simple mechanism are to be credited with the production of the Hutchinson pupil or other pupillary changes, the only lesion worthy of the place is disturbance, irritative or paralytic, of the intracranial fibres of the cilio-spinal tract ’.

The late Professor von Bergmann, from 70 cases, reports as follows :—

In 39 cases both pupils were markedly dilated (56 per cent.).
In 7 cases both pupils were markedly contracted (10 per cent.).
In 20 cases the pupil on the same side was dilated (30 per cent.).
In 4 cases the pupil on the opposite side was dilated (6 per cent.).

Parsons, in answering some queries in 1903, writes :—

‘ I should anticipate from cortical irritation bilateral pupillary dilatation, perhaps more marked on the opposite side : from pressure the opposite effects, so far as mere cortical paralysis goes, but this would be more liable to be vitiated by vascular changes—the complex condition seen in coma. It is very difficult to elicit pupillary constriction by cortical stimuli—very easy to elicit dilatation, but always bilateral though often more marked on the opposite side.’

In cases examined by me the following conditions were found :—

Pupils equal	46 per cent. of cases
Pupils constricted on the affected side . .	36 per cent. of cases
Pupils dilated on the affected side . .	18 per cent. of cases

From my experience, therefore, and from that of the authorities quoted above, it would appear that alterations in the size of the pupil are of very doubtful significance in the diagnosis of middle meningeal hæmorrhage, and that the ‘ Hutchinson pupil ’ is but rarely observed.

The results obtained by ophthalmoscopic examination are of much greater value. Such investigations should be carried out as a routine procedure. In the earlier stages of the hæmorrhage some œdema of the disk, together with dilatation of retinal veins and diminution in the calibre of the arteries, will be observed on the affected side. This affords a most valuable aid in the differential diagnosis as to the side on which the hæmorrhage is situated—not always such a simple matter as appears at first sight.

Treatment. Operation is indicated in all cases of middle meningeal hæmorrhage if the condition of the patient be compatible with such treatment. The earlier the operation is carried out the better.

Operation. *For Hæmorrhage from the anterior branch.* After the usual preparatory treatment, the 'site of election' for trephining

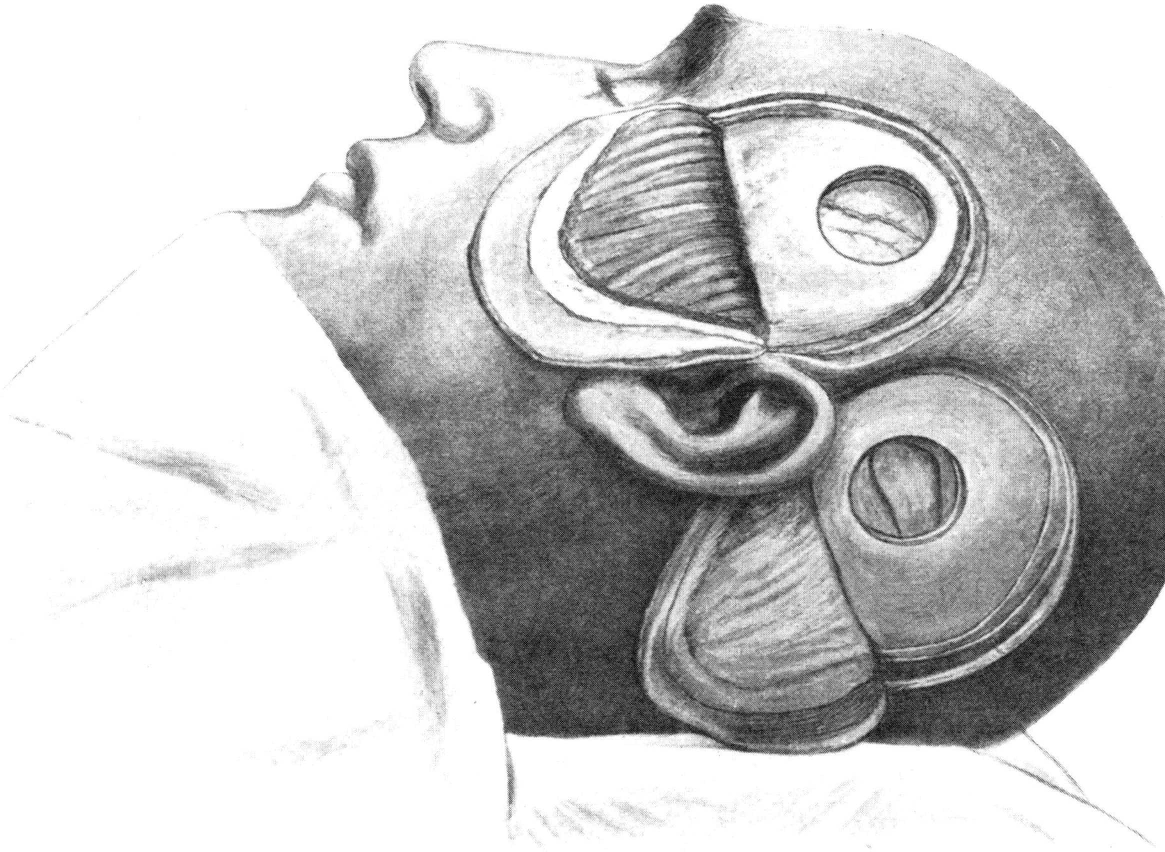

FIG. 52 A. EXPOSURE OF THE BRANCHES OF THE MIDDLE MENINGEAL ARTERY. *First stage.* Suitable scalp-flaps have been turned down, and the skull has been trephined over the 'sites of election' for exposure of both anterior and posterior branches.

is marked out on the scalp by taking a point which lies 2 inches posterior to the external angular frontal process, and the same distance above the zygoma. A bradawl may be introduced so as to indent the external table of the skull, thus aiding the subsequent accurate application of the trephine.

The incision commences immediately posterior to the external angular frontal process, curves upwards and backwards along the temporal crest, and terminates in front of the tragus of the ear.

The flap, comprising skin, temporal fascia and muscle, and pericranium, is turned to its zygomatic base and all bleeding-points secured.

The subsequent procedures vary according to the condition of the bone :—

If there be no fracture of the bone, the pin of the trephine is applied to the indented spot and the disk of bone removed. After the removal

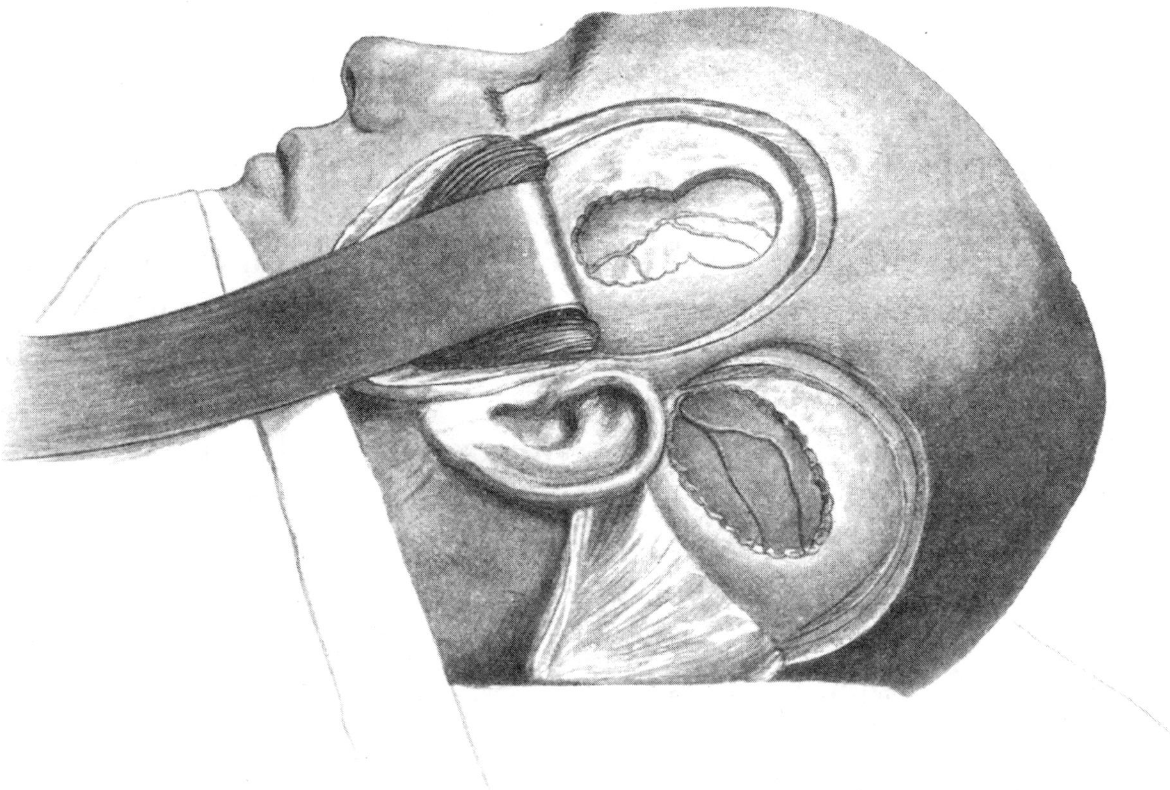

FIG. 52 B. EXPOSURE OF THE BRANCHES OF THE MIDDLE MENINGEAL ARTERY. *Second stage.* The trephine-holes have been enlarged with the craniectomy forceps in the required directions.

of the disk the clot will be exposed; but, in order to obtain full exposure, the gap must be enlarged with the craniectomy forceps, mainly in the upward and downward directions.

If a fissured fracture be found, the trephine is applied in close relation to the intersection of the line of the artery and the line of the fracture, the gap being enlarged in the required direction.

When the fracture is comminuted, the fragments of bone are either elevated or removed until sufficient room has been obtained.

The greater part of the clot can be removed with a Volkmann spoon, or with an ordinary teaspoon, and the region flushed out with hot saline solution.

To secure the bleeding-points. When the artery is injured beyond the limits of the gap, the bone must be nibbled away till the bleeding-point is exposed. In some cases it may be necessary to remove a considerable portion of the bone entering into the formation of the temporal fossa. In the meantime, hæmorrhage may be controlled by plugging towards the base of the skull with strips of gauze. Sufficient room having been obtained, the gauze is withdrawn, when smart sponging should enable the operator to determine the source of the hæmorrhage. At this stage of the operation, a head-lamp is useful. After the exposure of the bleeding-points, the following measures can be adopted whereby to arrest the bleeding :—

(*a*) The application of a ligature or of silver 'clips' (see Fig. VI) on either side of the bleeding-point.

(*b*) The vessel may be underrun on either side of the bleeding-point.

(*c*) The vessel may be seized with artery forceps and twisted.

(*d*) The hæmorrhage may be arrested by means of gauze plugs.

(*e*) The foramen spinosum may be occluded with bone or wooden pegs.

(*f*) The common or external carotid arteries may be ligatured.

Every effort should be made to control the hæmorrhage by means of ligature, silver clip, underrunning, or torsion. Gauze plugs may usually be relied on to stop the bleeding, but they possess the great disadvantage of exercising pressure on the cortex and preventing expansion of the brain.

Occlusion of the foramen spinosum and ligature of the carotid arteries complicate and prolong the operation. The foramen spinosum is occluded in the following manner: the dura mater is quickly stripped up with the fingers away from the base of the skull, the soft parts gently but firmly retracted and the foramen identified. Its occlusion may be effected by means of a sterilized wooden match or bone peg, by a small piece of bone derived from those osseous fragments which have been removed during the operation, or with the aid of a piece of catgut; in each case the occluding medium should be well driven into the foramen.

It is open to doubt whether ligature of the carotid arteries is ever necessary, though several cases have been recorded in which such a procedure was carried out. The external carotid should be tied in preference to the common vessel, further interference with the blood-supply of the brain increasing necessarily the risk of cerebral œdema, &c.

The hæmorrhage having been arrested by one or other of these methods, the cavity is thoroughly washed out with hot saline solution and drained, a small rubber drainage-tube being brought out through the scalp-flap. The tube should be removed after twenty-four to thirty-six hours, according to the circumstances of the case.

For hæmorrhage from the posterior branch. The 'site of election' for exposure of the posterior branch lies at the intersection of the two following lines:—

A line drawn backwards from the upper border of the orbit parallel to Reid's base-line.

A line drawn vertically upwards from the posterior border of the mastoid process.

The trephine is applied, the disk removed, and the gap enlarged with the craniectomy forceps in the forward and backward directions. The hæmatoma is evacuated and the bleeding arrested after the methods enumerated above.

Results. The ultimate result of operation for middle meningeal hæmorrhage depends on two factors—the time at which operation is carried out, and the question of brain lesion. There is every reason to believe that, when treated early and when uncomplicated by brain injury, the prognosis, both immediate and remote, is wholly satisfactory.

Wiesman[1] collected 257 cases, of which 110 were submitted to operation, with a mortality of 27 per cent. Of the cases in which no operation was performed 88 per cent. died.

Duchaine[2] reports 27 cases in which operation was carried out, with death in 6 cases only, a mortality of 22 per cent.

[1] Bergmann's *System of Surgery*, vol. i.

[2] *Ruptures de l'Artère méningée moyenne.*

Von Bergmann collected 110 cases treated by operation, with 74 recoveries and 36 deaths, a mortality of 32·27 per cent.

Blake only lost 3 cases out of a total of 42 submitted to operation.

Even when every allowance is made for the fact that operative measures were adopted in the more hopeful cases, the above statistics show conclusively that early operation affords great hope of cure.

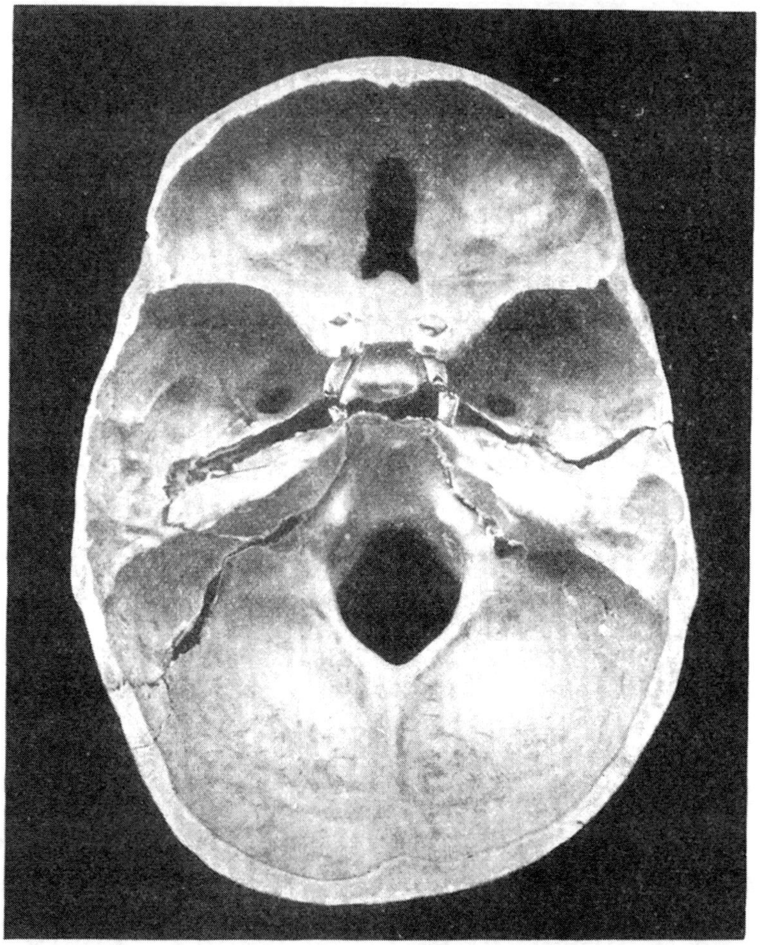

FIG. 53. A BASIC FRACTURE WITH LACERATION OF BOTH CAROTID ARTERIES.

Before passing on to **subdural hæmorrhage,** it will be convenient to discuss briefly the question of injury to the **internal carotid artery.**

This vessel, during its forward passage in the outer wall of the cavernous sinus, from the posterior to the anterior clinoid processes, crosses the line of the typical middle fossa fracture (see p. 84). The artery is loosely embedded in the sinus, it is protected by the third, fourth, ophthalmic division of the fifth and sixth nerves, and it is situated some distance above the level of the base of the skull. In spite of this degree of protection from injury, the artery may be lacerated in this part of its intracranial passage. The basic fracture is necessarily of a very severe nature. Two cases have come under my own care: one in which both arteries were torn across, the fracture passing from one middle fossa to the other, with such wide separation

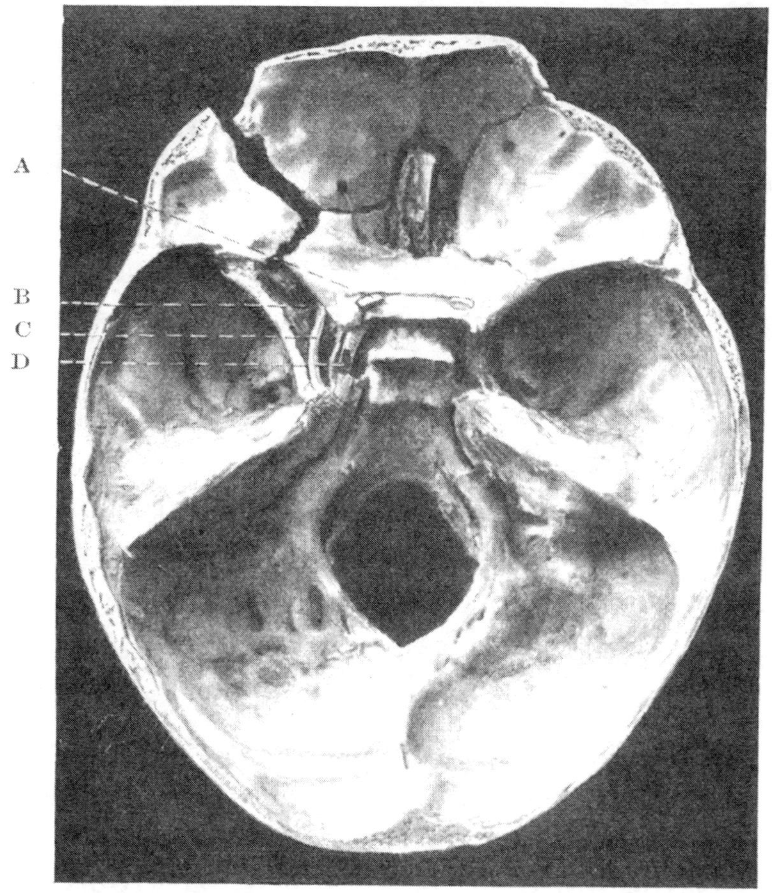

FIG. 54. A BASIC FRACTURE WITH LACERATION OF THE CAVERNOUS SINUS. A, The optic nerve; B, The cavernous sinus; C, The third nerve; D, The internal carotid artery.

of the anterior and posterior segments of the skull that the two were freely movable on one another (Fig. 53), whilst in the second case, the fracture, originating in the left frontal region, passed backwards across the anterior fossa, comminuting the base in the region of the cavernous sinus, lacerating that sinus and tearing the artery (Fig. 54).

In both cases death was almost instantaneous, blood pouring from the nose and mouth.

In some few cases the vascular lesion is confined to a minute tear in the coats of the vessel, a fistulous communication being formed between the artery and the cavernous sinus—arterio-venous aneurysm. This condition is discussed on p. 204.

II. Subdural hæmorrhage.

Hæmorrhage into the subdural space may be (*a*) diffuse, or (*b*) localized.

(*A*) **Diffuse subdural hæmorrhage.** The blood may be derived from one of the great sinuses of the brain or from superficial cerebral vessels (laceration of the brain).

The *superior longitudinal sinus* may be torn by the in-driving of fragments of bone in a comminuted depressed fracture of the vertex, or by wide separation along the line of the sagittal suture. Blood is diffused throughout the subdural space, on one or on both sides of the falx cerebri, but always tending to gravitate towards the lower limits of the supra-tentorial space.

In the event of the wound being compound, air may enter into the sinus. Insomuch, however, as the sinus pressure is, under normal conditions, positive, this complication is of rare occurrence, unless the patient is in a state of profound shock, from loss of blood, or suffers from urgent dyspnœa.

Allusion should also be made to the condition described by Stromeyer, as ‘ sinus pericranii ’, where a subpericranial hæmatoma communicates with a venous sinus. Such hæmatomata may pulsate, are more or less reducible on pressure, and are increased on straining or on the application of pressure to the internal jugular vein.

The *lateral sinus* may be laid open in any part of its course, more especially at the angle of junction between the lateral and sigmoid sinuses, in close relation to the occipito-mastoid suture, a region not infrequently involved in basic fractures. The blood effused will occupy the supra- or infra-tentorial spaces according to the situation of the rent in the sinus-wall.

The *cavernous sinus* is frequently involved in anterior and middle fossa fractures. The blood effused usually escapes into the nose and mouth.

Symptoms. The rapid diffusion of blood throughout the subdural space, and the usual coexistence of extensive injury to bone and brain, seldom permit of the development of such definite symptoms as might accurately define the localization of the hæmorrhage.

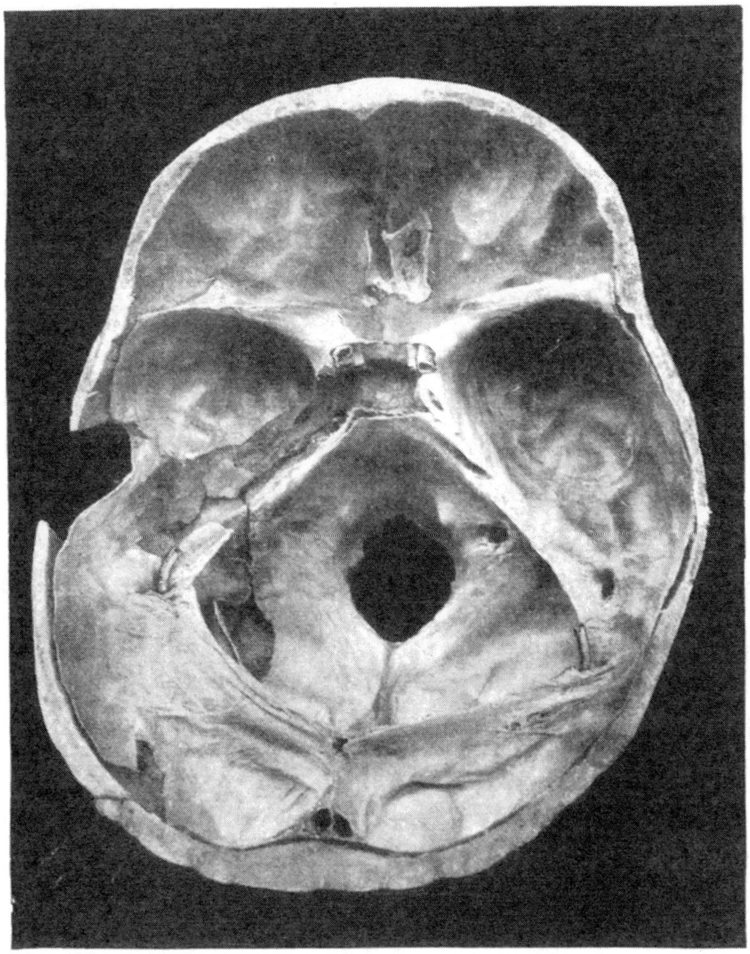

Fig. 55. A Comminuted Fracture of Vault and Base, the Basic Fracture Involving both Middle and Posterior Fossæ. The middle fossa fracture, on the left side, follows the usual course. The posterior fossa fracture resulted in laceration of both lateral sinuses—at the usual site, junction of sigmoid and lateral sinuses. Probes are inserted at each site of laceration. The resultant hæmorrhage was mainly intradural, but, as is seen in the figure, the dura mater of the posterior fossa is stripped away from the bone by an extra-dural extravasation.

The most important feature in the diagnosis lies in the fact that compression symptoms are early in onset and progressive in nature. The 'lucid' interval, so prominent a feature in middle meningeal extravasations, is either absent or of such short duration as to be difficult of recognition. The rapid development of symptoms pointing to brain compression, and the nature of the injury itself should enable the surgeon, in the majority of cases, to come to the conclusion that the patient is suffering from diffuse subdural hæmorrhage. In all cases of doubt, lumbar puncture should be carried out, the presence of blood-corpuscles in the cerebro-spinal fluid confirming the diagnosis.

Indications for operation. Whether one considers the case from the point of view of the more immediate prognosis or from the more remote aspect of the case, operation is indicated, if the condition of the patient is compatible with such treatment. In considering the advisability of adopting an active form of treatment, it must be taken into account that, if the patient recovers without operation, the presence of an extensive subdural blood-clot must necessarily interfere, as an after-result, with the functions of the cortex, and that the removal thereof affords considerable hope of permanent cure.

Operation. Operative measures may be considered as follows:—

The treatment of the fracture and of the dural rent.

The treatment of the subdural extravasation.

The treatment of the fracture and of the dural rent. A scalp-flap is framed, suited to the occasion and formed with due regard to existent scalp laceration. The fracture being fully exposed, depressed or comminuted fragments of bone are elevated or removed. Complete exposure of the sinus-wall, both in front and behind the site of laceration, is required, and for this purpose the craniectomy forceps may be called into requisition. In the event of copious bleeding during these procedures, strips of gauze should be inserted on either side of the sinus rent between the dura and the bone, thus compressing the sinus and stopping the bleeding.

The sinus rent may be treated after one or other of the following methods :—

1. It may be sewn up with mattress sutures of fine catgut, by which means it may be possible to stop the hæmorrhage without interfering with the sinus blood-stream.

2. The open mouth of the sinus may be puckered up by means of a purse-string suture.

3. The needle may be passed right round the sinus on either side of the rent, piercing the falx cerebri in the case of the superior

longitudinal sinus and the tentorium cerebelli in wounds of the lateral sinus. The two ligatures are then tightened up and the bleeding controlled.

4. The gauze plugs (see above) may be allowed to remain for twenty-four hours or more, and then carefully withdrawn.

The treatment of the subdural hæmorrhage. Though the complete evacuation of the clot is seldom practicable, much may be done to remedy the condition. The tenseness of the dura mater, the absence of pulsation, and the peculiar plum-colour imparted to that membrane by the presence of underlying blood-clot point to the nature of the trouble.

The dura mater is incised and the presenting clot removed, as far as circumstances permit, with the aid of a spoon and irrigation (hot saline solution at a temperature between 110° and 115° Fahrenheit). Free drainage must be supplied, and it is necessary, therefore, that a counter incision should be made at the most dependent part of the clot. A suitable region may present itself if the bone be extensively comminuted. Under other circumstances, a narrow channel may be cut in the bone, prolonged in the downward direction, till the lower limits of the clot have been reached (see Fig. 56).

A rubber drainage-tube may be inserted in the manner depicted in the same figure. Except at the point of emergence of the tube, the dura mater is sewn up (with fine interrupted catgut sutures).

(*B*) **Localized subdural hæmorrhage (subdural hæmatocele).** We are greatly indebted to Bowen [1] for our knowledge of subdural hæmatomata. That subdural hæmorrhage might take the form of a localized collection was a recognized fact, but the condition was but little understood, the typical clinical symptoms were not recognized, and surgeons hesitated to adopt surgical remedies. All these facts impeded advance in both diagnosis and treatment. Subdural hæmatoceles, even at this date, are often regarded as rarities, but, in the light of present knowledge, it would appear that wider recognition of the hæmorrhage in its clinical aspect will show that such ideas are erroneous.

In the preceding section it was shown that subdural extravasation resulting from sinus-injury tends to become diffused throughout the

[1] *Guy's Hospital Reports*, vol. lix.

subdural space. With respect to localized hæmorrhages our data are by no means complete, but all available evidence tends to show that subdural hæmatoceles are dependent on laceration of the pia-arachnoid vessels—a condition practically synonymous with superficial laceration and contusion of the cortex. The blood, derived from small cerebral veins and minute cerebral arteries, exercises primarily but slight pressure effect. Its force is expended on compressing and emptying the subjacent and surrounding cerebral vessels, producing, in other words, a condition of *local cerebral anœmia.* This pressure is insufficient to lead to the development of general compression, but suffices to produce certain rather indefinite symptoms. We have, therefore, before us a very different picture to that depicted in cases of middle meningeal hæmorrhage. In such extradural hæmorrhages some definite period of time must elapse before the dura mater is sufficiently stripped from the bone to allow of the formation of a clot of size sufficing to exercise both local and general compression effects. Pressure effects then become very manifest.

On the other hand, in localized subdural extravasations there is an immediate effect, for the brain is contused or lacerated. On recovering from the immediate effects of the injury—concussion of a greater or lesser degree of intensity—the patient does not regain complete mental and bodily convalescence. He suffers from symptoms suggestive of brain irritation—headaches, photophobia, mental irritability, insomnia, loss of appetite, the pulse accelerated, and the temperature slightly raised. Later on, more definite symptoms arise, but, intervening between the day of the accident and the time at which these more definite localizing symptoms develop, there is an unmistakable *latent* period—a period to be sharply differentiated from the previously mentioned *lucid* interval (see p. 139).

This 'latent' period lasts for a variable period of time—seldom less than a week or more than three months. At the end of that time the picture changes, and the patient evidences symptoms obviously referable to local brain compression. From a clinical point of view it is fortunate that subdural hæmatoceles tend to involve the fronto-parietal region with the consequent development of motor symptoms, especially paresis or paralysis of the contra-lateral side. Hence the name sometimes applied to the condition—traumatic late apoplexy.

The speech areas are implicated if the injury be situated on the left side. Paralysis limited to the lower extremity is exceedingly suggestive, such a palsy occurring only with the greatest rarity in extradural hæmorrhages (from the middle meningeal artery).

If the pressure be unrelieved by operation the patient passes from the excitatory to the paralytic stage of brain compression, gradually falling into a condition of coma, the pulse increasing in frequency and the respiration becoming more and more embarrassed.

In the study of this condition, the following are the points to which special attention should be paid :—

1. The comparative want of severity with respect to the injury received.

2. The absence of any 'lucid' interval, such as is present, for example, in middle meningeal hæmorrhage.

3. The presence of a definite 'latent' period.

4. The late development of symptoms pointing to general and local brain compression.

Finally, it may be stated in general that the more indefinite and the more deferred the pressure symptoms, the greater the probability that we have to deal with a localized subdural hæmorrhage. Lumbar puncture may materially aid in the differential diagnosis between extra-dural and subdural hæmorrhages.

The following case affords a typical example of subdural hæmatocele :—

An elderly man fell down, striking the right side of the head against the pavement. He lost his senses for a few minutes and was then brought to the hospital, dazed and complaining of headache (note the absence of any *lucid* interval). He was sent home in a cab and was assisted to bed by his wife. He kept to his bed during the next week, complaining of constant headache, and was exceedingly irritable (this is the 'latent' period). Towards the end of the third week his wife noticed that he seldom used the left upper and lower extremities. This paresis increased steadily, the face was drawn to the right side, and his condition became so serious that the wife brought him again to the hospital (this is the 'manifest' period).

When seen by me he was only partly conscious, the mental condition varying, however, during the day. He was exceedingly irritable, muttering to himself in a low tone, words being more or less unintelligible. The left upper extremity was paralysed, the face drawn to the right side, and the left lower extremity was but little used. The pupils were equal, the disks normal. The tem-

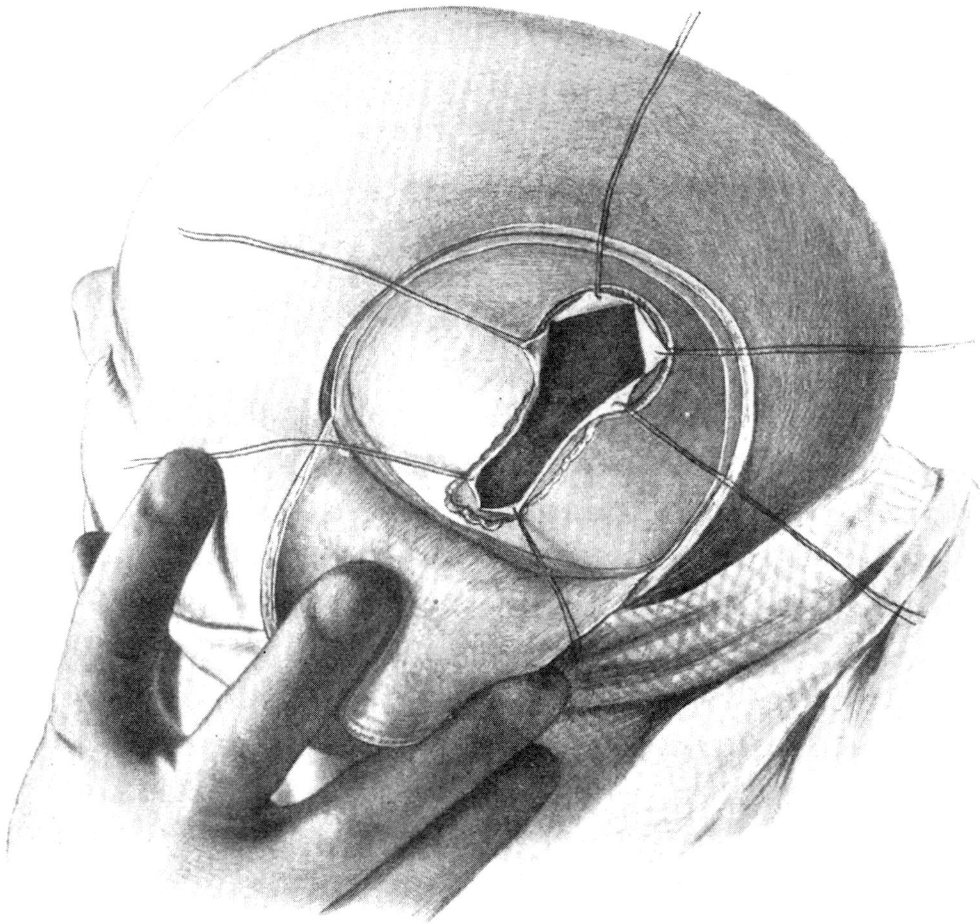

FIG. 56 A. THE OPERATIVE TREATMENT OF SUBDURAL HÆMORRHAGE. *First stage.* The skull has been trephined over the upper part of the clot and the bone cut away in the downward direction in order to reach the lower limits thereof. The dura mater has been incised, crucially in the upper part and vertically in the lower part.

perature in the left axilla was two degrees lower than on the opposite side.

The hæmatocele was exposed, cleared out, and the cavity drained. Recovery was rapid and complete. Two years later all was well.

Operation. The lesion is usually of so gross a nature that little difficulty will be experienced in determining the site for trephining. The protective gauze and scalp-tourniquet are applied as usual (see p. 14), and a bradawl introduced through the scalp so as to indent the external table and allow of the subsequent accurate application of the trephine. A scalp-flap, suited to the occasion, is

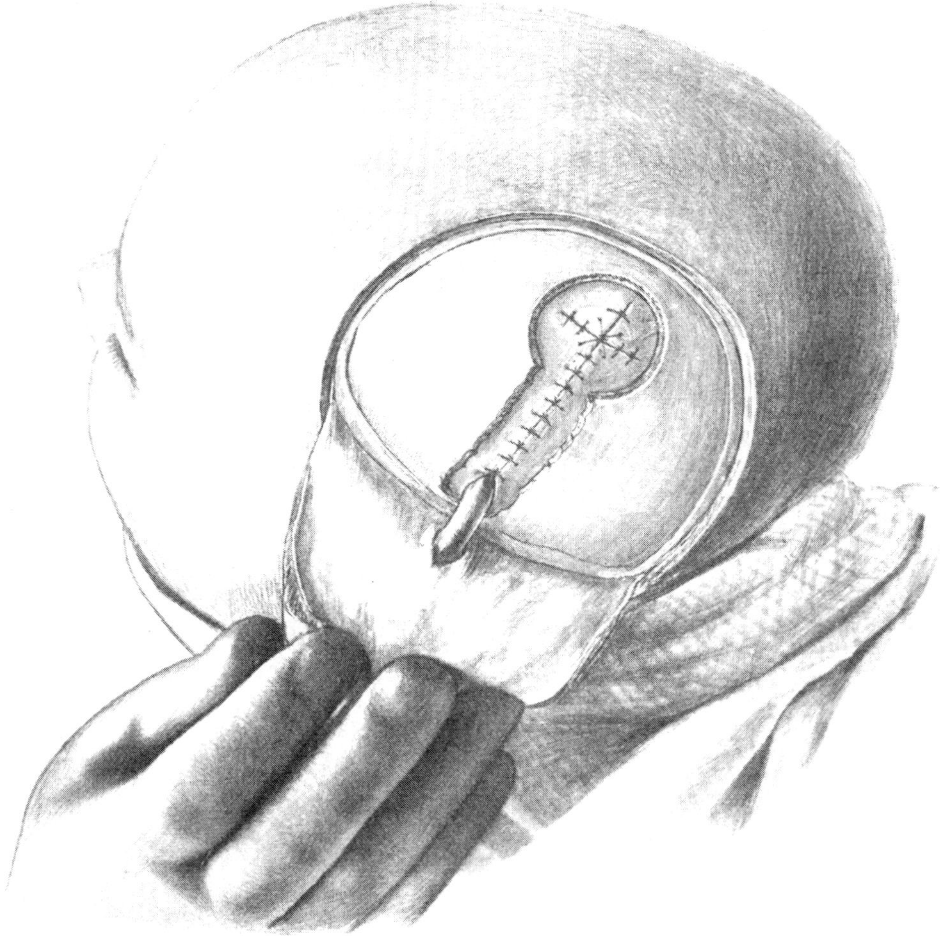

FIG. 56 B. THE OPERATIVE TREATMENT OF SUBDURAL HÆMORRHAGE. *Second stage.* The clot has been removed and the dura mater sewn up. A drainage tube has been inserted so as to drain the subdural region through the lower part of the scalp-flap.

framed, the skull trephined, and the disk of bone elevated and removed. The appearance of the dura mater now allows the operator to verify his diagnosis—the membrane is non-pulsatile, it bulges markedly outwards and presents a blue-purple colour. The bone is then nibbled away in the downward direction towards the lower limit of the clot, the scalp incision being prolonged according to requirements.

In the region of the trephine-hole the dura is incised in a crucial manner, and the four flaps held aside by catgut sutures passed through the apex of each flap. A blunt director is introduced beneath the dura, passing towards the lower limit of the clot, and the membrane slit up to within a short distance of the lower margin of the gap. All meningeal vessels that cross the line proposed for dural section must first be underrun on either side of that line. Retraction of the dura will now allow of adequate exposure of the underlying hæmatoma. Its removal can be carried out with the aid of a spoon, and by means of gentle irrigation (hot saline at a temperature between 110° and 115° Fahrenheit). It is usually impossible to remove the whole of the coagulum, but the greater portion can be got rid of in the manner described.

The dura mater is approximated above by the cross-union of the four apical sutures, whilst the downward prolongation is also sutured except at the most dependent point, where a rubber drainage-tube is inserted beneath the dura mater and brought out through the scalp-flap (see Fig. 56). This tube should be anchored to the dura mater with a single fine catgut suture.

The tube should be allowed to remain in position for at least thirty-six hours. In this the surgeon must be guided by the amount of discharge and the general progress of the case.

Results. The most complete results obtained by operative treatment are supplied by Bowen, who classifies a series of 72 cases as follows :—

Class A. Subdural hæmorrhage, apparently without other serious injury to bone or brain.

36 cases. 22 recovered after operation.
14 died—11 without and 3 after operation.

Class B. With serious brain-injury.

36 cases. 6 recovered after operation.
30 died—10 without and 20 after operation.

In other words, every case died in which no operative measures were adopted, whilst after operation 28 recovered and 23 died. My own experience is limited to 4 cases, 3 of which recovered.

Pia-arachnoid hæmorrhage. From evidence obtained at post-mortem examinations, it may be concluded that the great majority of cases of severe head-injury—especially those in which 'irritation' of the brain is a prominent feature—are associated with pia-arachnoid hæmorrhage. This is evidenced by the presence of a film of blood and serum over certain regions of the brain, not confined to the region subjacent to the skull area primarily involved, but also present over the opposite pole of the brain (injury by contre-coup).

Subpial hæmorrhage differs from the subarachnoid variety in that the blood follows the invaginations of the pia mater, lining, therefore, both major and minor cerebral sulci. Subpial and sub-arachnoid hæmorrhages are, however, generally co-existent, and the term—pia-arachnoid hæmorrhage—aptly describes the conditions commonly found.

The **symptoms** resulting from such blood extravasations are such as are described in the sections dealing with concussion and irritation of the brain (see p. 166).

INJURY TO THE BRAIN

Injury to the brain must always be regarded as by far the most important of the many complications associated with fracture of the skull. A fracture is not necessarily accompanied by brain-injury, and laceration of the brain may exist without a fracture. There can, however, be no question that the more severe cases of head-injury are almost invariably associated with some degree of brain-injury—varying from contusion to extensive laceration, cortical or central.

No part of the brain is exempt from injury, but two regions, the antero-inferior aspect of the frontal lobe and the antero-external aspect of the temporo-sphenoidal lobe, show a special liability to contusion and laceration.

The brain may be injured immediately subjacent to the site at which the blow is delivered (direct injury), or at the pole directly opposite that at which the blow was applied (indirect injury).

Direct injury results from the in-driving of comminuted and depressed fragments of bone, from the passage of a foreign body, and from the direct transmission and diffusion of forces through the subjacent cerebral substance.

The indirect forms of injury are less readily explained. Their frequency cannot be disputed. I drew attention to the subject in my Hunterian Lectures in 1904, there stating that indirect injury to the brain was more common than the direct form. My opinion is confirmed by Phelps,[1] who states that injury by indirect violence is of almost constant occurrence.

Three theories have been advanced in explanation :—

1. 'Their production has been ascribed to the change in form that is suffered by a skull in virtue of its elasticity when subjected to violence which causes distortion of the brain to the point of bursting.'

2. 'In the displacement of the cerebro-spinal fluid by the consecutive depression and bulging that is believed to follow a blow on the head; a momentary vacuum is formed at either axis of force, and the vessels of the brain and meninges rupture from lack of support.'

Neither of these theories are tenable, insomuch as they are based on an acceptance of the 'bursting and compression' theories (see p. 74) —theories which, in my opinion, it is impossible to accept.

3. The 'contre-coup' theory. According to this theory the injury is due to sudden and violent displacement of the brain against the opposing osseous barrier. This theory has been opposed by many—notably by Helferich—on the ground that the brain is said to completely fill the cranial cavity, and that 'shaking' from side to side is impossible.

This theory affords, however, the most satisfactory explanation of contralateral laceration. The following points may be advanced in its favour :—

(*a*) The frontal and temporo-sphenoidal lobes are more liable to contusion and laceration than any other parts of the brain, both regions possessing certain anatomical relations accounting for their ready injury. The frontal pole is related to the angle of junction between the horizontal and vertical plates of the frontal bone, the temporo-sphenoidal lobe to the cul-de-sac, at the anterior part of the middle fossa, that is overhung by the wings of the sphenoid bone.

(*b*) The lacerated area is almost invariably situated at that part of the brain which lies opposite to the region struck in the line of the transmitted force. Furthermore, brain lesions are most prevalent when the accident results from a fall from a height, a class of accident in which 'shaking' of the brain is most likely to occur, and least

[1] *Traumatic Injuries of the Brain.*

common when the basal fracture is dependent on a bilateral compression force.

(*c*) The statements that 'shaking' cannot take place, and that the soft cerebral substance cannot be driven forcibly and violently against the opposing bony barrier, so as to be locally bruised and torn, are incorrect.

That such violent displacement of the brain can and does occur is proved by the following case :—

A prize-fighter was knocked out by a blow on the right side of the head, dying a few hours later. The post-mortem revealed no fracture of vault or base, but a linear laceration of the brain on the mesial aspect of the right hemisphere which exactly corresponded to the free margin of the falx cerebri. In this case, therefore, conclusive evidence was obtained that the brain had been driven from right to left against a firm and resisting barrier, corresponding laceration resulting.

The lacerated area is usually cone-shaped, the base corresponding to the surface of the brain, the apex facing towards the lateral ventricles. In the most severe cases the anterior or lateral horns of the lateral ventricles may be involved at the apex of the cone, and, in the event of further cerebral softening, the horns of the ventricles may, as it were, bulge outwards, thus assisting in the formation of those traumatic cephaloceles that communicate between the lateral ventricle and the surface of the brain.

On the other hand, if the degree of laceration be slight and the injury compatible with life, organization and partial resolution takes place, with the formation, in nearly all cases, of adhesions between the cortex and the membranes, of false membranes, arachnoid cysts, and of blood cysts. In the more serious cases cerebral fibrosis results, in direct proportion to the degree of cerebral destruction, with corresponding degeneration, both of the cerebral cortex and of the tracts that evolve therefrom.

Symptoms. Certain regions of the brain may, when injured, give rise to localizing symptoms. More generally, however, all localizing features are obscured by an overpowering element—the presence of concussion, irritation, or compression of the brain.

Still, in some cases, the localizing features are sufficiently marked, at some period of the case, to allow of a more definite diagnosis. The symptoms, therefore, must be considered under the two heads, (A) *localizing*, and (B) *general*.

A. Localizing symptoms.

Localizing to the frontal lobes. Phelps,[1] from a series of 130 cases, arrived at the following conclusions—that, 'in nearly every case in which consciousness was retained or regained, and the mental faculties not perverted by general delirium, laceration of the left frontal lobe was attended by default in intellectual control, and that the lesion was usually of the anterior region and implicated its inferior surface.' 'Subcortical disintegration was characterized by abrogation of mental power, and superficial laceration by aberration in its manifestations.' And secondly, that, 'in nearly every instance in which laceration was confined to the right side, the mental faculties remained unaffected, except as they were obscured by delirium and stupor occasioned by coincident general lesion.'

Although the above statements have not altogether been confirmed by cases that have come under my observation, yet, coming from such a source, they must be accepted unless refuted.

Bianchi states that, after extirpation of the frontal lobe of the ape, the whole intellectual life of the animal is changed. Perception, attention, inhibition, and in particular memory and association are enfeebled. The psychical tone is lowered; the ape lacks initiative, courage, and spirit.

Laceration of the under aspect of the lobe may, by direct involvement of the olfactory region, interfere with the faculties of smell and taste.

Localizing to those parts that minister to the function of speech. The condition of the patient usually prevents one from obtaining early information as to the power of speech. Isolated lesions of the posterior part of the third left frontal convolution result in *motor aphasia*, a condition characterized by the inability on the part of the patient to speak, in spite of the fact that comprehension is unimpaired. The brain-injury is, however, seldom so defined as to

[1] *Traumatic Injuries of the Brain*, p. 138.

be characterized by loss of speech without other phenomena. In very close relation to the area responsible for speech is the *writing* centre, situated at the posterior end of the middle frontal gyrus, near the centre for the movements of the hands and fingers. Injury to this centre results in *agraphia* and *alexia.*

Word-deafness results from lesions implicating the upper temporo-sphenoidal lobe, and *word-blindness* from injuries to the supra-marginal and angular gyri (see Fig. 57).

Phelps pointed out that the lesion must be an extensive one if the symptoms included under the term *sensory aphasia* (word-blindness,

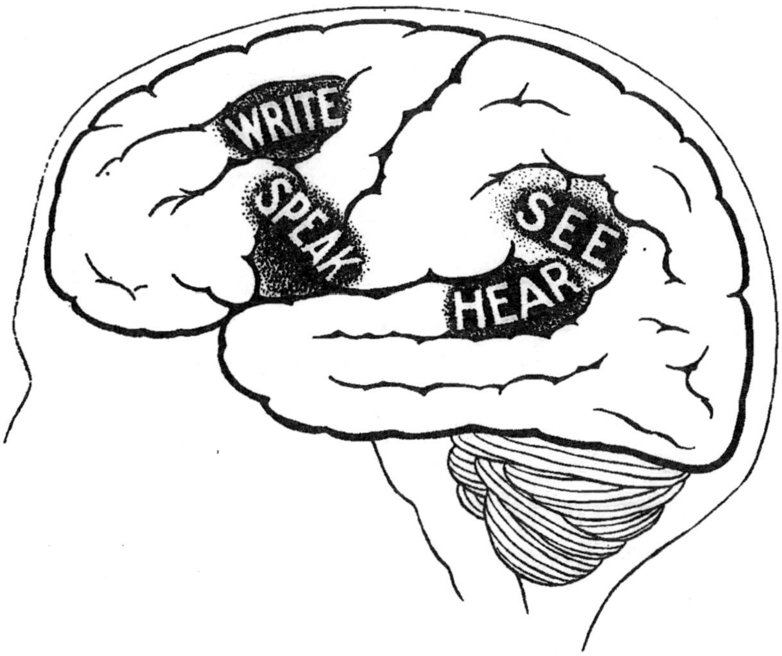

FIG. 57. THE AREAS CONCERNED IN SPEECH EXPRESSION.

word-deafness) are to be evolved. No localized injury to any small area suffices, and the cortex must be deeply involved. Lacerations of the brain are usually of so gross a nature that further differentiation is seldom to be obtained. Here it might be noted that the cortical centres responsible for speech and its accessories, word-seeing, word-writing, and possibly word-hearing, are all situated on the left side in normal right-handed individuals. The corresponding areas on the right side may be regarded as 'silent' areas, and may be utilized, if desired, for decompression purposes. No operation, with that purpose in view, should be carried out, however, unless the surgeon is assured that the patient is right-handed in his actions. A case has recently come to my knowledge where a right-parietal decompression operation was carried out with disastrous results.

Localizing to the temporo-sphenoidal lobe. The relation of sensory aphasia to lesions of the temporo-sphenoidal lobe has already been mentioned. The anterior poles of this portion of the brain, a region frequently involved in head injuries, may lead to the development of impaired smell and taste, especially if the lesion includes the uncinate lobe and be situated on the left side. In other respects, the temporo-sphenoidal lobe may be regarded as a 'silent' area of the brain.

Localizing to the pre- and post-central convolutions. Injury to the pre-central or motor area usually leads to the development of definite symptoms—twitchings, convulsions, or paralysis of the face and extremities on the contra-lateral side. In the earlier stages reflexes are abolished. Later on, as the result of degenerative changes in the pyramidal tracts, spasticity, contractures, and rigidity, with increased reflexes will be observed in the affected limbs. On the other hand, the muscles do not show any reaction of degeneration. Babinski's sign is generally present.

Injury to the post-central convolutions might be expected to lead to various alterations in tactile and muscle sense, in stereognosis, and in sense of pain and temperature, but the general condition of the patient seldom permits accurate demonstration. Such sensory disturbances are more frequently observed as late results of head-injury.

Localizing of the occipital lobes. Laceration of the occipital lobes may lead to homonymous hemianopia, for which defect it is probable that the degree of laceration must be considerable, involving mainly the mesial aspect of the occipital lobe (see Fig. 69). Schäfer has shown that the greater portion of the occipital lobe may be removed in monkeys without producing loss of vision, and it is only when the lesion involves the parieto-occipital fissure and passes into the occipito-temporal convolutions that loss of vision is permanent.

Slighter degrees of occipital injury may lead to subjective symptoms, such as flashes of light, colour changes, &c.

Localizing to the cerebellum. Lesions of the cerebellum rarely permit of the development of such localizing symptoms as are observed in cerebellar tumours. Inco-ordination of movement, ataxia, and other symptoms observed in cerebellar tumour formation are, from the general condition of the patient, incapable of demonstration in cerebellar laceration. It is necessary, however, to draw attention to the significance of yawning and gaping. This symptom has been

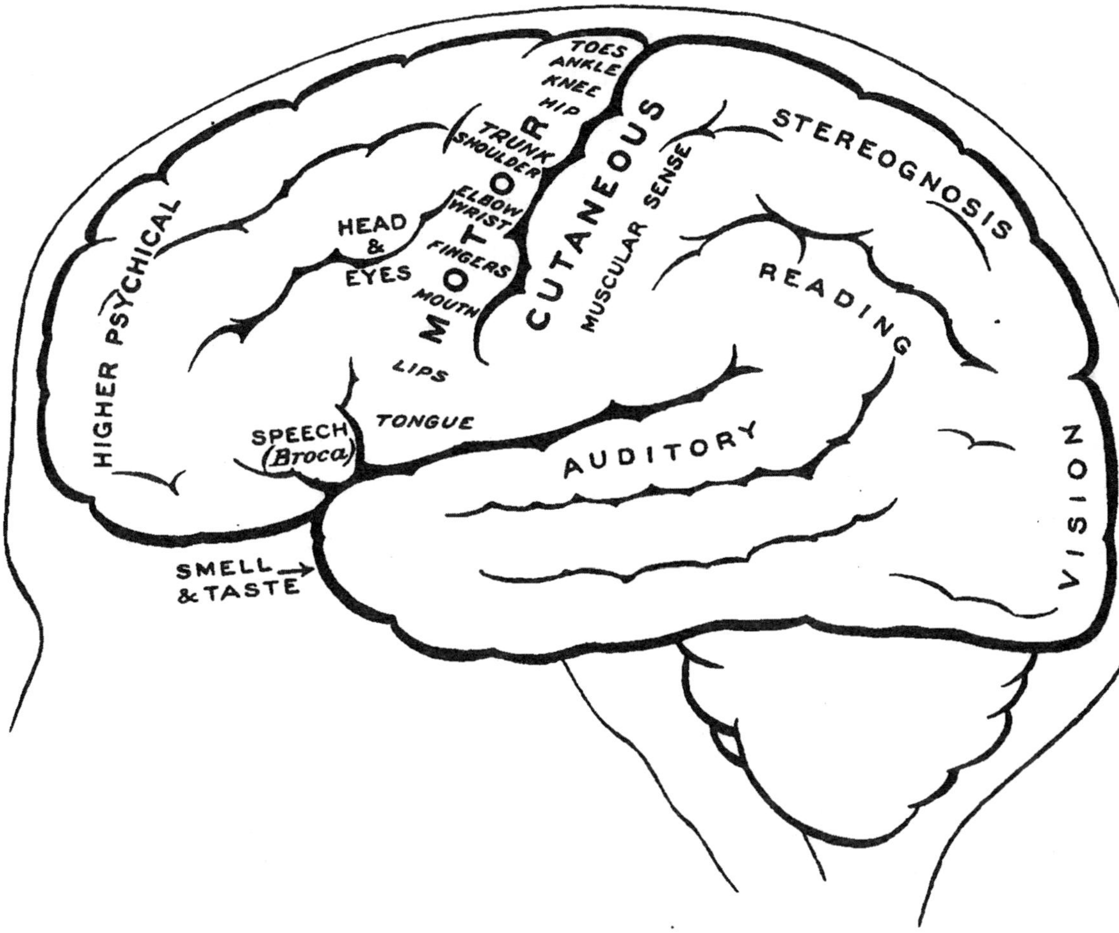

FIG. 58. THE CORTICAL MOTOR AND SENSORY AREAS.

observed in several recent cases, and, as far as my observation goes, is only present in cerebellar lesions.

In the consideration of these localizing symptoms, it must be borne in mind that brain lacerations are of an exceedingly gross nature, and that there may be—as the late Professor von Bergmann [1] pointed out—'notwithstanding the severest brain symptoms, not the slightest discoverable anatomical alteration in the brain. On the other hand, notwithstanding the absence of all brain symptoms, extensive and striking destruction of the brain substance.'

[1] *System of Surgery*, vol. i, p. 179.

B. General symptoms.

Concussion or cerebral shock.

Its pathology. Concussion used to be regarded as implying a 'molecular disturbance' of the brain—a definition so unsatisfactory that it may be relegated to a desired obscurity. At the present day, though some difference of opinion exists as to whether the condition is or is not necessarily dependent in its development on associated cortical or subcortical lesions, macroscopical or microscopical, concussion is regarded as implying a condition of *acute cerebral anœmia* through sudden inhibition or paralysis of the vasomotor centre.

With respect to the existence of visible lesions of the brain, Kocher maintains that such lesions—hæmorrhages and the like—are necessarily present, proposing that the term 'brain concussion' should be eliminated in favour of 'brain contusion'. On the other hand, the late Professor von Bergmann pointed out that such a course was not possible, instancing the many cases of concussion where contusion could not possibly have existed.

There cannot, in my opinion, be any question as to which is the correct view. It is unreasonable to ask one to believe that the milder cases of concussion, cases in which the patient merely suffers from loss of consciousness for a few minutes, from which he rapidly recovers and is discharged from treatment within a few days, and from which he suffers in the future from no remote ill effects whatsoever, it is unreasonable to ask one to believe that such cases have experienced so severe a lesion as brain contusion or laceration. Both these conditions would require a long period of convalescence, and would tend to leave in their train very serious after-results.

It is obvious, therefore, that there exists a degree of concussion from which the patient can quickly and entirely recover. It is also clear that in many cases the patient passes through a long and serious illness, whilst, in some cases, a fatal termination may ensue—and that too within a few hours. It is consequently clear that we have to deal with varying grades of concussion, some of which are of so mild a nature as to be clearly unassociated with definite cerebral lesion, whilst others are of so serious a nature that death may take place within a few hours, and in such cases the gravest cerebral lesions may be found at the autopsy.

In other words, it would appear that concussion is more or less dependent in its severity on the degree of associated cerebral change.

It is, however, to the milder type of case that we should turn in order to determine what is exactly meant by concussion. In such cases the patient merely suffers from a mild degree of *cerebral shock*, a condition closely resembling shock in general. 'Shock' is defined as a 'condition resulting from fall in blood-pressure, due to inhibition or paralysis of the vaso-motor centre'. The afferent impulses that pass up the various sensory paths inhibit or paralyse the vaso-motor centre, a centre that has for its main function a tonic constricting influence on the peripheral arteries. Hence, these vessels dilate atonically, the blood collects in the great splanchnic area, and, insomuch as the cerebral arteries possess no separate vaso-motor apparatus, they passively follow the changes in the general circulation. The brain is consequently in a state of arterial anæmia, the arteries relatively emptied, the veins passively engorged.

Clinically, concussion or cerebral shock differs from ordinary shock in one manifestation only—sudden loss of consciousness. This development is readily explained on the ground that concussion results from a violent blow applied in the near neighbourhood of the vaso-motor centre, with consequent *sudden* vaso-motor depression and *acute* anæmia of the cerebral cortex. This leads to immediate great fall of blood-pressure, loss of consciousness, and lack of muscular control.

Statements have recently been brought forward to the effect that concussion is in reality a mild type of compression. This view received at first sight some confirmation from the experiments of Koch and Filehne, who, from the application of consecutive slight blows to the heads of dogs, showed that each blow resulted in bulbar stimulation followed by bulbar depression. The blows being continued, the degree of stimulation decreased and that of depression increased until exhaustion and death resulted. During the periods of stimulation the pulse-rate slowed, during those of depression it increased.

It should be noted, however, that concussion, as observed in the human being, results from one sudden and violent blow. It may,

I think, safely be assumed that, in such cases, the stimulating effect of the blow is entirely abolished in favour of an acute depression. And, as Archibald[1] says, 'their records of respiration, pulse, and blood-pressure resemble far more closely the course of an increasing compression, with its gradual slowing of pulse and respiration and steady rise of blood-pressure, than that of concussion with its sudden standstill of pulse and respiration and fall of blood-pressure.'

In *favourable cases* the injury being of a comparatively mild nature, the vaso-motor centre soon recovers tone, and, as the result of previous depression, the vascular conditions are now reversed—*the stage of depression* giving place to the *stage of reaction*. The blood-pressure rises, the carotids pulsate forcibly, the face is turgid and flushed, the skin hot and moist, whilst the temperature rises, and the general cerebral hyperæmia is evidenced by headache, restlessness, and perhaps by delirium.

In the *more severe cases* the vaso-motor depression is unduly prolonged, or persists till death, the patient remaining concussed for a considerable period of time, or dying in that condition. In these fatal cases the post-mortem examination *usually* reveals brain laceration, but *always* evidences considerable engorgement of superficial cerebral veins, increase of cerebro-spinal fluid and œdema, both of the pia-arachnoid region and of the brain substance itself. These latter phenomena are accounted for by the fact that, insomuch as the venous pressure and cerebro-spinal tension are equal, the greater the engorgement of the cerebral veins the more extensive is the transudation of fluid into the pia-arachnoid and cerebral systems. In a fatal case of concussion—recently under my care—the surface of the cortex, when exposed by operation, was obscured by a layer of œdematous pia-arachnoid $\frac{1}{4}$ inch in depth.

Arguing from the presence of the very definite pathological changes observed in all fatal cases—contusions, lacerations, hæmorrhages, and œdema—one may arrive at the conclusions (1) that lesions of a similar but less serious nature are existent in the serious but non-fatal cases, and (2) that the prolongation of the stage of depression is directly dependent on the presence of such lesions.

On investigating the numerous cases that come under the care

[1] *American Practice of Surgery*, Bryant and Buck.

of the surgeon, certain features present themselves which are not always readily explained on the definition of concussion as given above. Thus, the variability of the symptoms evinced in cases of concussion admitted into hospital are well exemplified by the following table, compiled from a consecutive series of 50 cases admitted into St. Bartholomew's, diagnosed and treated as concussion :—

12 *cases in the hospital for* 7 *days or less* (*cerebral shock only*).

Temperature on admission : 8 subnormal.
2 normal.
2 slightly raised.

Pulse on admission : 3 subnormal.
3 normal.
6 accelerated.

26 *cases detained for* 7 *to* 10 *days* (*probably cerebral shock only*).

Temperature on admission : 6 subnormal.
9 normal.
11 slightly raised.

Pulse on admission : 4 subnormal.
12 normal.
10 accelerated.

9 *cases detained for* 14 *to* 21 *days* (*probably cerebral contusion*).

Temperature on admission : 2 subnormal.
3 normal.
4 slightly raised.

Pulse on admission : 6 subnormal.
1 normal.
2 accelerated.

3 *cases detained for* 21 *to* 30 *days* (*certainly cerebral contusion*).

Temperature on admission : 1 normal.
2 slightly raised.

Pulse on admission : 1 subnormal.
1 normal.
1 accelerated.

Still, when all is considered, concussion and compression are but ill-defined from one another, both in their clinical and pathological aspects. The more indefinite cases of concussion are probably such as border on compression, the increasing œdema gradually carrying the patient across the border line between the two conditions.

In the present state of our knowledge respecting concussion or cerebral shock it may, I think, be accepted (1) that concussion is dependent on an acute inhibition or paralysis of the vaso-motor centre; (2) that the milder cases are unassociated with any pathological visible changes; (3) that the prolongation and severity of the depression stage are directly proportionate to the extent of the brain lesion, such lesions varying from œdema and contusion to extensive hæmorrhages and lacerations.

Its symptomatology.

The stage of depression. The symptoms are evoked immediately on the receipt of the blow, the patient falling to the ground from lack of muscular control and loss of consciousness. The muscular system is completely relaxed, the limbs, when raised, falling helplessly to the ground. The face is deathly pale, the eyes usually open, fixed, and expressionless, the pupils equal, commonly dilated and responsive to light. The patient *may* be aroused by strong stimuli—pinching, shouting in the ear, pressure over the supra-orbital nerves, &c.

The pulse is small, slightly accelerated, and occasionally intermittent. The respiration is weak, shallow, and often irregular. The temperature is lowered, sometimes to such an extent that it cannot be registered on the thermometer. The surface of the body is cold and clammy, beads of sweat standing out on the brow. The deep reflexes are abolished. Some attempts may be made at swallowing when fluids are placed in the mouth.

Urine is often expelled at the time of the accident, and, more rarely, fæces may also be passed involuntarily.

The condition either gives place to that of reaction or the state of unconsciousness and collapse becomes more profound, in which case the prognosis is most unfavourable.

The stage of reaction. Weak, purposeless movements are observed and the patient may sigh heavily, mutter, or groan. This is followed by profuse vomiting, after which the temperature begins to rise, the body becomes warmer, and the patient recovers his senses either entirely or in part. The heart beats strongly, the pulse being full and slightly accelerated in rate. The carotid arteries are seen to pulsate forcibly, the face is flushed and moist. The patient is restless, and complains of severe headache, due in all probability to intradural hypertension. Under efficient treatment these symptoms of cerebral hyperæmia abate, the patient recovering quickly or slowly, according to the severity of the blow. Retrograde amnesia is often a conspicuous feature in the more severe cases, varying greatly in depth and character, seldom permanent.

In the more serious cases—those associated with severe cerebral injury—the pupils dilate fully and do not react to light. Corneal reflex is absent. The medullary centres gradually become exhausted, the pulse becoming smaller, increasing in rapidity, and finally unrecognizable. Respiration becomes weaker and often Cheyne-Stokes in character. Respiration ceases before the heart gives out.

Cerebral Irritation.

Its pathology. Sufficient evidence is supplied, both by clinical symptoms and by post-mortem examination, to show that brain irritation is dependent on definite brain lesions, these varying from 'bruising' to minor degrees of laceration. Bruising or contusion of the brain—evidenced by pia-arachnoid hæmorrhages and by cortical and subcortical hæmorrhages—is most prevalent in the frontal and temporo-sphenoidal regions. The same may be said with respect to laceration.

Its symptomatology. From the initial stage of concussion the patient passes into that of irritation, the reaction being of a rather violent type and accompanied by considerable rise of blood-pressure.

The patient lies curled up in bed, the lower extremities flexed at the hip and knee, the upper limbs bent across and partially covering the forwardly flexed head. He is exceedingly restless. Restraint is usually required. The eyes are tightly closed, and all attempts at pupillary examination are strenuously resisted. The patient groans, mutters, and uses language, perhaps suited to the occasion but not adaptable to polite society. Headache is severe, often referred to the frontal region. The skin is hot and dry—burning—the body temperature is raised whilst the pulse is accelerated and its tension increased. Both urine and fæces may be passed into the bed, not so much from loss of bladder and rectal control as from transitory moral perversion.

The state of irritation subsides or merges into that of cerebral compression.

Compression.

Its pathology. A compression force—whether foreign body, blood extravasation, abscess or tumour—must act on the brain substance or on the fluid constituents of the skull. The brain, however, is itself incompressible. It may be squeezed like a sponge, but its actual structure is unalterable. Consequently, the compressing force exercises its main influence on the fluid contents, driving out the cerebro-spinal fluid, depleting the cerebral veins and emptying the arterioles, producing in other words a state of brain anæmia.

Experimentally, it has been ascertained that from 3 to 6 per cent. of the cranial capacity can be taken up by a foreign body without producing compression symptoms—probably owing to the escape of cerebro-spinal fluid into the spinal canal, and the recession of the medulla and cerebellum into the foramen magnum. Furthermore, it would appear that the incidence of compression symptoms is associated with depletion of those cerebral veins which are in closest relation to the compression force. As this force increases—for example, in middle meningeal hæmorrhage—the pressure exercised on the surrounding regions increases proportionately, to the level of the capillary pressure, and even to that of the smaller arteries. A state of cerebral anæmia results, first localized to the region primarily involved, then invading more widely and finally affecting both supra- and infra-tentorial spaces.

With regard to the continuity of pressure between these three spaces, there is but little pressure discontinuity between the two supra-tentorial spaces, whilst, between the supra- and infra-tentorial regions, there is less ready communication.

A slight degree of compression in the supra-tentorial space will act on the corresponding space only, greater degrees will involve all three. On the other hand, a rise of infra-tentorial pressure is not of necessity associated with a corresponding elevation in the other two regions. For example, a cerebellar tumour readily affects the medullary centres, whilst the higher cortical regions are for the time being totally unaffected. Again, a tumour situated in the frontal pole does not necessarily produce any of those symptoms of cerebral compression which are regarded as referable to an increase of sub-tentorial pressure—slow pulse, vaso-motor disturbances, subnormal pressure, and deep rhythmical respiration.

Returning once more to the vascular effects of a localized compression, it is obvious that whilst the compressing force is producing a surrounding anæmia—depleted veins and arterioles—yet that the neighbouring but more distant brain is venously engorged—from venous retardation. Insomuch, moreover, as the venous tension and cerebro-spinal pressure are equal, it is obvious that, as the result of venous engorgement, there is some surrounding serous transudation into the perivascular, pia-arachnoid, and cerebral regions. The brain bordering on the anæmic arca is therefore œdematous, the œdema diminishing and fading away in direct proportion to the distance of the area involved from the primary focus of compression.

If the compression force is of a progressive nature, the engorged area becomes in turn anæmic, and still more distant regions become engorged and œdematous. This state is known as that of *progressive œdema.* Its complete development is largely dependent on brain infection—abscess of the brain, &c.

Thc rapidity with which the symptoms of compression develop are largely dependent on the producing cause. Thus, three examplcs may be cited :—

(1) Compression of slow development, requiring weeks or months before typical symptoms are observable—e. g. tumour formation.

(2) Compression of medium development, requiring days only : c. g. absccss, subdural hæmatocele, and some forms of middlc meningeal hæmorrhage.

(3) Compression of acute development, almost immediate : e. g. diffuse subdural hæmorrhage, some cases of middle meningeal hæmorrhagc, depressed fractures, and intracranial foreign bodies.

The special symptoms of compression arc, as Leonard Hill pointed out, referable to the effects produced on the bulbar centres. That such is the case is suggested by the following facts :—

(1) The same compression symptoms result wherever the compressing force acts.

(2) Experimentally, an increased pressure in the posterior fossa produces compression symptoms earlier than when the compressing force is exercised in some more distant region of the brain.

(3) A fracture involving the posterior fossa gives rise to compression symptoms earlier than a fracture in some more distant region.

(4) A far smaller body kills in the bulbar region than in the cerebral chamber.

(5) The general pressure effects are in no way due to excitation of the part of the brain pressed on, for, after division of the mesencaphalon, the pressure was just as active in calling forth changes in respiration and circulation (Sir Victor Horsley).

Leonard Hill also pointed out that the first effect of anæmia of the bulbar region was in the nature of stimulation, the vaso-motor centre being influenced in such a manner as to produce a general rise of blood-pressure. A further degree of compression may again produce the same result, the arterial pressure rising considerably above the normal. Later on, the medullary centres—and more especially the vaso-motor—become exhausted, with consequent grave fall in blood-pressure. The pulse, previously slow and full, becomes rapid, small, readily compressible, and irregular in rhythm, whilst the respiration, previously deep and regular, becomes gasping, irregular, and Cheyne-Stokes in character.

The sequence of events may be depicted in another manner. In cerebral compression, the battle—as pointed out by Schüster—largely resolves itself into a life and death struggle between the attacking compression force on the one hand and the defending vaso-motor centre on the other.

Up to a certain point the vaso-motor centre holds the whip-hand. The capillary anæmia as producd by the compression force—cerebro-spinal tension, &c.—brings about a condition which not only acts as a stimulus to the vaso-motor centre but also exercises a marked effect on the vagus and respiratory centres. The blood-pressure rises, the pulse is slowed in rate, and its tension markedly increased, whilst the respiration is slightly irregular both in depth and rhythm. The vaso-motor centre thus attacked sends out further impulses so as to raise the blood-pressure to slightly above requirements. The bulbar centres are again flushed with blood, the vaso-motor centre 'slacks off', and the blood-pressure falls again.

The compressing force is, however, still active and full of fight. A further capillary anæmia results. The vaso-motor centre again responds and the blood-pressure rises higher than ever, the pulse-rate is further slowed, and the respiration is deeper, less regular, and even stertorous.

This combat continues, and, in the presence of an active compression force, there is that rhythmic activity of the vaso-motor centre which is represented by the well-known Traube-Herring curves; again, the height to which the vaso-motor centre drives the blood-pressure may be taken as representing the activity of the compression force.

When the compressing force rises above a certain limit the *débâcle* occurs—the vaso-motor centre retires from the fight, there is a rapid fall in blood-pressure, the medulla is emptied of blood, and both cardiac and respiratory centres share in the defeat (rapid pulse of poor volume and Cheyne-Stokes respiration).

These being the effects as exercised by compression on the bulbar centres, one must not omit to consider the results produced on the higher cortical centres. Anæmia is the feature and unconsciousness is the ultimate result, preceded by headache and drowsiness progressing on to stupor and coma. Intermediate between the stages of sleepiness and coma, one observes occasionally a stage of irritation —such as is pictured in many cases of typical middle meningeal hæmorrhage.

In fatal cases the respiratory centre gives out first, the heart often beating for some time after all attempts at respiration have ceased. In a case recently under my care, respiration ceased during the process of trephining. The patient was kept 'alive' for three hours by means of artificial respiration, and under such mechanical breathing the patient retained a good colour and the heart worked well. So soon, however, as efforts were rclaxed, the pulse became weaker and weaker until further artifieial respiration again restored the balanee. This proeess was kept up till it was realized that the respiratory eentre was ‘ dead ’.

From these faets, it may be assumed that the special symptoms of eompression are dependent (*a*) on anæmia of the bulb—with eorresponding eardiac, respiratory, and vaso-motor ehanges; and (*b*) on anæmia of the cortex—with unconseiousness.

Its symptomatology. According to Kocher, the following are the four stages of eompression :—

1. *The stage of compensation.* A mild degree insuffieient to seriously eompromise the circulation. Cerebro-spinal fluid escapes into the spinal canal and some of the venous radieles are eompressed. Some venous engorgement. Some headaehe, possibly some focal symptoms. Some mental dullness.

2. *Stage of beginning compression.* Beginning failure of the cireulatory eompensation. Headaehe pronouneed, vertigo, restlessness, exeitement or delirium. Objective symptoms of venous stasis—dilatation of the veins of the eye, both external and internal, œdema of the disk. Affeetion of the medullary centres, shown by a slowed pulse and a slight rise in temperature.

3. *Stage of fully-developed compression.* Widespread capillary anæmia. Medulla affected markedly. The period of vaso-motor regulation has set in with its high blood-pressure, and this, with its vagal quality, gives the pulse its bounding eharaeter. The rise in blood-pressure shows a definite rhythm. Also rhythmieities in respiration whieh may aequire the Cheyne-Stokes character. Rhythmie alterations in the size of the pupils, with alternate inerease and deerease in the depth of stupor, so that the ‘ up-wave ’ eauses the patient to moan, beeome irritable, and thrash about, whilst the ‘ down-wave ’ sees him eompletely eomatose. Pulse is markedly slowed and the disks evidenee pronounced ‘ ehoking ’. Reflexes are abolished, eyanosis extreme, respiration snoring.

4. *Stage of paralysis.* Irregular eardiae and respiratory efforts, pulse grows rapid, coma deepening, museular relaxation, pupils widely dilated, and permanent fall in blood-pressure. Respiratory paralysis.

Treatment.

(*a*) *Of concussion.* In considering the treatment of concussion, it has to be remembered that we are treating a condition dependent on vaso-motor depression, and that we are ignorant—at any rate for the time being—as to the nature and extent of a possible cerebral lesion. It is obvious, therefore, that although we are clear as to the general lines on which treatment is to be carried out, yet that our earlier methods must be expectant and our subsequent methods symptomatic. In other words, we must be prepared, at any moment, to change the method of treatment according as symptoms demand.

The more general treatment—applicable to all cases, of whatever severity—consists in putting the patient to bed with the head low, in the application of warmth to the body and extremities, and in the administration of hypodermic injections of morphia, a drug of great value in the more severe cases of concussion. It must, however, be administered with caution, lest important symptoms be masked.

Strychnine and brandy are practically useless. They merely whip the willing horse—the heart is doing full duty and cannot be further stimulated by such measures.

In *mild and moderately severe cases* this form of treatment will suffice to tide the patient over the collapse stage and induce the stage of reaction. So soon as this *commences*, the rising temperature and vomiting heralding the change, the head of the bed should be lowered, hot bottles and blankets removed—the patient being covered with a linen sheet only—and all forms of stimulant avoided.

Calomel should be given by the mouth, 1 to 5 grains, according to the age of the patient. Headache may be relieved by applying ice-bags to the head, by tying round the forehead a handkerchief soaked in a weak solution of eau-de-Cologne, and by the administration of various drugs, more especially aspirin (10 grs.), antipyrin (10 grs.), and hyoscin (gr. $\frac{1}{100}$).

In *more severe cases* more radical measures must be adopted to combat the severe vaso-motor depression, with its consequent splanchnic congestion and cerebral anæmia. No method is more desirable than infusion. This method, with its attendant advantages and disadvantages, has been detailed on p. 118. It is merely necessary to add that infusion must not be carried out in a haphazard manner.

Its application is based on scientific principles, and its results must be noted with the greatest care. The surgeon must keep a watchful eye on the temperature and blood-pressure, and he must be prepared at any moment to change his plan of campaign.

(*b*) *Of irritation.* The patient should be kept in a darkened room and should not be worried more than is absolutely necessary for diagnostic purposes. An attendant is usually required, whose methods should be persuasive rather than forcible. Great tact is required.

Morphia is of the greatest value in the treatment of this condition. It relieves the headache, acts as a damper on the hyperæmic brain, and keeps the patient from threshing about in bed and injuring himself. Sleep is essential for an early recovery and cure.

In the *more severe cases* venesection should be carried out, and operative measures will be required if the rising temperature and slowed high-tension pulse herald the advent or indicate the presence of compression of the brain.

(*c*) *Of compression.* The various operations carried out for the relief of compression of the brain are discussed elsewhere. They include such operations as are conducted for localized hæmorrhages, whether subdural or extra-dural (see Chap. V), and such also as are described as 'decompression' operations (see p. 121).

With regard to the general indications for adopting active surgical measures, the surgeon is, of course, guided in his estimation of the case by the general condition of the patient—depth of unconsciousness, &c.—but more especially by the temperature changes and alterations in blood-pressure. In my own practice I am guided very largely by the temperature changes—as described on p. 114. On the other hand, some surgeons pin their faith more especially on the blood-pressure changes. Thus Archibald writes: 'If the blood-pressure be 130 mm. Hg. on admission, an hour later 150, still later 200 or 250, we are immediately in possession of the fact that the available intracranial space is being steadily, dangerously reduced, and that the vaso-motor centre is straining every nerve to stave off defeat.'

I am, of course, ready to concede the great value of blood-pressure tracings, but, in my experience, the temperature changes have been even more consistent, so much so that I base my treatment of a case very largely on such changes. One word of warning—the temperature must be taken every half-hour, and active surgical measures adopted *so soon as* the rising temperature, slowing high-tension pulse, and deepening unconsciousness point to advancing compression.

There is undoubtedly a growing tendency amongst those who have carefully studied the effects of trauma on the skull and brain to carry out exploratory and decompression operations at an early period, even in cases which present no symptoms of special localizing significance. The pathological conditions so commonly found and the excellent results that have been obtained prove that the adoption of early surgical treatment is founded on a very sound basis.

Points in the differential diagnosis between traumatic and other forms of coma. The previous history of the case, the nature of the accident, and the lesions found may enable the surgeon to arrive at ready diagnosis. Often, however, it is impossible to exclude non-traumatic forms of coma without an exhaustive examination of the patient. In the process of examination, it is convenient to have in one's mind a simple memoria-technica. Thus,

A stands for Alcohol and Apoplexy.
E ,, ,, Epilepsy (post-epileptic coma).
I ,, ,, Injury.
O ,, ,, Opium poisoning.
U ,, ,, Uræmia.

To this list must be added Diabetic Coma.

Having these conditions in mind, the patient is examined from head to foot in the following manner :—

The *vault of the skull* is first examined and all evidence obtained as to the presence and extent of external injury.

The *ears and nose* are investigated for escaping blood or cerebrospinal fluid, important symptoms in the diagnosis of fracture of the base.

The *eyes* are next examined. Ocular palsies suggest injury or apoplexy; hæmorrhages—subconjunctival or palpebral—point to injury; whilst the condition of the pupils and disks may offer valuable information. Thus:

In concussion, the pupils are equal, dilated, but responsive to light.

In irritation, they are equal but contracted.

In compression, they are either equal, dilated and fixed, or unequal.

In alcohol, they are more or less normal, except in the deeper stages of intoxication, when they are dilated and irresponsive to light.

In apoplexy, dilated and fixed, or unequal. Pin-point in pontine hæmorrhage.

In epilepsy, usually equal and responsive.

In opium, immovably and symmetrically contracted.

In uræmia, dilated and sluggish.

In diabetes, equal but dilated. React to light.

In doubtful cases an examination of the disks may clear up the diagnosis. The presence of albuminuric retinitis, optic neuritis and atrophy (diabetes and uræmia), retinal hæmorrhages (injury), offer material diagnostic aid.

The *tongue* should be examined for such biting as is observed in epilepsy. The odour of the *breath* is investigated—the sickly smell of alcohol, the sweetish odour of uræmia, the peculiar smell of opium, the chloroform-like smell of diabetes.

The appearance of the *face* may be suggestive. The unilateral facial palsy of trauma and apoplexy; the stertorous respiration, puffing out of the cheeks, and general turgidity of compression, uræmia, apoplexy and deep alcoholism; the quiet breathing and pale face of concussion, opium poisoning, and of post-epileptic and diabetic coma.

The *urine* should be examined for albumen and sugar, and the body and lower extremities for œdema.

The *extremities* are investigated with respect to unilateral palsy, a condition only present in trauma and apoplexy. General convulsions point to injury, uræmia, and epilepsy. Resistance to manipulation is suggestive of alcoholic excess. Unilateral palsy may be associated with corresponding alteration in the deep reflexes.

The *pulse*-rate and the condition of the arteries supply valuable evidence. The coats may be atheromatous, whilst the slow, full pulse is strongly suggestive of compression, apoplexy, and alcoholism.

The *temperature* should be taken on both sides of the body. A rise of temperature is usually dependent on brain injury, apoplexy, and alcoholism. In opium poisoning, uræmia, and epilepsy the temperature is more likely to be normal or subnormal. In pontine hæmorrhage, hyperpyrexia is commonly observed.

Some difference in the temperature on the two sides of the body points to injury or apoplexy.

The *depth of the coma* is often of the greatest assistance in the differential diagnosis. Thus, in concussion, alcohol poisoning, and in the minor grades of epilepsy and uræmia, the patient may often be sufficiently aroused by shouting in the ear, digital pressure over the supra-orbital nerves, or by the application of the battery, as to give some account of the accident, &c. In compression, in the deeper states of uræmic and diabetic poisoning, and in the status epilepticus, the patient can seldom be aroused from the deep coma into which he is sunk.

In all cases of doubt the patient must be kept under careful observation.

CHAPTER VI

THE REMOTE EFFECTS OF HEAD-INJURY

General considerations. It is often stated that a patient who has received a severe head-injury is 'never the same man afterwards'. Before accepting such a sweeping statement—the gravity of which is obvious—it is essential that an extensive survey should be made into the remote effects of head-injury, and, in their consideration, the surgeon must not be biased by those cases that seek hospital relief. It is the unfavourable cases that present themselves for examination, the more favourable are usually lost to view. Furthermore, whether the early results are completely satisfactory or not, but little guide can be obtained into the more remote results unless, as a routine procedure, an attempt be made to trace all such cases in their after-history. The more remote results can then be estimated at their true value.

The difficulties attendant on all attempts at following up hospital cases are considerable, and consequently we are greatly indebted to Crisp English[1] for his tabulation and discussion on the after-history of 300 cases treated at St. George's Hospital—300 cases personally investigated at periods varying from one to twenty years subsequent to the time of the injury.

English's conclusions have been compared with those derived from my own personal experience, with the result that they were found to coincide so closely that they may be accepted as affording an accurate guide into the remote results of head-injury in general.

English classified his cases into three series—each 100 in number—according to the severity of the lesion.

Series 1. Fracture cases.
Series 2. Cases of concussion, contusion, and laceration.
Series 3. Miscellaneous cases.

[1] *Hunterian Lectures,* February 1904.

The remote results as observed in the first and second series were as follows :—

Series 1.	No effects	31
	Slight effects	50
	Marked effects	19
Series 2.	No effects	48
	Slight effects	42
	Marked effects	10

In the 200 cases, therefore, that come under Series 1 and 2, 79 experienced no ill effects from the injury, 92 developed slight effects, and definite defects were present in 29 cases.

Before alluding further to the mental and bodily condition of the patients subsequent to the accident, including their wage-earning capacity, it is necessary to enlarge on the fact that the depreciation in mental and physical faculties depends, not only on the severity of the injury, but also on the age, disposition, and status of the patient.

The effect of age. All evidence tends to prove that head-injuries in the young and the old are more serious than when the accident occurs during middle life. In the old, the power of repair is impaired ; in the young, the developing faculties are impeded in their progress.

The effect of disposition. The temperament of the patient must always be taken into consideration, the neurotic type seldom recovering so quickly or so completely as the more plethoric.

The effect of status. A complete recovery is far more likely to occur when the status of the patient allows of complete rest, bodily and mental, for some considerable time subsequent to the accident. A premature return to work, with possible added family troubles, invariably acts as a deterrent to complete recovery. In the milder cases a few weeks suffice to allow of restoration to health, in other cases an interval of at least one year should be allowed before the patient again takes up his duties. It is obvious, therefore, that family troubles and business emergencies influence to a marked degree the completeness of recovery. It might be anticipated that the financial necessities of the case would cause the various after-results of head-injuries to be more marked amongst the labouring classes. The personal equation, however, enters largely into the question, and due allowance must be made for the greater financial and social losses entailed when the injury involves one who occupies a high social sphere. It must also be borne in mind that those occupying such spheres may not benefit from the Workmen's Compensation Act.

On referring again to English's cases, it was found that the wage-earning capacity of the patient afforded a valuable clue in the estimation of the remote results in general. Thus in Series 1 and 2 the following results were obtained :—

Series 1. 86 cases :

52 carried out the same work at the same wages.
13 carried out lighter work.
7 could do but little work.
8 had to take to other work, less dangerous.
6 were totally disabled.

Series 2. 78 cases :

51 carried out the same work at the same wages.
12 worked as before, but without much interest.
6 were compelled to undertake lighter work.
4 could do a little work.
2 gave up their trade for another, less dangerous.
3 were totally disabled.

Thus 59 per cent. in Series 1 and 80 per cent. in Series 2 were able to do the same work at the same wages as previous to the accident.

It will be of interest to compare English's results with those obtained by other investigators. Thus, in 48 cases examined by Graf, the following results were obtained :—

In 9 cases, no bad results.
10 cases, slight troubles or impaired work-power.
12 cases, limited power of work.
17 cases, complete incapacitation from work.

Thus 35 per cent. of cases were completely incapacitated from work, results far more serious than according to English's investigations.

Again, Crandon and Wilson made inquiries into the after-effects in 38 cases, with the following results :—

	Yes.	*No.*
Headache	13	25
Eye troubles	17	21
Dizziness	15	23
Deafness	16	22
Paralysis	1	37
Faints	4	34
Fits	2	36
Loss of memory	4	34
Troubled by the sun	13	25
Troubled by alcohol	6	32

On investigating those cases reported by English, in which the patient was compelled to take on lighter work or change his vocation, one at once encounters a diversity of symptoms, some so indefinite as to be included under the term traumatic neurasthenia, others so distinct as to fall naturally under certain well-recognized groups, such as traumatic cephalalgia, epilepsy, &c.

Traumatic neurasthenia. All those cases characterized by the indefinite nature of their complaint require the most careful sifting—to separate the wheat from the chaff—for there is always a certain proportion of malingerers, such as realize the pecuniary advantages of their position. When these are excluded, a large class remains in whom the injury must undoubtedly be regarded as the *fons et origo mali.* A curious and interesting train of symptoms supervene after the accident, indefinite from a localizing point of view, but quite definite from the standpoint of the patient himself. Mental irritability, with a ready tendency to fly into a passion—Kaplan's explosive diathesis—may be regarded as an almost constant symptom. The patient is changed in his manner towards those near and dear to him, restless, irritable, and intolerant of noises, morose, and incapable of managing his financial affairs.

The change may be insidious in origin, but, in the absence of appropriate treatment, steadily progressive. The mental changes, unless checked in time, tend to merge into definite insanity, not infrequently of a homicidal or suicidal character.

Insomnia, with terrifying dreams, loss of appetite, emaciation, headache, vertigo, nervousness, amnesia, lack of power of mental concentration, and mental depression are all noticeable features. All such symptoms are aggravated by indulgence in alcohol, exposure to the sun, &c.

From a localizing point of view the symptoms are obscure, but they are probably none the less dependent on pathological changes—thickening of the meninges, effusion into the subdural and sub-arachnoid spaces, œdema of the cortex, &c. Furthermore, it will usually be found that, during the height of the attacks, the pulse-rate is slowed, the temperature raised, and the respiration embarrassed—symptoms suggestive of cerebritis and alterations in the intracranial pressure.

In exploratory operations conducted in cases of this nature, I have been particularly struck by the fact that in a large proportion of cases one finds what appears to be a condition of local œdema—some fluid beneath the dura mater, and a greater excess of the same in the pia-arachnoid meshwork. This œdema is a manifest condition readily demonstrated to onlookers. I am not an advocate of ventricular puncture in these cases, mainly on the ground that it complicates the operation and brings no added benefit in its train, but in such cases as it has been carried out the jet of cerebro-spinal fluid proves the added existence of an increased intraventricular pressure. From Leonard Hill's experiments it would appear that this œdema is dependent on chronic vascular changes—arterial anæmia, venous congestion, and cerebro-spinal and serous accumulation.

At a later date the meninges may become thickened and adherent to one another and to the surface of the brain, whilst false membranes and arachnoid cysts may develop.

Treatment. For these more general and indefinite remote results of head-injury the treatment comprises REST, bodily and mental, light diet, fresh air, cheerful but quiet surroundings, and encouragement. Potassium iodide and mercury (preferably by inunction) often do good, whilst phenacetin and antipyrin are perhaps the best drugs for relief of headache. For sleeplessness potassium bromide is perhaps the best remedy.

I have found in some cases that Turkish baths and massage have brought about considerable improvement. In advising such energetic treatment the surgeon must be guided by the case before him, these measures being more or less restricted to the less serious and more chronic cases.

In the more serious cases, especially when slowing of the pulse during the height of the attacks and some blurring of the disks point to a probable increase of intracranial pressure, operative measures must be considered. The greatest circumspection is required in determining the class of cases in which operation may be proposed, and the surgeon must be most guarded in his prognosis. So far as my personal experience goes, the operation has invariably brought about some amelioration in the condition of the patient, whilst now and again a complete cure may be anticipated. Those cases which on exploration evidence an œdema of the brain are the least favourable; those in which the surgeon finds a subdural cyst or hæmatoma offer the best prognosis.

With respect to the details of the operation, two courses are available: (1) examination of the meninges and brain at the seat of injury, and (2) a 'decompression' operation. The former course should be adopted whenever the local conditions are favourable, that is to say, whenever depression or absence of bone, localized headache, &c., suggest a localized lesion. Under other circumstances Cushing's intermusculo-temporal method of decompression should be carried out. This operation should be conducted first over the right temporal region, thus avoiding all possibility of inclusion of Broca's area, a similar operation being done on the left side at a later date in the event of incomplete success.

Traumatic cephalalgia. Of all the after-results of head-injuries, headache is the most constant symptom, either localized to the region primarily involved or diffuse. Even when diffuse, however, the aching is frequently referred to the frontal region. Localized headaches are the more acute. The patient can place his finger over the site of the trouble with accuracy and constancy. Examination on the part of the surgeon causes him to wince or cry out. Percussion with the tip of the finger not only leads to marked exacerbation but also induces a dull aching sensation, which lasts for some time afterwards. Whether acute or dull, exacerbations are of frequent occurrence, and during these attacks the patient is entirely incapacitated, desiring nothing more than to be left alone.

In some cases the pain is referred along the course of one of the superficial nerves, in which case it is probable that the affected nerve is caught up in the scar.

Headache, of whatever nature, is increased by exertion, indulgence in alcohol, exposure to the sun, &c.

Crisp English considers that many cases of localized headache are dependent on a localized chronic osteitis, and recommends trephining and removal of the affected bone. There can be no doubt that the mere removal of a disk of bone will occasionally bring about a cure, but, from my own experience, I take a different view with respect to the pathological lesions present. I have operated on over a dozen cases of chronic cephalalgia, and I have found in nearly every case definite pathological lesions—depression of internal table, thickening of the meninges, subdural cysts and subdural hæmatomata. The mere removal of a disk of bone may relieve the symptoms by reducing the local pressure or by removing a source of meningeal irritation, but such treatment seldom brings about permanent relief. The dura mater should be opened in nearly every case, the frequent discovery of a subdural complication—cyst or hæmatoma—showing that such a course is necessary.

These patients suffering from chronic headache are often pitiable subjects, spending their time in wandering from doctor to doctor, from hospital to hospital, seeking relief. They are only too eager to obtain benefit from surgical intervention. The greatest care is required in deciding as to operative procedures. Injudicious surgical measures are not only disappointing to both surgeon and patient, but also discreditable to this branch of surgery. On the other hand, it must be acknowledged that remedies other than surgical are generally inefficacious. The surgeon, therefore, takes considerable responsibility on his shoulders when he states that an operation is inadvisable. Though guarded in my prognosis, I generally advise operation on the ground that it is impossible to foretell the cause of the headache, and brilliant results may be obtained.

Treatment. When the headache is diffuse, REST, aided by the administration of phenacetin, &c., may exercise some effect. Operative treatment should not be recommended unless the intensity of the attack, blurring of the disks, and slowing of the pulse suggest that there is some increase in the general intracranial pressure. Under such circumstances, exploration should be carried out over the region at which the injury was received. In the absence of evidence with respect to external injury, a subtemporal decompression operation is the operation of election.

When the pain is localized to some special region, the outlook is more favourable. Operative measures should then always be carried out over the painful spot. A scalp-flap is framed according to the region which it is desired to expose, the disk of bone removed, and the meningeal territory examined. For detailed operative technique, see p. 20.

When the pain is referred along the course of one of the scalp nerves, it may be relieved by alcohol injections (see p. 314), or by exposure of the nerve, followed by removal of at least 1 inch of its trunk.

Traumatic epilepsy. When epilepsy arises after a head-injury, it is almost the invariable rule that the attacks should partake *at first* of the focal or Jacksonian type. A case of traumatic epilepsy should, therefore, possess the following characteristics :—

1. The fit should be preceded by some sensory or motor aura—the aura corresponding to the region of the brain primarily involved.

2. The fit should always start by twitchings of the parts supplied by the motor area which is in direct relation, or in close proximity, to the site of dural or osseous lesion.

3. The fit may remain localized to the region first affected, or, as is more commonly the case, may spread to other regions. In the latter case the various motor areas are affected in a certain definite order, according to their cortical arrangement. Thus, a fit arising from irritation of the right cortical face-area leads first to twitchings, then to convulsions, and perhaps finally to paralysis on the contralateral face-muscles, the movements then spreading from the face to the upper extremity, and from the arm through the trunk to the lower extremity. When the fits become generalized, spreading to the opposite side of the brain, the cortical areas are affected in the reverse order.

4. The patient should retain consciousness throughout the attack.
5. The fits should not be succeeded by any paresis or paralysis.

Later on, when the fits become more frequent and severe, they lose their typical Jacksonian characters, the various regions being affected so rapidly one after the other that all focal symptoms tend to be obscured. The fits are then often associated with definite loss of consciousness, and succeeded by paresis or paralysis of the parts primarily affected. The patient also usually complains of lassitude or headache, this lasting some hours after the termination of the fit.

Traumatic epilepsy does not always partake of the typical Jacksonian type. Sometimes the fits are so sudden in onset and violent in character that, from the first, the more typical features are absent. Again, fits of the focal or Jacksonian type do not necessarily imply that some pathological causative agent will be found on exploration. Ordinary epilepsy sometimes partakes of the focal type. I have myself operated on three cases of focal epilepsy, deceived by their Jacksonian characteristics, and found nothing abnormal. On the other hand, in all these cases definite and permanent improvement was observed subsequent to the surgical procedures.

It might also be added that encouraging reports are to hand, not only in cases of idiopathic epilepsy with focal symptoms, but also in cases without focal symptoms. A decompression operation is carried out on the basis of Kocher's statement to the effect that the fit is immediately preceded by a rise of intracranial pressure, for which a safety-valve must be supplied—such as is afforded by an intermusculo-temporal operation of decompression. Whether Kocher's statement is correct or not, the fact remains that some cases of idiopathic epilepsy, without focal symptoms, benefit considerably from operation.

The localizing symptoms of traumatic epilepsy. When the cause of the trouble is situated over the motor area—the pre-Rolandic cortical strip—the fits should commence by twitchings of the fingers, toes, corners of the mouth, &c., according to the site of the lesion. The fits are seldom preceded by any sensory auræ, though occasionally such may be the case, for even at the present day some doubt exists as to whether the precentral area should be regarded as purely motor or sensori-motor. In other cases, the patient, without being able to state definitely his sensations previous to the onset of the fit, may be able to foretell its immediate development, and still more rarely he may be capable of aborting the fit or diminishing its intensity by grasping firmly or massaging the region of the body in which the fit first develops.

When Broca's motor speech-area is primarily involved, the fits are preceded by difficulty in phonation, mumbling of words and incoherence, grinding of the teeth, &c., the fits then rapidly spreading to the parts responsible for the movements of the muscles of face and upper extremity.

When the fits arise from a post-central source of irritation, they are usually preceded by well-marked sensory auræ—tinglings, burning and painful sensations—again according to the region affected.

When preceded by sensations of taste and smell, the lesion is probably situated over the anterior part of the temporo-sphenoidal lobe.

When by visual impressions—flashes of light, &c.—the lesion is probably situated over the occipital lobe of the brain.

Pathology. The pathological conditions responsible for the development of fits are various, resolving themselves, when fully investigated, into two main groups: those associated with meningeal changes only, and those accompanied by definite cortical scarring and tract degeneration.

In the event of osseous deficiency the scalp is usually more or less adherent to underlying structures, and the gap in the skull filled with dense fibrous tissue, which is itself adherent to the membranes of the brain and perhaps to the brain itself.

In the absence of osseous deficiency, the cerebral irritation is usually dependent on depressed fragments of bone, on subdural hæmatomata and cysts, and on meningeal thickening.

In the event of cerebral degenerative changes it may be presumed, whether there is a deficiency in the bone or not, that considerable matting of meninges and cortex is existent with pyramidal degeneration.

In the absence of evident signs of external injury, cases of focal epilepsy in the young require careful investigation, inquiry being made as to difficult labour, for, as Harvey Cushing points out, 'When we consider the widespread lesions associated with those cases that later on are recognizable as Little's disease, and that presumably an enormous number of children receive at birth some trifling injury which, from lack of symptoms, is overlooked, may it not be that many cases of so-called idiopathic epilepsy dating from childhood can be safely attributed to the effects of early traumatism ?'

In all these, and in other doubtful cases, before undertaking surgical procedures, the surgeon should obtain the services of a skilled neurologist.

The clinical course of the case. If a typical case of Jacksonian epilepsy can be observed from beginning to end, many curious and interesting features will be observed. The fits, at first typically Jacksonian, gradually lose their typical character, becoming more frequent and less focal in nature, the patient losing consciousness during the fit, and the fits succeeded by weakness or paralysis of the parts primarily involved. The general mental state of the patient suffers proportionately—he becomes morose, despondent, irritable, homicidal, or suicidal in tendency. How far these retrograde symptoms are dependent on degenerative processes in the brain, and how much they result from the moral effect of the frequent epileptiform seizures, are questions that can only be determined by observing the effect of treatment, surgical or otherwise. Some cases respond readily to treatment, others are too far advanced to experience any material benefit, some end their days in the lunatic asylum.

In any case, surgical treatment, if adopted at all, must be carried out before definite brain-degeneration arises—such changes being evidenced by spasticity of the limbs, exaggerated knee-jerks, &c. When such pathological changes are existent, there can be but little hope of benefiting the patient.

Further points in the clinical course of the case, and such also as throw further light on the pathological conditions present, will be obtained by a survey of 21 cases that have come under my own care or close observation.

Time elapsing between the date of the accident and the first fit.

Between 1 and 19 years	9 cases
Within 8 months	9 cases
After a few days	1 case
Uncertain	2 cases

Age at time of accident.

Before 15, 12 cases. Youngest, 3 years.
After 15, 9 cases. Oldest, 55 years.

Sex.

Males 20. Females 1.

Conditions found on external examination and on operation.

External examination: Depression of bone and scar, 6 cases.
Deficiency of bone, 3 cases.
Scar only, 5 cases.
Nil, 7 cases.

At operation: Sclerosis of bone, 1 case.
Tuberculous mass, 1 case.
Subdural cyst or hæmatoma, 8 cases.
Scalp adherent to dura, 3 cases.
Scar in brain, 1 case.
Œdema of brain, 3 cases.
Nil found, 1 case.

Some lesion, such as might be accepted as responsible for the development of the fits, was discovered in 17 out of 18 cases. Duret's experience tends to bear out the view that some pathological lesion will be found in almost every case. In 67 cases reported the following conditions were found :—

Depression of bone, 27 cases.
Splinters of the internal table, 15 cases.
Cysts, subdural, 4 cases.
Thickening of membranes, 7 cases.

Operation. When the localization of the trouble is suggested by the presence of focal symptoms, and by a corresponding scalp- or bone-injury, no difficulty need be experienced in determining the site of exploration. When the fits are associated with definite focal symptoms, but without the supplementary evidence obtained by visible signs of external injury, exploration should be conducted over that region of the brain from which the fits appear to emanate. In the absence of all localizing brain symptoms, operative measures should be carried out over the site of scalp or bone lesion.

Whatever the circumstances of the case, the preliminary details are identical. The scalp is shaved, cleansed, the head enveloped in gauze, and the scalp-tourniquet applied.

The formation of the scalp-flap. When the scalp is adherent to the bone, the incision, carried throughout down to the bone, is made in such a manner that the flap will not only allow of the detachment of the scar, but will also permit of the complete exposure of the neighbouring portion of the skull.

When the scalp is adherent to dura or brain, as the result of osseous deficiency, the edge of the knife should be directed towards the under aspect of the flap, and the flap carefully peeled away from the region of the gap.

The examination of the bone.

When no fracture is found, the operator should trephine over the cortical area from which the trouble appears to emanate.

When a fissured fracture is found, trephining is carried out where the line of fracture cuts across that region of the brain which appears to be involved.

When a depressed fracture is found, the trephine is applied in such a manner that the circle just includes the outer segment of the depression. After removal of the disk, the dura mater should be peeled away from the under surface of the bone, and the whole of the depressed area cut away with the craniectomy forceps.

When there is osseous deficiency and when the gap is filled in with fibrous tissue, adherent to the margins of the gap and probably to the dura or brain as well, it is essential that this fibrous tissue should be freely removed. All evidence goes to substantiate the statement that meningeal irritation is the main cause of the fits, &c.

The removal of this tissue is best carried out by beginning at the most promising part of the gap, detaching the tissue adherent to the most prominent portion of the bone, and exposing the underlying dura mater. The central mass of scar tissue should then be seized with forceps, lifted up and detached as completely as possible, both from the margins of the gap and from the underlying dura or brain. In the more complicated cases, where the scar tissue is adherent to dura and brain, the most careful dissection is required, and in many instances it is necessary to include that part of the dura mater which is incorporated with the scar. The cerebral substance should be carefully protected (see below).

The treatment of the dura mater. When the dura has not been injured during the process of exposure, pulsating freely, and presenting a normal appearance, preparations can be made to close in or protect the gap in the skull.

When the membrane bulges outwards, and when, in other respects, the indications point to an increase of intradural pressure, the dura must be incised in a crucial manner, and further investigation carried out in the search for a subdural hæmatoma, arachnoid cyst, or other lesion. A hæmatoma is washed out and drained, an arachnoid cyst shelled out or treated by excision of the parietal wall (see p. 204).

When the dura is thickened, matted, and adherent to the brain, it is picked up at the least adherent part and carefully dissected away, exposing the pia-arachnoid region. The surface of the brain being so brought into view, the scalpel and dissecting forceps may be required to remove all tags and shreds of matted tissues, this process being continued till a reasonably healthy region has been brought into view.

The treatment of a cortical scar. There is no reason why a superficial scar should not be freely removed, but, unfortunately, this procedure is necessarily followed by the formation of another scar, at least as extensive as the original fibroid condition. The removal of cortical scars has therefore justifiably fallen into disrepute, and most surgeons content themselves with an exposure of the pia-arachnoid region, the actual cerebral substance being left intact. All bleeding must be arrested, blood extravasation merely favouring the formation of fresh adhesions.

The prevention of fresh adhesions between the dura and the brain and between the scalp and the dura or brain. 'It is useless to talk about the prevention of fresh adhesions; they form in spite of anything that may be done' (English). With this statement, I am in complete accord. It has been recommended that fresh egg-albumen, gutta-percha tissue, silver foil, &c., should be inserted beneath the dura or between the scalp and the brain. Experience shows, however, that all these substances are useless, being invaded or surrounded by granulation tissue, and, later on, absorbed by or enclosed in dense fibrous tissue.

The formation of adhesions between the scalp and the dura or brain can, however, be effectually prevented by the insertion of plates, &c. (see below).

The closure or protection of gaps in the skull.

Indications for operative treatment. Large defects, post-operative or traumatic.

Small defects situated over exposed portions of the skull or over the more important regional areas.

Both large and small defects associated with chronic headache, insanity, Jacksonian epilepsy, &c.

Certain congenital defects in the vault.

Small defects, unless situated in exposed regions or associated with symptoms, seldom demand protection.

Methods.

(*a*) *The formation of bone-flaps, derived from neighbouring parts of the skull, from some other bone of the patient, or from the bones of a freshly-killed animal.*

(*b*) *The interposition of plates of some foreign material between the scalp and the bone, or the insertion thereof into the osseous deficiency.*

(*a*) *Bone-flaps. The osteoplastic method of König and Müller.* Two flaps are framed in the manner described below, and the two interchanged in position. A ∩-shaped flap, comprising the whole thickness of the scalp, is turned down so as to expose the region of the deficiency, the margins of the incision lying about ½ inch outside the margin of the gap. The flap is dissected from underlying structures to which it may be adherent, care being taken to avoid injury to the blood-vessels entering at the base of the flap.

A second flap is framed from the scalp immediately to one side of the first flap. This second flap corresponds in size and shape to the one already framed, but differs in that its base points in the opposite direction. It is also peculiar in that it consists of the whole thickness of the scalp plus the external table of the skull. The scalpel is carried down to the bone, and the margins of the incision retracted in such a manner as to allow of the application of the hammer and chisel. The external table is cut through along the line of the scalp incision and split away from the rest of the bone. The two flaps are now interchanged in position and sewn down with a few salmon-gut sutures.

The osteoplastic flap is by no means easy to frame, the external table tending to split up during the process of separation ; moreover,

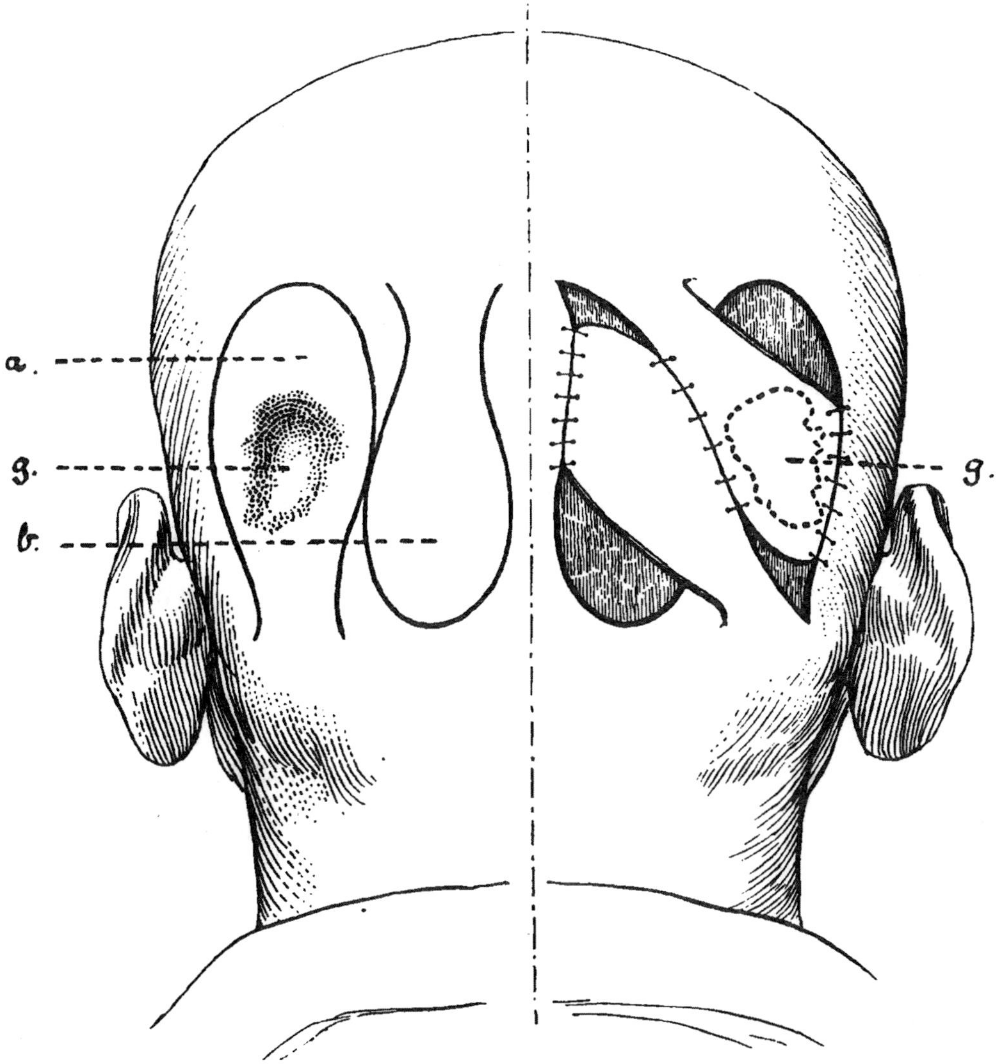

FIG. 59. THE KÖNIG-MÜLLER OSTEOPLASTIC FLAP. *a.*, The scalp-flap ; *b.*, The osteoplastic flap ; *g.*, The gap in the skull.

its formation is confined to the upper-occipital and parietal regions of the skull, regions where the two tables are separated by diploic tissue. In the temporal and cerebellar regions this method cannot be adopted, and in the frontal region the deformity and scarring act as a bar to such operative procedures.

In suitable cases, however, good results may be obtained by this method. Asepsis is essential to success.

Bone-flaps derived from some other bone of the patient (e. g. the tibia), or from the bones of a freshly-killed animal (e. g. the scapula of a dog), seldom yield satisfactory results. The gap in the skull is first exposed, the margins refreshed, and the size and shape estimated. The bone-graft is then cut from the other bone, suited in every respect to the deficiency, inserted in the gap and sewn into position. The graft, however, seldom retains its vitality, being invaded by granulation tissue, and converted, in the course of time, into dense fibrous tissue. Furthermore, in the event of the slightest failure of aseptic technique, it acts as foreign body and must be removed.

The attendant difficulties and the frequent failures of these auto- and hetero-transplantations of normal bone lead to the utilization of decalcified, calcined, and boiled bone-plates. Between these there is very little to choose, for, whether due to the absence of calcium salts or the destruction of bone-cells, they merely act as scaffolding media for the formation of fibrous tissue and are more or less completely absorbed.

(*b*) *Plates of some foreign material.* The following method has been found to give the most satisfactory results. Plates of pure annealed silver are utilized, $\frac{9}{1000}$ inch in thickness (No. 2 Birmingham metal gauge). The plates are light and of fair malleability. Supposing now that it is required to protect a deficiency in the vault—irregular in shape, round or oval, it matters not—the maximum antero-posterior and vertical diameters are measured and a piece of silver cut out, which is about $\frac{1}{2}$ inch greater in both diameters. The convexity of the skull in the region of the gap is estimated and the plate hammered into corresponding shape. This is readily carried out by placing the plate on a heavy leaden base and hammering to the required convexity. The convexity is regulated by the site of application of the blows, the heavier being applied to the central or apical portion of the plate, the weaker to the periphery. A rough general convexity is so produced. The edges of the plate are smoothed with the file, and a few holes bored to allow of the escape of any blood or cerebro-spinal fluid that might tend to collect beneath.

The plate is then boiled and applied as follows. The osseous defect is exposed by a scalp-flap—not including pericranium—the margin of the scalp-flap lying *at least* 1 *inch* external to the margin of the gap.[1] The flap is dissected down so that its base is situated *not more than* $\frac{1}{2}$ *inch* below the lower limit of the gap. The pericranium is then stripped away towards the periphery. The plate is applied so that it rests below against the base of the scalp-flap, lies

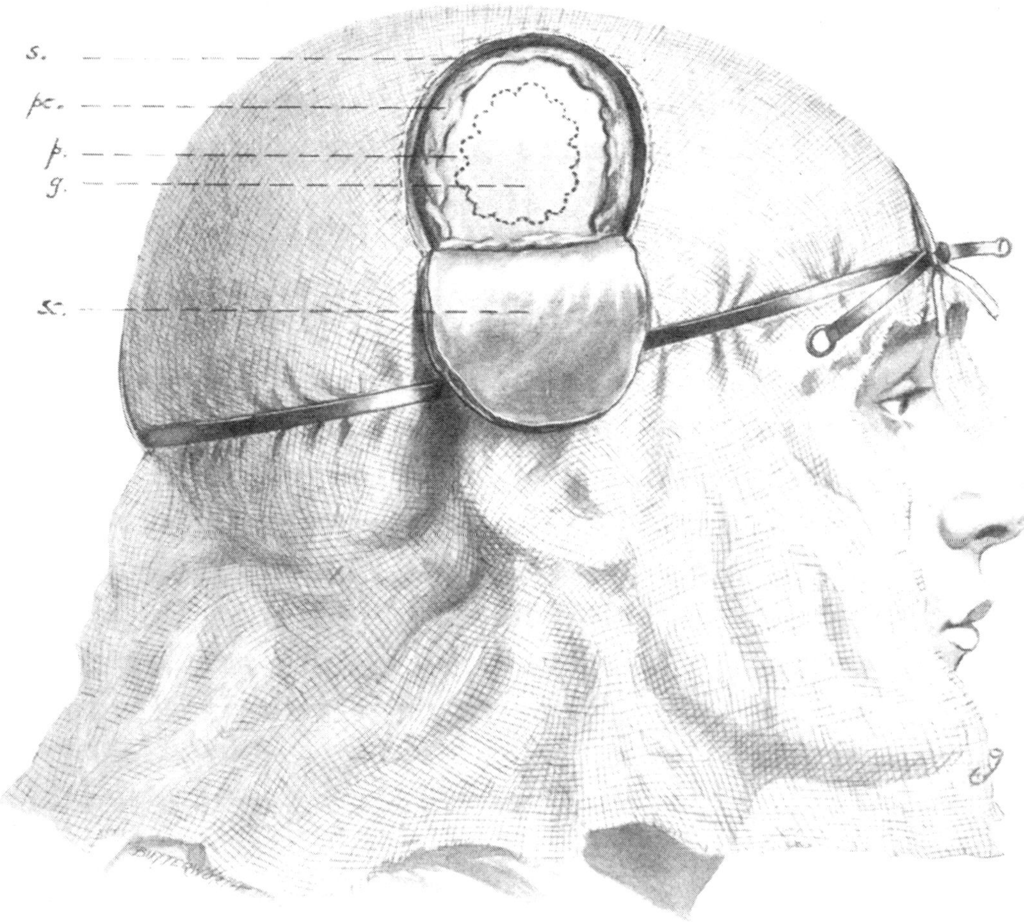

FIG. 60. THE AUTHOR'S METHOD OF COVERING IN A GAP IN THE SKULL. *s.*, The scalp ; *pc.*, The pericranium ; *p.*, The plate ; *g.*, The gap in the skull (inside the irregular dotted line) ; *sc.*, The scalp-flap.

throughout between the scalp and bone, and overlaps the margins of the gap by about $\frac{1}{2}$ inch. The pericranium is heaped up around and over the margins of the plate, and the scalp-flap replaced. The plate is maintained in position by the support received from the base

[1] It is absolutely essential that the scalp incision should lie some distance away from the outer margin of the plate. Failure to adopt this procedure impedes the healing of the wound and adds to the risk of infection.

of the flap, marginally by the pericranium, and generally by the reposition of the scalp-flap.[1] In the process of time, new bone is formed by the pericranium, this and fibrous tissue developing along the line of the scalp incision fixing the plate accurately and firmly in position.

Needless to say, absolute sterility of the field of operation and of all media is essential. In the event of failure in cleanliness, however slight, it will become necessary to reopen the wound and remove the plate. In such cases a second attempt may be made at a later date.

Results. The results attained by operative treatment must always be considered under two headings: the immediate and the more remote.

The immediate results are almost always of a satisfactory nature, the fits being more or less completely controlled, or so diminished in quantity and quality as to satisfy both surgeon and patient. Such early results may be regarded as the general rule, and some enthusiasts believe that the ultimate results are equally satisfactory. However, in following up these cases, it will be found that, in a considerable proportion of cases, the more remote results are by no means so satisfactory. A complete and permanent cure is seldom obtained, though the great majority of cases evidence considerable improvement, the fits recurring, though less frequent and less intense than previous to the operation.

The results which may be obtained should therefore be considered as follows:—

Cases of complete and permanent cure.

Cases of definite amelioration.

Cases in which no benefit is derived.

In 20 cases that have come under my own care, the following results were obtained:—

Complete cure in 2.

Marked improvement in 14.

No change in 4.

Cushing reports on 128 cases of traumatic epilepsy, operative

[1] If desired, the plate may be anchored in position by means of a few small silver-plated screws.

measures being adopted in 58, 40 cases of focal epilepsy and 18 exhibiting no localizing feature. The results were as follows :—

12 cases were free from attacks for from 1 to 5 years.

30 were greatly improved or showed some improvement.

17 exhibited no change.

2 died in status epilepticus.

Traumatic insanity. Traumatic insanity is closely allied to traumatic epilepsy, occurring, as a general rule, late in the history of the case, when the frequency of the fits and the associated disturbance of the higher faculties breaks down the mental and moral control of the patient.

The particular form of insanity varies according to the circumstances of the case. Kraft Ebbing reported on 42 cases, the disease partaking of the following types :—

18 cases of mania.
13 cases of dementia.
5 cases of dementia with epilepsy.
3 cases of general paralysis.
3 cases of melancholia.

Of 104 cases reported by Christian,

16 were of dementia.
29 of mania.
47 of general paralysis.
12 were of epilepsy.

Mania—of a violent type—usually develops within a short time of the accident—a few hours or days. Its development is probably dependent on an *acute cerebral œdema*—the result of a most severe grade of vaso-motor depression—and it is often, though not necessarily, associated with extensive cerebral injury. There is marked engorgement of the cerebral venous system, and considerable increase of cerebro-spinal fluid, both on the surface of the brain and in the ventricular spaces.

When insanity develops at a later date, of whatever variety, it is probably dependent on definite pathological changes. Ll. Powell, Duret, and others, after investigating the conditions, came to the conclusion that the injury was comparatively superficial—subdural cysts and hæmatomata, pachymeningitis, osteosclerosis, ossification of the dura mater, &c. They also maintain—an opinion that I also hold—that the nervous phenomena are, in most cases, due to reflex meningeal irritation.

Ll. Powell reports on 67 cases submitted to operation, with the following results :—

In 41 there was mental recovery.
12 there was marked mental improvement.
5 there was slight mental improvement.
4 there was no change.

Death resulted in 5 cases.

The results obtained by surgical treatment are largely dependent on the time that has elapsed since the accident. Lapse of time is no bar to operation, but the sooner this procedure is carried out the better for the patient.

Treatment. I think that it must be accepted that, without surgical interference, the prognosis is of the most unfavourable type. These cases, if left to themselves, drift into the public and private lunatic asylums, there remaining to the end, hopeless wrecks.

If such is the case—and I think that refutation is impossible—and if it be accepted that definite pathological changes are usually present, then it is obvious that surgical interference offers the only hope of cure or alleviation. The surgeon must be guided by the case before him, but, in the absence of hereditary taint, exploration should be carried out, preferably at the site of the original injury, and as early as possible before the advent of definite cerebral and pyramidal degenerations.

The operative details vary according to the necessities of the case. Thus, in acute mania, acting on the supposition that the development is dependent on an acute cerebral œdema, the surgeon should carry out a decompression operation. Personally, I hold the view that Cushing's subtemporal decompression operation (see p. 121) should be carried out on both sides of the skull, with or without lumbar puncture.

In the more chronic cases, operative procedures are conducted over the region injured in the anticipation of discovering depressed bone, subdural cysts, hæmatomata, &c. The operative details peculiar to all of these conditions are discussed in other sections.

With special reference to general paralysis of the insane, Dr. Claye Shaw holds the opinion that a general increase of intracranial pressure is commonly present. At his instigation, and on other occasions, I have carried out decompression operations, but I have not been able to satisfy myself that the patients have experienced any benefit other than temporary. There was on each occasion a considerable excess of cerebro-spinal fluid with surface œdema of the brain, but the ultimate results were certainly disappointing.

MENINGEAL CYSTS

Amongst the pathological conditions responsible for the development of epilepsy, chronic cephalalgia, &c., meningeal cysts must be regarded as of frequent occurrence.

Traumatic meningeal cysts are varied in size, site, and structure. They may be classified as follows :—

1. *Cysts within the calvarium.* Between the dura and the bone.
Between the dura and the brain.
Within the brain-substance.
2. *Cysts projecting through a gap in the calvarium* (traumatic cephaloceles). For a description of these cysts the reader is referred to p. 40.

Cysts within the calvarium. Traumatic cysts within the calvarium, whatever their situation, may be divided into two definite groups :—

1. Where the cyst possesses fibrinous walls (in which hæmatoidin cysts may be deposited) and contains a grumous material. These cysts are usually subdural in position, are dependent on the previous existence of a hæmatoma, and are known as 'blood-cysts'.
2. Where the cyst—often of considerable size—is lined by a thin, shiny, membranous wall. The contained fluid is almost colourless, closely resembling cerebro-spinal fluid, but albuminous and having no sugar-reducing reaction. The fluid is at high tension, spurting out when the cyst is punctured. The cyst usually lies in relation to the arachnoid membrane. Hence the name, 'arachnoid cyst'.

To account for the development of these 'arachnoid cysts' two theories have been advanced. Firstly, that they arise as the ultimate result of a long-continued circulatory disturbance of the vessels of the membranes or of the cortex, with consequent local cystic accumulation of cerebro-spinal fluid or serum; and secondly, that shrinking of the brain occurs in the region of an injury as the result of sclerotic changes in the cerebral substance, any contraction tending to lead to the formation of a vacuum which becomes filled with fluid derived from the surrounding membranes. According to this latter theory, arachnoid cysts are in reality 'cysts ex vacuo'.

As regards symptomatology, little need be said. Occasionally 'arachnoid cysts' of considerable size have been discovered at post-mortem examinations which appeared to have exercised no local or general pressure effects during life. More often the cysts, whether 'blood-cyst' or 'arachnoid cyst', lead to the development of Jacksonian epilepsy, chronic headache, and the like, and are discovered during the exploratory operation carried out for such conditions. Occasionally they may be shelled out entire, but it is more usual for the surgeon to remain content with the removal of the parietal wall (see p. 195). The results obtained by surgical treatment are sufficiently gratifying.

TRAUMATIC ORBITAL ANEURYSM

(*Pulsating Exophthalmos*)

This condition was first investigated by Rivington in 1875. Since that date many other cases have been reported, and the following remarks are based on the examination of the records of 26 cases, 2 of which have come under my own care.

The nature of the trouble, the results obtained by operative treatment, and the direct evidence supplied by post-mortem examination furnish sufficient proof to justify the statement that the symptoms are dependent on the formation of an arterio-venous aneurysm, the internal carotid artery and the cavernous sinus intercommunicating by means of one or more fistulous channels. That such a lesion may arise from direct violence—the introduction of some sharp weapon along the upper and inner portion of the orbital cavity—is readily comprehensible. Such injuries are, however, of rare occurrence, and the formation of the aneurysmal communication is usually the result of indirect violence—the application of severe blows to the antero-lateral and lateral aspects of the head.

In explanation, the following preliminary facts may be accepted :—

In the great majority of cases the blow was applied to the temporal region, the patient was rendered unconscious, bleeding freely from the ear, nose, and mouth, and remained under treatment for some considerable time. From these facts it may be assumed that the patient suffered from a fracture of the base of the skull—anterior or middle fossa, or both fossæ. Evidence has already been brought forward to show (1) that the majority of fractures involving both anterior and middle fossæ traverse the body of the sphenoid, and (2) that the cavernous sinus is very susceptible to injury. It was also demonstrated that the internal carotid artery is only liable to injury in that part of its intracranial course where it is embedded in the outer wall of the cavernous sinus. Two instances of such a lesion have been described in the section dealing with injuries to intracranial vessels (see p. 148, and Figs. 53 and 54).

From these facts and from the post-mortem evidence supplied by the few cases that have come to autopsy, it may, I think, be concluded (1) that traumatic orbital aneurysm implies a condition of arterio-venous aneurysm with direct communication between the internal carotid artery and the cavernous venous sinus, and (2) that the aneurysmal formation is dependent on a basic fracture which traverses the region of the body of the sphenoid bone.

The exact nature of the communication between the two vascular channels may be estimated from the fact that proptosis—usually the first symptom to make its appearance—seldom becomes apparent till one or two months have elapsed after the accident. It would appear, therefore, probable, that the artery is not ruptured but merely weakened at the time of the injury, the weakened arterial wall gradually giving way before the force of the blood-stream till a definite communication is formed between the two channels.

The male sex, by reason of its greater liability to severe injuries, is generally the one involved, especially between the ages of 20 and 30.

Symptomatology. 1. *Proptosis*—usually the first symptom to develop—seldom makes its appearance till after the lapse of one to two months. The eyeball is protruded in the downward and outward direction, the main pulsating tumour presenting at the upper and inner quadrant of the orbit. Proptosis is generally steadily progressive, and, in the most marked cases, the globe may be almost pushed out of its socket. In any case the 'whites' of the eye are unduly prominent.

2. *Aneurysmal symptoms.* The tumour pulsates synchronously with the heart's beat, whilst compression of the common carotid of the same side results in cessation of pulsation and great diminution in the size of the aneurysmal swelling. On releasing the compression force the tumour regains its original size in two or three beats of the heart, and, for a short time, pulsates more forcibly than before. A definite thrill is imparted to the examining finger, and, on auscultation, a loud murmur is heard, not only over the tumour itself, but also widely conducted over the bones of the vault, especially along the line of the superior longitudinal sinus. The free collateral circulation between the angular and ophthalmic arteries permits of the involvement of vessels in the inner orbital and upper nasal regions. This is well shown in the case depicted in Fig. 61.

3. *Pressure symptoms.* The impairment of venous flow in those radicles which drain into the cavernous sinus is evidenced by the marked engorgement of palpebral, conjunctival, episcleral, and retinal veins. Obstruction to lymph flow is shown by a hazy cornea, chemosis, and œdema of the parts surrounding the orbit. The danger thus incurred by the cornea is rendered more serious by the inability on the part of the patient to close the eyelids over the protruded globe. Keratitis and sloughing of the globe are to be feared. From muscular involvement, squints and diplopia are frequently observed. The pupil may be fully dilated through paralysis of the third nerve.

4. *Subjective symptoms.* Defect in vision is experienced at an early date, but perhaps the most prominent subjective symptom lies in 'noises in the head', compared by the patient to the thud of a steam-hammer, the whirring of wheels, the buzzing of bees, &c. These noises are more or less constant, most annoying to the patient, and increased on bending down, straining, &c.

All these symptoms tend to become more severe as time lapses, though cases have been recorded in which the symptoms remained *in statu quo.* In the event of failure at relief or cure, the patient runs considerable risk of losing his sight from corneal ulceration, whilst repeated hæmorrhages and secondary infection may place the patient in imminent danger of his life.

Treatment. In the consideration of the treatment of this condition, the results obtained in the 26 cases investigated will afford a valuable guide.

In 4 cases an expectant attitude was adopted, the patient being kept quiet, restricted in diet, and dosed with potassium iodide. One case improved, two experienced no material benefit, and the fourth, dissatisfied, discharged himself from the hospital.

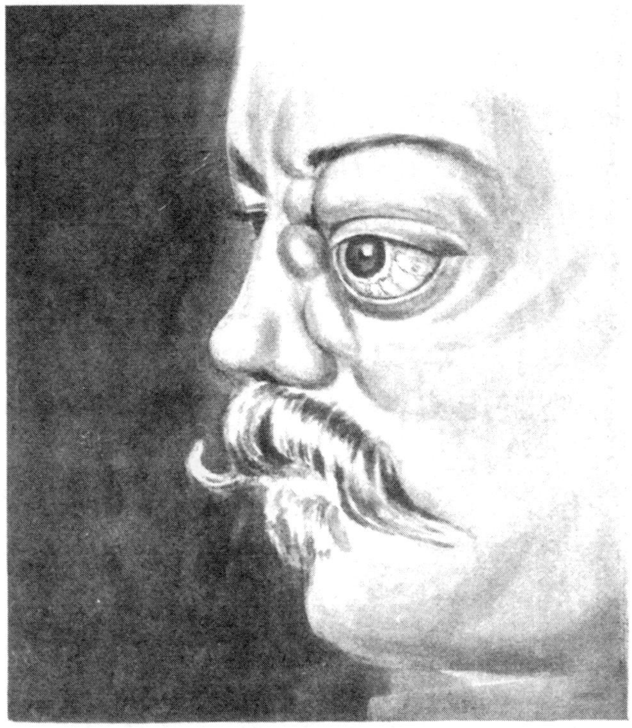

FIG. 61. A CASE OF TRAUMATIC ORBITAL ANEURYSM.

In 10 cases compression was applied to the common carotid artery, with the result that in 3 cases the conditions remained stationary whilst in the remainder, either on account of the pain produced or from complete failure to bring about any improvement, this mode of treatment was abandoned in favour of ligature of the common carotid. In some cases the carotid compression was carried out by means of tourniquets, in others intermittent digital pressure was utilized by means of relays of assistants.

In 18 cases the common carotid was ligatured, in 12 cases as a primary measure, in 6 after failure of other methods. The immediate and remote results were in all cases as satisfactory as could be anticipated. Proptosis at once diminished, the globe receding in some cases to the normal position, and the distressing subjective symptoms were almost entirely relieved. In many cases the patients were enabled to return to work.

Some defect in vision commonly persists, dependent on muscular paresis (on account of the previous stretching), retinal thrombosis, or corneal changes. The longer radical treatment was deferred the greater and more distressing were the after-effects of the lesion.

According to Sattler, however, the results obtained by ligature of the common carotid are less favourable than as stated above, and by no means devoid of danger to life. Fifty-six cases were collected with results as below :—

39 cases recovered and showed marked improvement.

11 cases experienced no benefit.

8 cases died.

It has been urged that ligature of the *internal* carotid artery would suffice to bring about equally satisfactory results, combined with less danger to life and diminished risk of secondary cerebral degeneration. Such, however, does not seem to be the case, for the anastomosis between the angular arteries and between the terminal branches of the ophthalmic is so free that the results obtained by ligature of the internal carotid appear to be unsatisfactory. Indeed, even when the larger trunk was tied, secondary operations have been occasionally required in order to excise some large anastomotic channel in the region of the inner canthus of the eye and over the bridge of the nose.

From these data, the following conclusions can be drawn :—

1. That by means of rest, careful dieting, and administration of potassium iodide in large doses, the progress of the case can sometimes be arrested, but that much patience is required and the ultimate result is entirely problematical.

2. That compression—digital or instrumental, intermittent or continuous—is painful, tedious, and usually quite inefficacious.

3. That ligature of the common carotid affords the best chance of cure or alleviation.

When should the common carotid artery be ligatured ? How soon after the development of symptoms ? This depends largely on the severity of the accident that produced the arterio-venous communication. If the blow was severe and the depth and duration of the stage of unconsciousness of a prolonged character, it may be presumed that the brain was injured. Under such circumstances early ligature of the common carotid presents an appreciable danger by reason of the development of hemiplegia on account of the further interference with the arterial supply to the brain. In such cases the patient should be confined to bed or kept quiet for not less than two months, the operation being carried out when the general condition warrants surgical interference.

In the event of early operation being imperative, periodic digital compression of the common carotid, for a few minutes at a time, may be carried out with the object of accustoming the brain to the proposed new form of circulation. In ordinary cases the sooner the common carotid is tied the better is the ultimate result.

CHAPTER VII

TUMOURS OF THE BRAIN

Tumours of the brain. Tumours may develop in any part of the cerebrum and cerebellum, from the sheaths of the efferent nerves, from the vascular tissues, and from the membranes of the brain. Tumours arising from the bones of the skull are considered elsewhere (see p. 325).

The regional distribution of these tumours may be estimated by reference to the following table[1]:—

Cerebellum	33 cases.
Deep or subcortical	32 „
Precentral	30 „
Post-central	25 „
Extra-cerebellar	19 „
Pontine	15 „
Temporo-sphenoidal	13 „
Multiple	7 „
Fourth ventricle	5 „
Third ventricle	4 „
Pituitary	2 „

Schüster,[2] from an investigation of 1,000 cases, showed that cerebellar tumours are relatively more common than cerebral, the comparative size of the two regions being taken into account. An examination of Paton's table shows that cerebellar and extra-cerebellar tumours together form rather more than 25 per cent. in 202 cases of brain-tumour formation.

Pathology. Gliomata, sarcomata, and endotheliomata are the

[1] Paton, *Brain*, vol. xxxiii, p. 67.

[2] *Pyschische Störungen bei Hirntumor*, 1903.

three commonest types of tumour formation. Other forms are fibromata, tuberculomata, syphilomata, cysts, and carcinomata.

Gliomata occur with almost equal frequency in cerebrum and cerebellum. They are generally primary and single, the boundaries

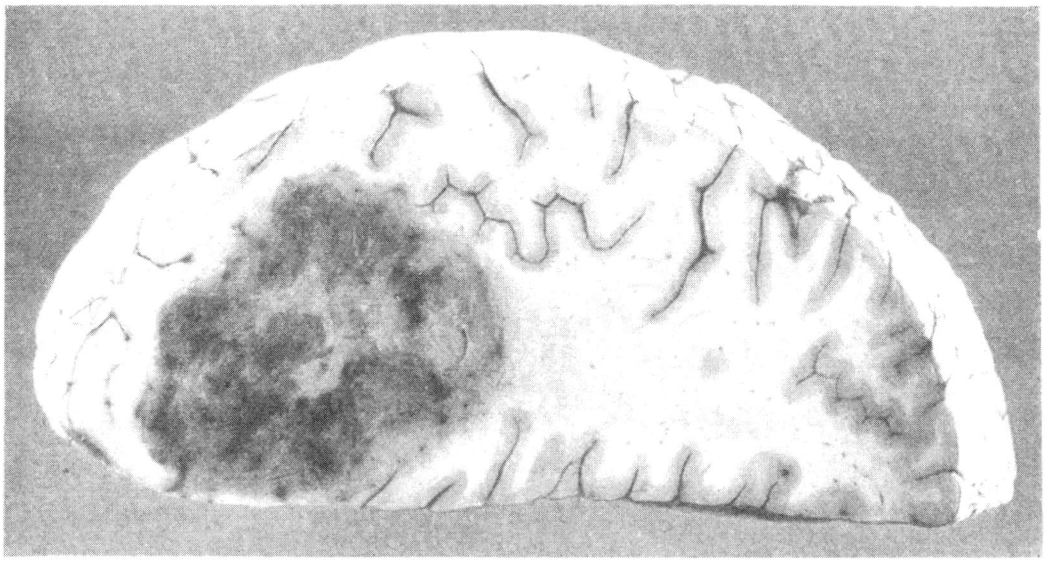

FIG. 62. A GLIOMA OF THE BRAIN.

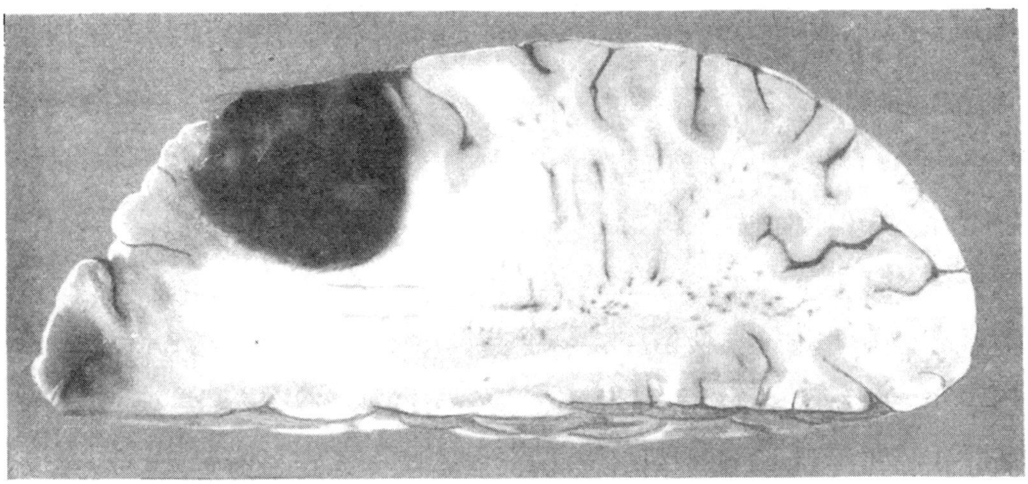

FIG. 63. A SARCOMA OF THE BRAIN.

but ill-defined, and the tumour is seldom amenable to radical surgical procedures.

Sarcomata grow from the meninges, periosteum of cranial bones, and from the sheaths of nerves and vessels. They are either primary and then single, or secondary and then multiple (sarcomatosis).

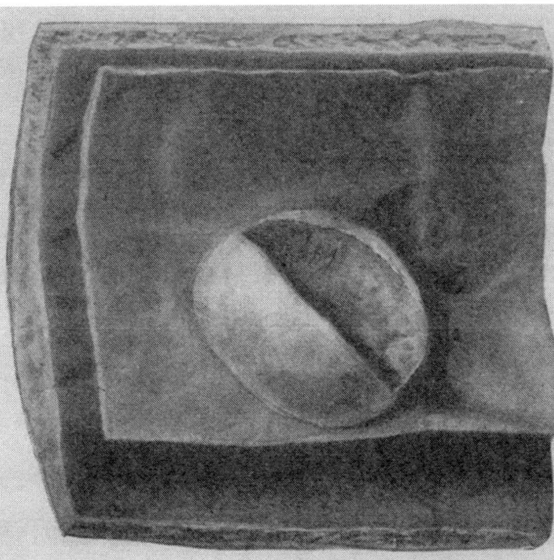

FIG. 64. AN ENDOTHELIOMA OF THE DURA MATER.

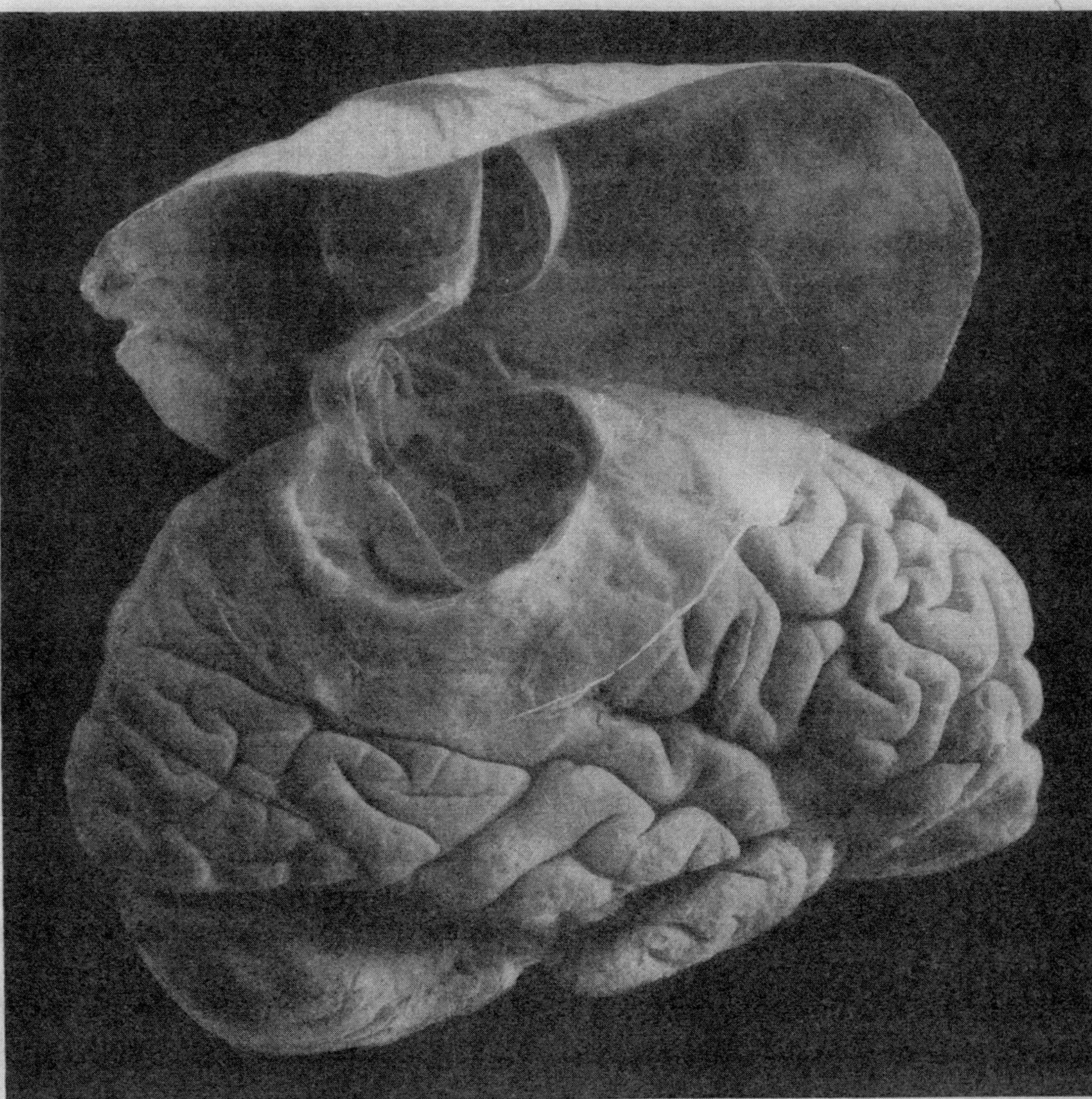

FIG. 65. A FIBROMA OF THE DURA MATER. Indenting the cortex and attached to the pia-arachnoid by fine filaments.

Sarcomata are often more or less encapsuled, tending in the first instance to exercise a compression force, and only in the later stages to invade the surrounding regions. It is during this early stage of development that the tumour is capable of removal.

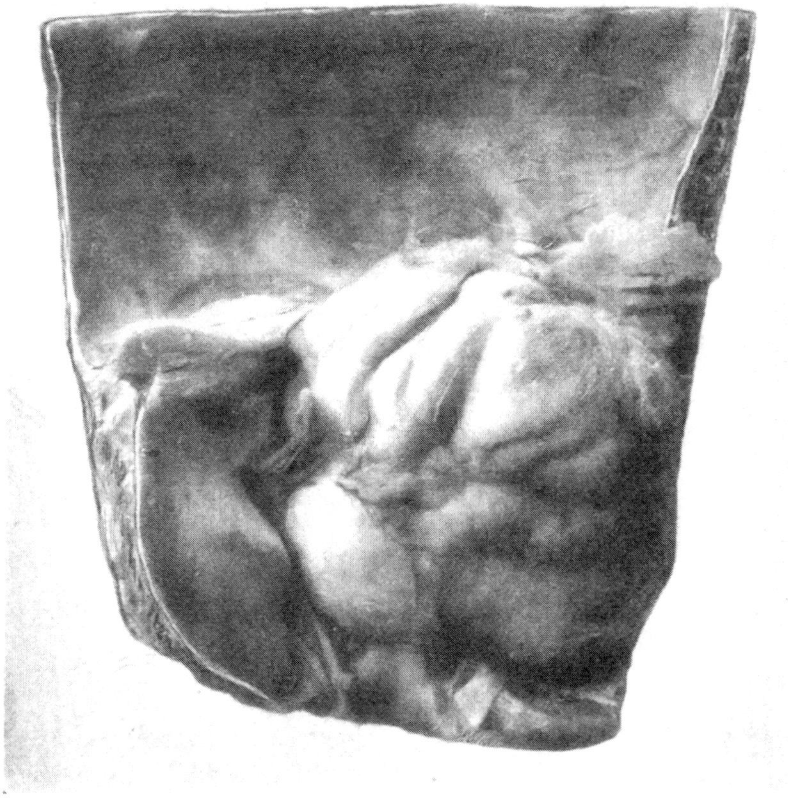

FIG. 66. AN ACOUSTIC TUMOUR. Attached loosely to the seventh and eighth nerves.

Endotheliomata grow from the meninges of the brain. They are hard, nodular, and, in their early stages, definitely non-infiltrating, and, when accessible, removable.

Fibromata are especially prone to originate in the cerebello-pontine angle, usually possessing a narrow stalk representing an atrophied nerve-trunk or vascular bundle. From the frequency with which these cerebello-pontine tumours are attached to the eighth nerve they are often designated *acoustic* tumours. They may be as small as a pea or as large as a hen's egg. In their early stages they are probably pure fibromata, appearing as pink-red lobulated tumours.

They are of slow growth, primarily compressing the brain-substance without invasion. Later on degenerative changes are prone to occur, with invasion of the cerebellar substance and extension into the internal auditory canal. Whether growing in the cerebello-pontine angle or in other parts of the skull, fibromata are often readily removed.

Tuberculomata are most commonly situated beneath the tentorium. They are often multiple. They cannot be considered as

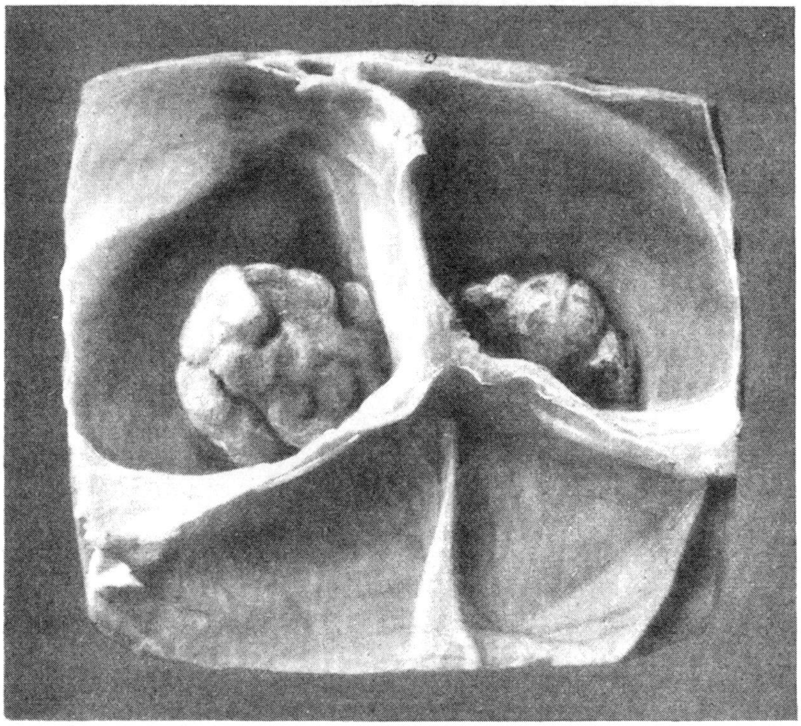

FIG. 67. SYMMETRICAL TUBERCULOMATA. Situated on either side of the falx cerebri above the tentorium cerebelli.

favourable tumours from the surgical point of view, insomuch as they are frequently associated with tuberculous lesions in other parts of the body and complicated by a tuberculous infiltration of the meninges.

Syphilomata occur with greater frequency in the cerebrum than in the cerebellum. Sometimes they are totally unaffected by antisyphilitic remedies, and, under such conditions, appear as densely hard and definitely encapsuled tumours. These more chronic gummata are usually cortical or subcortical in position, and, when accessible, are readily removable.

Cysts are of frequent occurrence. They may be (1) of traumatic origin, containing a grumous material characteristic of the incompletely absorbed blood-clot; (2) of parasitic origin (e. g. echinococcus); (3) due to cystic degeneration of a sarcomatous, carcinomatous, or gummatous mass; or (4) simple arachnoid cysts (see p. 203). Many of these cysts are amenable to surgical treatment.

Carcinomata are always secondary to cancer in other parts of the body—more especially carcinoma mammæ. They are usually multiple, and quite unsuited to surgical procedures.

Any of these tumours may be complicated by the presence of internal hydrocephalus, this condition being dependent on the pressure exercised by the tumour on the veins of Galen, or on the interference with the normal transudation of fluid from one ventricle to another.

Symptomatology. The symptoms resulting from tumour formation may be considered under two headings:—

1. *General symptoms*, dependent on the general increase of intracranial pressure.
2. *Localizing symptoms*, dependent on local compression.

Previous to discussing the symptomatology of brain tumours, it cannot be too forcibly urged that the surgeon is seldom justified in embarking on an extensive operation for tumour removal except after consultation with a neurologist. Ill-planned and ill-timed operations are usually disastrous in their results, and little creditable to craniocerebral surgery in general. On general grounds also, the symptomatology of brain tumours, as given below, must be accepted in the light in which it is offered, not representing the complete neurological aspect of the case, but affording an index to general diagnosis. For further information the reader is referred to more extensive works on brain tumours.[1]

I. General Pressure Symptoms

Headache.
Mental disturbances.
Optic neuritis, &c.
Vomiting.

[1] *Lettsomian Lectures*, by the late Dr. Charles Beevor; Duret, *Tumours of the Brain*; Nothnagel, *Tumours of the Brain*, &c.

Alterations in pulse, respiration, and blood-pressure.

Alterations in temperature.

Headache. Headache is an almost constant symptom, and presumably dependent on general or local dural tension. It may be general or localized, intermittent or continuous, intense or comparatively mild in character. It is the more intense when the tumour develops in the confined space of the subtentorium, and when the tumour is of considerable size. In young subjects, before the skull is synostosed, some compensatory enlargement of the skull may postpone the development of headache, or diminish its intensity.

The diagnostic value of a localized headache is rather problematical, but, when constantly referred to some particular region and when associated with definite tenderness on percussion, the localization of the headache assumes considerable importance in the regional determination of the tumour. Still, too much stress must not be placed on the site of the pain. A cerebellar tumour may give rise to frontal headache, and vice versa.

Mental disturbances. In the earlier stages of tumour development the patient is irritable, depressed, or apathetic, shows his objection to his fellow mortals on all possible occasions, is unable to concentrate his attention or exhibits impairment of memory. As has rather quaintly been observed, he appears in every sense to 'have a weight on his mind'. Inquiry amongst relatives will show that he has 'changed in every way', or 'is not the same man'.

Mental changes vary according to the site and size of the tumour. For example, it has been stated that a general air of elation or exhilaration (Witzelsucht) may be regarded as almost diagnostic of tumours situated in the anterior part of the frontal lobe.

As the tumour increases in size, somnolence becomes the marked feature, progressing on to stupor and coma. In rare cases, mania may develop.

Optic neuritis. Optic neuritis must be regarded as one of the most constant and valuable symptoms in the diagnosis of intracranial tumour formation. The degree to which it progresses depends more on the site of the tumour than on its size. In general, it may be stated that it is most constantly associated with tumours of the temporo-sphenoidal and cerebellar regions, less common in frontal tumour formation, still less frequent in post-central tumours, and perhaps least common in tumours of the pons. In this last-mentioned case optic neuritis is always late in development, and not infrequently absent throughout the whole stage of the illness.

Primary optic atrophy only occurs when the tumour exerts direct compression on the optic chiasma and tracts—for example, pituitary tumours.

Paton,[1] from a series of 252 cases treated at the National Hospital, of which 202 were accurately diagnosed, found that optic neuritis or atrophy was present in 81·2 per cent. cases. The fundus change, though usually bilateral, may be confined to the ipso- or contra-lateral side. Considerable discussion has taken place as to the localizing value of unilateral disk changes. For instance, it has been stated that a unilateral neuritis indicates that the tumour is situated on that side of the brain, and that when disk changes are bilateral the side which evidences the higher grade of inflammation is the side on which operation should be conducted. In the light, however, of the most recent research it would appear that unilateral symptoms are not to be relied on in establishing the localization of the tumour. Gowers[2] lays stress on the statement that with strictly unilateral neuritis one should always suspect a general rather than a local exciting cause.

The actual cause of the neuritis is still a matter of doubt. It is possible that the same cause is not present in every case. Still, sufficient evidence is to hand to justify the probability that neuritis is dependent on the general increase of intracranial pressure—there is, at any rate, a close relationship between the two. The cerebro-spinal fluid is forced into and dammed up within the vaginal sheaths of the optic nerve, leading, in the first instance, to an œdema, and later on, to compression of the lamina cribrosa and interference with the circulation.

The increase of intraventricular pressure may also act directly on the optic tracts and chiasma—the anterior boundaries of the third ventricle—the pressure being then transferred directly to the nerve tracts.

[1] *Brit. Med. Journal*, March 1, 1908. [2] *Lancet*, July 10, 1909.

Furthermore, the great intensity, great frequency of occurrence, and rapid development of optic neuritis when the tumour is subtentorial in position may be explained on the hypothesis that the rigid enclosure of the cerebellum permits of the ready application of pressure to the veins of Galen or to the iter, thus leading to an increase of intraventricular pressure, this pressure being then transferred to the optic region.

The alternative theory states that the old tissue destruction and the new tissue formation sets free certain toxic substances which act on the optic nerve-fibres, leading to œdema and inflammation. Paton, however, comes to the conclusion that 'the nature of the tumour does not play any part in determining the onset of neuritis except in so far as the nature determines its localization'.

Whatever be the localizing value of optic neuritis, it is generally accepted that it commences in the upper nasal quadrant.

Visual acuity is but little impaired in the earlier stages of optic neuritis, but so soon as atrophic changes develop, diminution in the field of vision occurs.

The pupillary changes associated with tumours of the brain are closely connected with these fundus changes. In the early stages, the pupils may be contracted with the object of protecting the inflamed surfaces exposed to light, whilst, when atrophy develops, the pupils may steadily dilate, becoming fully dilated and fixed as the atrophic changes become fully developed.

These pupil changes must therefore be taken into consideration in estimating the value of pupillary changes in general.

Vomiting. Vomiting is dependent on stimulation of the medullary vomiting centre, or on irritation of the dura mater in the immediate neighbourhood of the tumour. The dura is supplied by branches of the fifth cranial nerve, the stimulus being referred to the vagus centre in the floor of the fourth ventricle.

Vomiting is of the so-called 'cerebral' type. It is of frequent occurrence, generally irrespective of ingestion of food and seldom preceded by any nausea and retching. The attacks are often associated with exacerbation of headache, and more rarely with some slight elevation of temperature. The more severe the vomiting the more likely is the tumour to be subtentorial in position.

Alterations in pulse, respiration, and blood-pressure. In the early stages there is but little alteration in pulse and respiration. Later on, the increasing intracranial pressure acts as a stimulus on the vagus and vaso-motor centres, the pulse becomes slowed and the blood-pressure raised. When the pressure is considerable, the slow pulse and deep, even stertorous, respiration evidence the effect produced on the medullary centres. In the terminal stages the imminent exhaustion of these centres is heralded by progressive acceleration of the pulse, by great fall in blood-pressure, and by the advent of Cheyne-Stokes respiration.

The more marked the alterations in pulse and respiration the more likely is the tumour to be subtentorial in position.

Alterations in temperature. The temperature tends to remain subnormal throughout the progress of the case, except during the terminal stages when pyrexia is often observed. Occasional elevations of temperature during the course of the illness may be explained by transient attacks of ependymitis or cerebritis.

Differences of temperature on the two sides of the body may occasionally be observed, especially when the tumour involves the basal ganglia.

II. Localizing Symptoms

(*A*) To the non-excito-motor frontal region (anterior frontal).

Headache tends to be localized to the frontal region, *vomiting* is seldom a conspicuous feature, and *optic neuritis* is not only rather later in development, but also less progressive than when the tumour is placed in other situations. If the tumour occupies the orbital aspect of the lobe, primary optic atrophy (from pressure) may be existent on the affected side with optic neuritis of the contralateral fundus.

The *mental condition* is often profoundly altered and, according to some writers, more especially so when the tumour is situated on the left side. The quality of mental change varies considerably in individual cases. In some there is an attitude of general suspicion, the patient following all points in his general examination with a curious air of suspicion, in others moral perversion is the rule, whilst in a third group of cases a state of elation and exhilaration is the predominant feature, a condition which, as previously stated, is said to be pathognomonic of a tumour frontally situated.

Anosmia—uni- or bi-lateral—may be present, but, on account of the general condition of the patient, considerable difficulty is experienced in endeavouring to demonstrate the existence of this symptom.

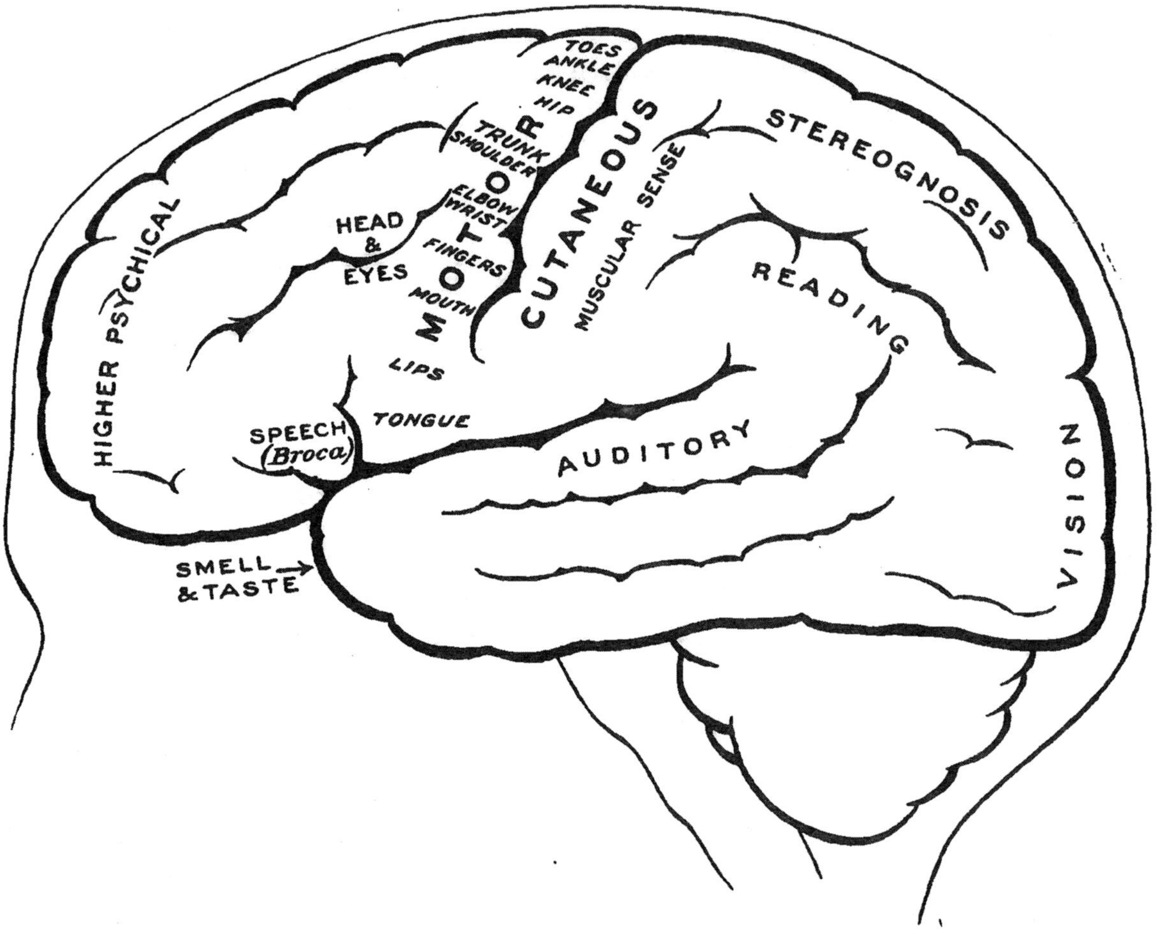

FIG. 68. THE CORTICAL MOTOR AND SENSORY AREAS.

Incontinence of urine has been observed, independent of the condition of the patient—in other words, without a sufficient degree of coma to account for the state.

When the tumour is of considerable size, some degree of *paresis* of the contralateral side of the body may result, due to backward pressure exercised by the tumour on the corona radiata preceding from the pre-Rolandic motor area. Associated with this paresis the deep *reflexes* may be increased with extensor plantar reflex (Babinski) and some diminution of superficial reflexes. The more posterior the tumour the greater the degree of paresis, and the more exaggerated the reflexes. When the tumour is situated on the left side the *motor speech* centre may be affected.

Fine tremors may be noticed, usually involving the muscles of the upper extremities, and best demonstrated by asking the patient to hold his arms horizontally with the palms downwards.

Paresis on the contralateral side may be preceded by or associated with *fits*, these partaking of the Jacksonian type and accompanied by conjugate deviation of the eyes towards the side opposite to that on which the tumour is situated. This association of fits suggests that the tumour occupies the second frontal convolution.

(*B*) **To the excito-motor frontal region.** In the early stages symptoms of irritation predominate, the patient suffering from *fits* of a focal or Jacksonian type (see p. 189), whilst, later on, *paresis* of a progressive type, involving the face or extremities unequally, becomes evident. In children, however, the rapid transference of impulses from one motor area to another causes the fits to soon lose their focal character, *general convulsions* taking their place.

If the tumour occupies the left side of the brain (in right-handed individuals) the *motor speech* centre of Broca may be involved, with difficulty in or failure of the power of speech.

Apraxia may be present, a condition characterized by inability on the part of the patient to perform certain familiar purposive movements, such as sewing, turning a key in the lock, &c.

The contralateral *pupil* may be contracted from irritation, or dilated from paralysis; the ipsolateral is variable, more commonly dilated.

In the event of extensive tumour formation and when the growth is associated with tract degeneration, the deep *reflexes* will be increased on the contralateral side, with well-marked extensor plantar response.

(*C*) **To the post-central, angular, and marginal convolutions.** Attacks of focal *epilepsy* are frequently observed when the tumour occupies the post-central convolution, such developments being probably dependent on forward pressure effects. These epileptiform attacks, however, are almost invariably preceded by some *sensory auræ*. Furthermore, the fits will usually be followed by ' some degree of anæsthesia or analgesia, a loss of tactile sensation over half the body, affecting mostly the hand and foot, with loss of power and astereognosis (inability to recognize the form and consistency, and to name objects placed in the affected hand)' (Beevor).

When situated in the left angular gyrus, *word-blindness* may result—inability to appreciate the meaning of written words, &c.

When the tumour presses on the optic radiation, *hemianopia* results, with ipsolateral temporal and contralateral nasal blindness.

(*D*) **To the temporo-sphenoidal lobe.** When the tumour occupies the anterior part of the temporo-sphenoidal lobe, more especially when it is situated on the internal aspect of that lobe, the degree of *optic neuritis* is intense. Perversion or loss of *smell* may be noticed—a symptom of difficult determination on account of the general condition of the patient.

As the result of pressure exercised on the optic tracts *hemianopia*—with hemianopic pupillary reaction (the pupil not reacting to light)—may be observed. Pupillary reactions, however, are complicated by possible paralysis of the third nerve.

Some *weakness of the face muscles* on the contralateral side is a fairly constant symptom, presumably dependent on the upward pressure exercised on the lower motor areas.

A tumour involving the more posterior and central portions of the lobe may bring about a certain degree of *word-deafness*, whilst objects may be incorrectly named or named with difficulty, the patient being more or less aware of his mistakes and evidencing considerable annoyance of the same.

In whatever part of the lobe the tumour be situated, certain sensory auræ may be present. Not infrequently the patient falls into the so-called 'dream-state'. When sensory auræ are associated with crude sensations of smell and taste, with chewing or spitting movements, the tumour is probably situated on the antero-internal aspect of the lobe.

(*E*) **To the occipital lobe.** *Headache* may be localized to the back of the head, and *optic neuritis* is usually both early in onset and intense in degree. Perhaps the most important localizing symptom is *homonymous hemianopia*—blindness in the temporal half of the retina on the same side as the lesion and in the nasal half of the opposite eye. This is explained by the fact that the fibres of the optic radiation, passing forwards from the affected occipital region, supply those retinal areas. The reaction of the pupil will be unaltered, for the pupillary nerve-fibres, in their course towards the third nerve nucleus, are only directed backwards as far as the anterior corpora quadrigemina. Consequently, an interruption of optic fibres between retina and third nerve nucleus brings about a loss of pupillary reflex when light is thrown on the blind portion of the retina, whilst if the lesion be situated further back, pupillary reaction is unaltered. This is Wernicke's sign.

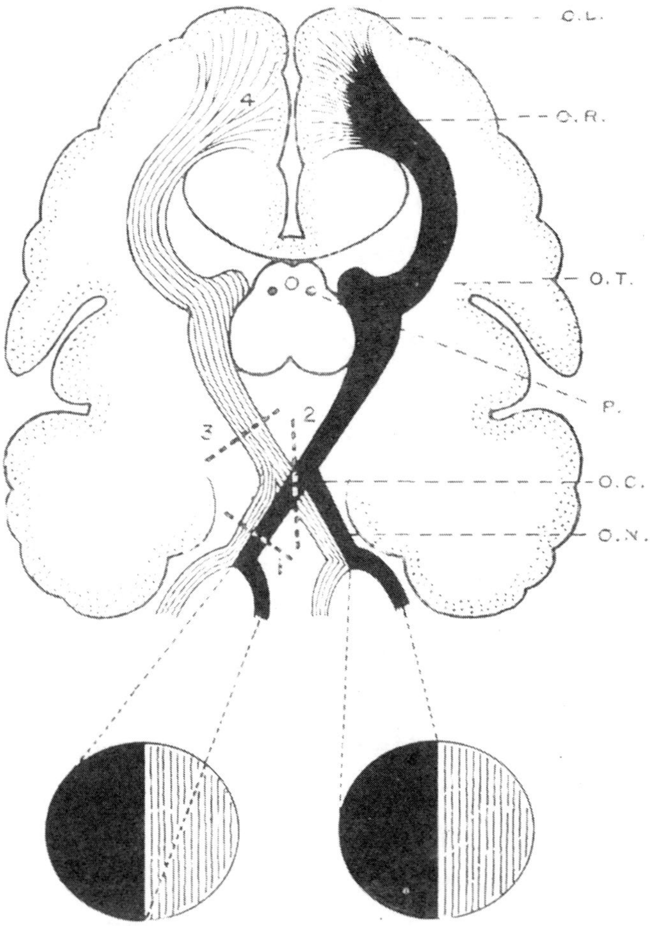

FIG. 69. THE VISUAL PATHS. O.L., Occipital lobe ; O.R., Optic radiation ; O.T., Optic tracts ; P., Pupillary fibres from optic tract to third nerve nucleus ; O.C., Optic chiasma ; O.N., Optic nerve ; 1, Blindness of affected eye ; 2, Bitemporal hemianopia ; 3, Bilateral homonymous hemianopia, with hemianopic pupillary reaction ; 4, Bilateral homonymous hemianopia, pupillary reaction normal.

(*F*) **To the subtentorial region.** Certain symptoms are more or less common to all subtentorial tumours, whether they arise within the cerebellar substance (intra-cerebellar) or immediately outside the brain-substance (extra-cerebellar). *Headache* is very severe, and in about 50 per cent. cases, localized to the back of the head, perhaps associated with stiffness of the neck muscles and retraction of the head. *Optic neuritis* is early in onset and intense in degree. It is more constant in cerebellar tumour formation than in tumours located in almost any other part of the brain. The choking of the disk is marked and hæmorrhages are frequent. *Vomiting* and other symptoms referable to increased subtentorial pressure—slow pulse, altered rhythm of respiration, &c.—are usually well marked.

Vertigo is most apparent when the patient is suddenly changed in position or tries to stand or walk. It appears in two forms, either as a definite sense of movement of self (subjective vertigo) or of objects (objective vertigo), or merely as a giddy feeling. In objective vertigo the sense of displacement of objects is more commonly from the side of the tumour towards the sound side.

Vertigo is dependent on the influences exercised by the tumour on the cerebello-vestibular apparatus, and on irritation of those branches of the fifth nerve which are distributed to the dura mater in the immediate neighbourhood of the tumour, the impulses being then transferred to the bulbar nuclei of that nerve and thence to the pneumogastric nucleus.

Ataxia and inco-ordination of movement are also prominent symptoms. Ataxia results from one or more of the following causes: (1) co-existent vertigo, (2) asthenia of the muscles of the affected side, the muscular contractions being irregular in their nature, ill-timed in their action, and often in excess of actual requirements, and (3) involvement of the spino-cerebellar tracts and their terminations.

The patient, when standing with the eyes shut and one foot advanced in front of the other, is unable to maintain his balance, staggers and tends to fall. No great diagnostic value can be attached to the direction in which he sways or falls, though, from my own experience, it would appear more probable that he should lurch towards that side on which the tumour is situated. In walking, however, there is occasionally a definite tendency to deviate towards the opposite side, probably due to over-correction of the weakened muscles on the affected side. The gait should present the typical appearance of cerebellar ataxia, and the patient may walk with the head drawn down towards the shoulder of the affected side, the chin being tilted in the opposite direction.

Inco-ordination of movement is rendered most obvious during active movement of the limb, decreasing towards the termination of that movement, and ceasing so soon as the object is attained. This is most readily demonstrated by the well-known 'finger-to-nose' test.

Nystagmus is one of the most frequent symptoms of cerebellar tumour, usually lateral, the movements coarse or fine, and most marked when the eyes are directed towards the side of the lesion.

In the more differential diagnosis between *extra- and intra-cerebellar* tumours, the following points should be noted :—

Extra-cerebellar tumours situated in the cerebello-pontine angle tend to lead to compression of the eighth nerve (with deafness and tinnitus), of the seventh nerve (with paralysis of the face muscles), of the fifth nerve (with anæsthesia of the parts supplied by that nerve), and more rarely of the sixth nerve (with paralysis of the external rectus). The ninth, tenth, eleventh, and twelfth nerves are but rarely involved.

Intra-cerebellar tumours seldom give rise to pressure effects on isolated cranial nerves. On the other hand, one expects ipso-lateral paresis or paralysis, with exaggerated reflexes (see Fig. 78). Conjugate deviation of the eyes to the side opposite to that on which the tumour is placed is a fairly frequent symptom, the deviation being associated with well-marked lateral nystagmus. When the tumour is of considerable size, or placed nearer the central portion of the cerebellum, pressure may be exerted on the pyramidal fibres with paresis or paralysis on the contra-lateral side of the body.

In addition, allusion should be made to Dana's symptom—'cerebellar fits'—said to be almost pathognomonic of an extra-cerebellar tumour (or abscess) situated in the cerebello-pontine angle. In such cases, there may be sudden attacks of tinnitus, vertigo, and apparent loss of consciousness, during which the patient falls to the ground as if struck with lightning. The final stage of falling is said to be dependent, not so much on actual loss of consciousness, as from the absence of cerebellar innervation and a total loss of equilibrium. These attacks are brought about by sudden alterations in position.

(*G*) **To the pituitary region.** Considerable research has recently been carried out, and much knowledge obtained as to the functions of the pituitary body and the symptoms that result from lesions of the gland.[1] As is well known, the pituitary body consists of two portions, an anterior (derived from upgrowth of buccal epiblast) and a posterior (formed from neural epiblastic downgrowth).

Complete removal of the body in animals invariably terminates fatally, the patient exhibiting a definite train of symptoms—cachexia hypophyseopriva—and dying within a few days or weeks, the younger

[1] Crowe, Cushing, and Homans, *Johns Hopkins Bulletin*, May 1910.

animals living longer than the older. The symptoms of apituitarism are as follows: fall of body temperature, lowering of blood-pressure, increasing feebleness, muscular tremors, a curious attitude resembling that of defæcation, coma, and death.

On further investigation it was proved that all these symptoms were observed when the anterior portion of the gland was alone removed, whilst, on the other hand, extirpation of the posterior half created no great change in the animal's general health.

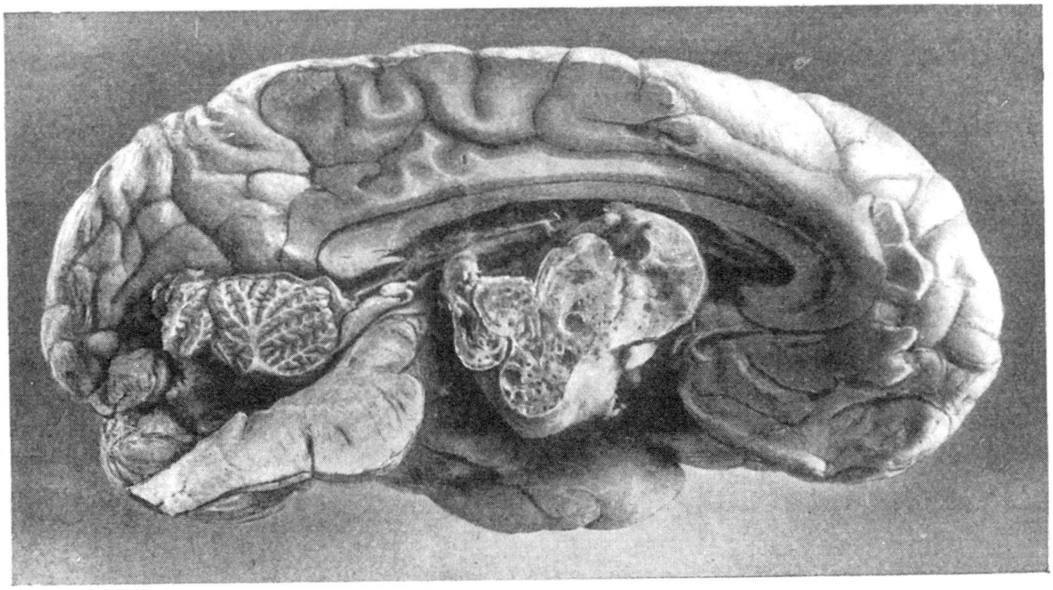

FIG. 70. A PITUITARY TUMOUR.

In the human being it would appear that the symptoms resulting from the development of pituitary tumour formation may be classified into two groups, those of hyper-pituitarism and those of hypo-pituitarism.

In the former case the secretion being superabundant, acromegaly and giantism are observed. Keith[1] considers that one of the substances secreted by the gland is of the nature of a hormone, rendering the osteoblasts hypersensitive to the various stresses that fall upon the human skeleton during life, and that the osteoblasts, at the origins and insertions of muscles, become increasingly sensitive to the traction of muscles. Muscular impressions and processes of the skeleton become exaggerated by the new bony matter, and if the

[1] *Lancet*, April 15, 1904.

epiphyseal lines be still open, the osteoblasts of which appear to be specially affected, giantism is produced. The skull and skeleton of the giant O'Brien are regarded as typical examples of the results due to over-secretion of the gland.

Hypo-pituitarism leads to a striking and rapid development of fat (adiposity), loss of sexual power and amenorrhœa, persistence of sexual infantilism (if the patient be attacked when young), harsh skin and œdematous tissues, subnormal temperature, and psychic disturbances.

In any case, whether the secretion of the gland be increased or decreased, the developing tumour tends to compress those cranial nerves with which it is in close anatomical relation. For instance, the gland, being situated immediately behind the optic chiasma, tends to compress the mesial nasal optic fibres producing bilateral temporal hemianopia, with primary optic atrophy as a final result. In some cases optic neuritis is observed with secondary atrophy. The third, fourth, and sixth nerves may also be affected, with consequent squints, ptosis, and perhaps complete opthalmoplegia.

In addition, it should be noted that glycosuria and albuminuria have been observed.

In the *general diagnosis* of brain tumours, reference must be made to *Lumbar puncture* and *X-ray investigation.*

Lumbar puncture. With respect to the desirability of carrying out lumbar puncture in brain tumours and the value of the information obtained, considerable difference of opinion exists. Lumbar puncture supplies information as to the tension of cerebro-spinal fluid and as to its bacteriological and cytological character. The evidence so obtained as to tension is of little value in view of the proved increase of intracranial pressure as evidenced by the mental condition of the patient, the headache, optic neuritis, &c. On the other hand, bacteriological and cytological examination of the fluid may point to the tuberculous or syphilitic composition of the tumour, thus offering help from the point of view of treatment. Still, information of almost equal importance can be obtained by tuberculin, Wassermann, and other tests. There is also considerable risk attendant on the process. The rapid withdrawal of cerebro-spinal fluid has been followed by disastrous results, the medullary stem being suddenly forced downwards into the foramen magnum, with corking up of that aperture, and complete upset of the medullary centres. Such a disaster is the more likely to occur when the tumour is subtentorial in position. Looking at the question from the broadest point of view, it would appear that the performance of lumbar puncture in cases of suspected brain tumour is fraught with considerable peril.

X-ray examination. X-ray examination should always be carried out. More commonly the results are negative, the nature of the tumour seldom permitting sufficient shadow formation. Occasionally the firmer and denser tumours allow of a more definite result. When the tumour arises from the bone, or is so situated as to change the shape of the part with which it is in contact, valuable information will be obtained. For example, the hollowing out and general enlargement of the sella turcica in pituitary tumour formation.

Treatment.

Indications for operation. The indications for operation must be considered under two groups :—

Those for radical operation aiming at the removal of the tumour.

Those for palliative operation aiming at the alleviation of symptoms.

For the radical operation. According to Risien Russell,[1] the following are the main indications :—

(1) Cases in which the tumour can be accurately diagnosed.

(2) Cases in which the tumour is situated in an accessible position. The more favourable sites are the surface of the cerebrum, the lateral lobe of the cerebellum, and the cerebello-pontine angle.

(3) Cases in which there is reason to believe that the tumour is simple, and of such a nature that it can be removed from its bed.

(4) Cases in which there is reason to believe that the removal of the tumour will not greatly imperil the patient's life, and, furthermore, will not result secondarily in the development of fits, paralysis, aphasia, &c.

For the palliative operation. The following are the main indications for operation :—

To prolong life.

[1] *Brit. Med. Journal,* October 26, 1906.

To alleviate the severe and persistent headache.

To stop fits.

To save the sight.

And, in general, to benefit the patient by reducing the increased intracranial pressure, *even though it may be quite impossible to remove or even locate the tumour.*

Of all the considerations enumerated above, for which palliative measures are indicated, there is no symptom which more urgently demands alleviation than optic neuritis. This question of sight-saving may be accepted as a basis on which to estimate the value of palliative measures in general. It is obvious that no mere 'decompression' operation will save the sight when the optic inflammation has progressed to atrophy, and even in the earlier conditions of neuritis cases must be carefully chosen. Herbert Bruce[1] admirably clinches the matter in the following words: 'As to the prediction of improvement of vision after trephining, everything depends on the condition of the disks. Yellowish white patches of exudate or white atrophic changes, especially when associated with macular changes, all indicate that the secondary changes in the disks will be permanent. In proportion to this development will the vision be impaired, whilst when the loss of vision has been dependent on the swelling of the disks, then not only will the sight be saved but largely improved. In other words, one might say, therefore, that when the neuritis has not progressed on to atrophy the sight would be saved.' Even in the event, however, of the ocular conditions being unfavourable for palliative operation, other factors in the case still remain—the terrible and persistent headache, the fits, the emaciation from vomiting, &c., all of which require the most careful consideration, and all of which can be remedied by an efficient decompression operation.

Radical operation for cerebral tumours. After the usual preparatory treatment and the application of the scalp-tourniquet, the skull is opened either by craniectomy or craniotomy. The two methods—with their relative advantages and disadvantages—have already been described (see Chapter II), but there can be no question that a brain tumour should be exposed by the formation of an osteoplastic flap. Such a procedure is called for on the ground that the

[1] *Annals of Surgery*, 1907, p. 543.

exact localization of the tumour is always a matter of very great difficulty, and that it is impossible to foretell with certainty as to whether it will be feasible to remove the tumour or not.

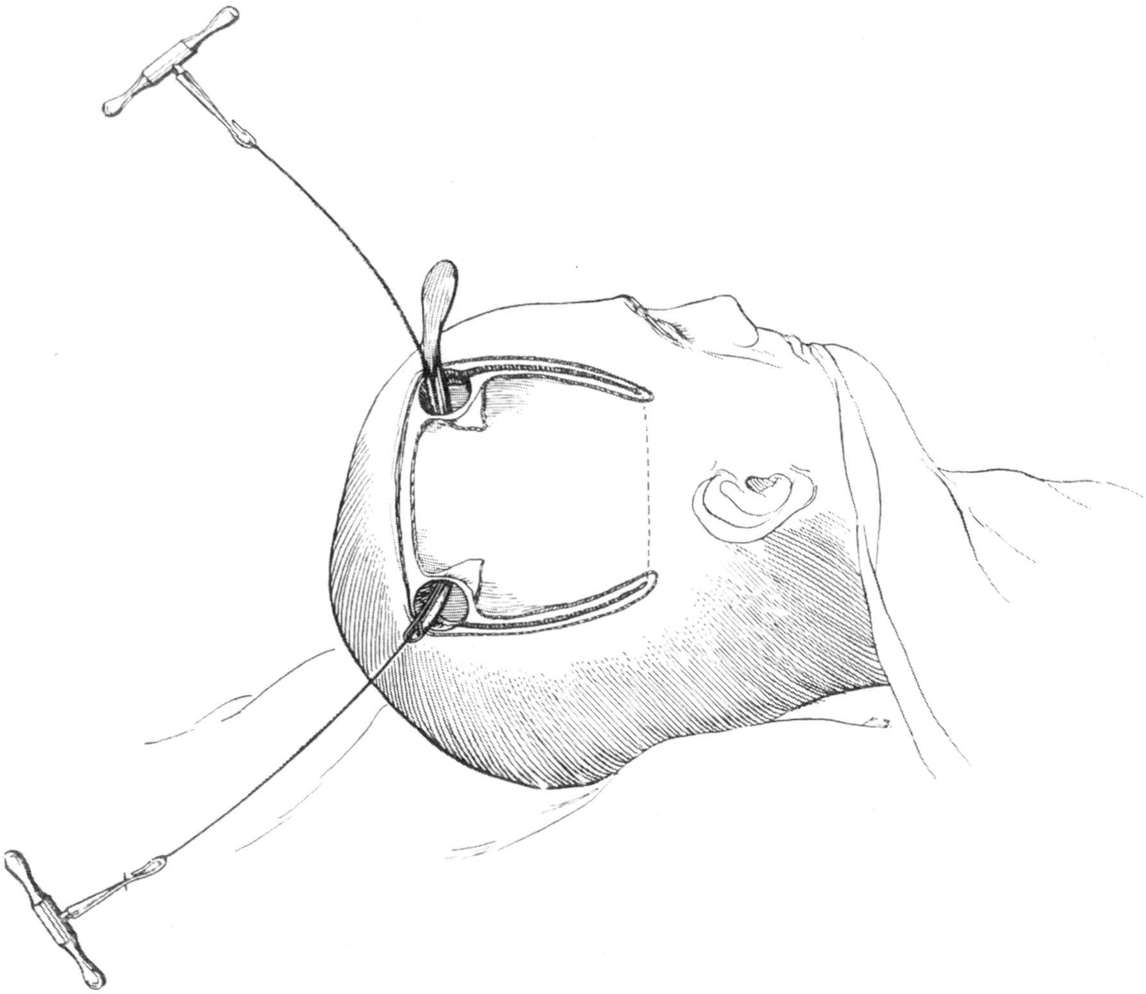

Fig. 71 a. First Stage in the Formation of an Osteoplastic Flap. Gigli's saw, protected from the dura mater by the special director, passing between the two trephine holes. For further description, see text.

A bone-flap is framed suited to the occasion, and permitting adequate exposure of the dura. The question then arises as to whether the dura should be incised, the brain explored, and an attempt made at the removal of the tumour, or whether these procedures should be postponed till the patient shall have recovered from any shock attendant on the first stage. The two-stage operation—first advocated by Horsley—is insisted on by some surgeons. By others it is maintained that it is preferable to complete the operation at one

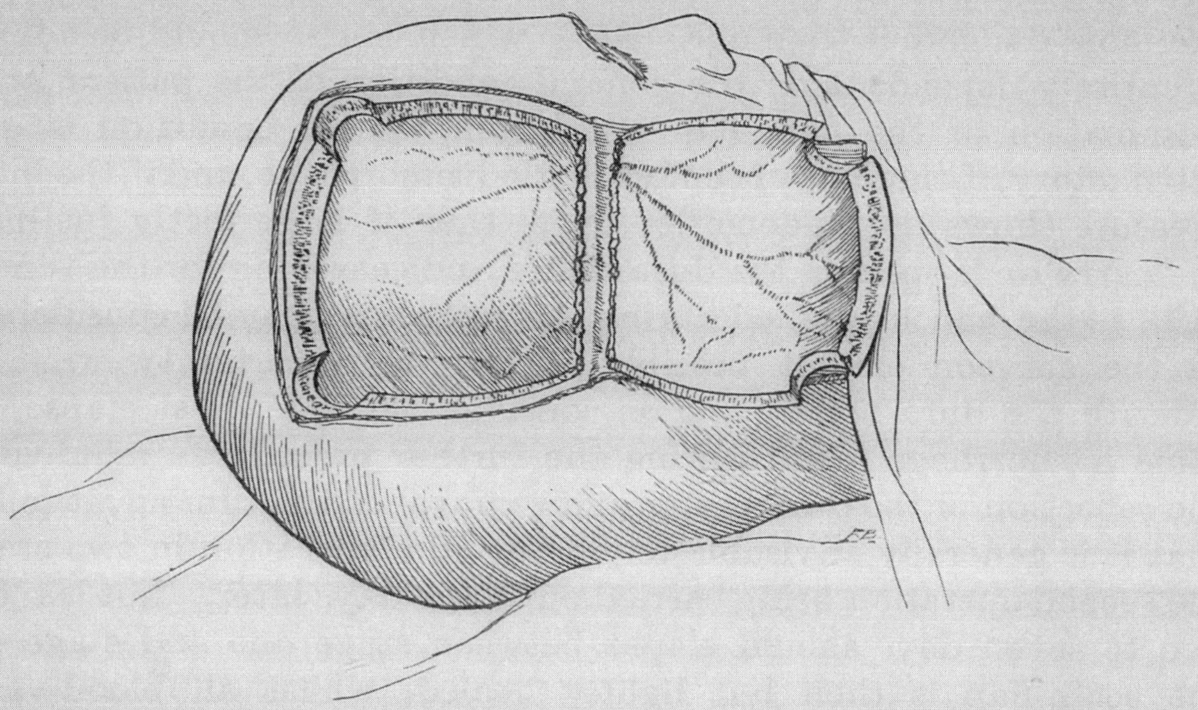

FIG. 71 B. SECOND STAGE IN THE FORMATION OF AN OSTEOPLASTIC FLAP. The bone-flap turned down and the dura mater exposed.

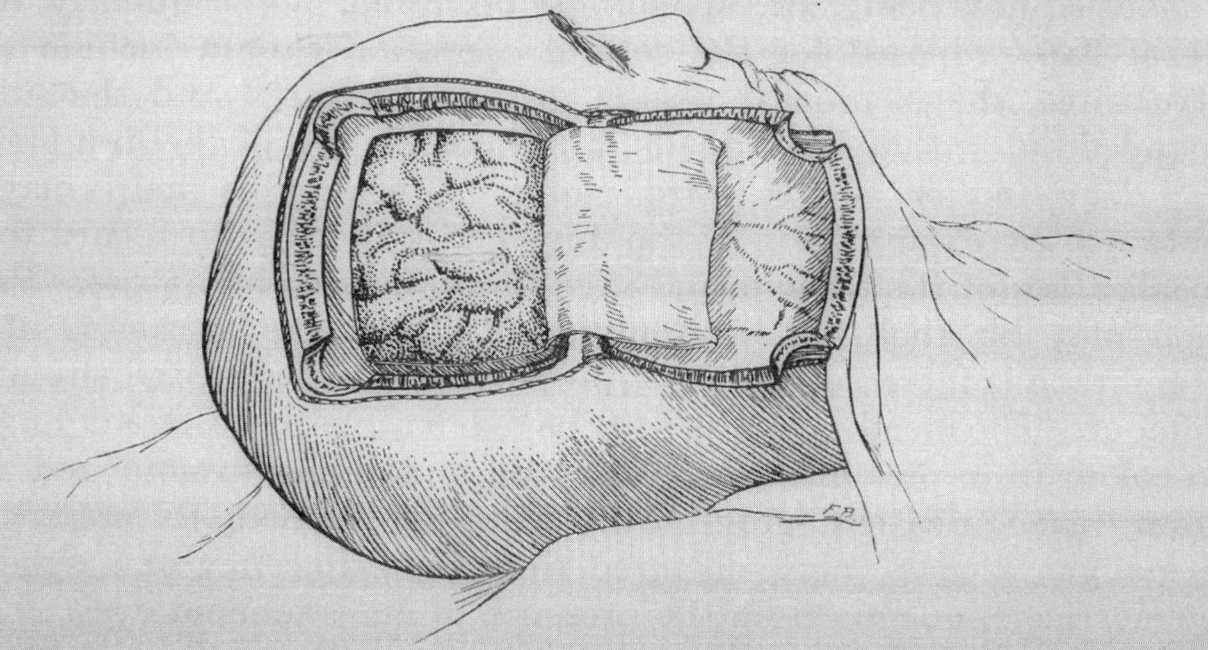

FIG. 71 C. THIRD STAGE IN THE FORMATION OF AN OSTEOPLASTIC FLAP. The dural flap turned down and the brain exposed. Note the relation of the scalp, bone, and dural incisions to one another.

sitting, mainly on the ground that two anæsthetics and two operations are more dangerous than one. As to which course should be adopted is entirely dependent on the general condition of the patient at the termination of the bone-flap formation. If his condition is quite satisfactory, if there has been but little hæmorrhage, and if the blood-pressure shows no tendency to drop, then it is perfectly justifiable to 'carry on', opening the dura mater and searching for the tumour. Still, as the shock entailed during the first stage may be considerable, as the surgeon cannot possibly foresee with certainty what lies beneath the dura mater, and as considerable time must elapse, and some hæmorrhage result during the further procedures required for the reflection of the dura mater and removal of the tumour, it follows that it is generally advisable to conduct the operation in two stages, the second operation being carried out some days later. Not less than five to seven days should elapse between stage one and stage two, the scalp-flap is then but lightly healed, whilst all blood-vessels should be sealed. The patient also will have entirely recovered from any shock attendant on the first stage.

At the second stage, the dura may be more or less covered with a film of coagulated blood, meningeal arteries and the outline of venous sinuses being correspondingly obscured. Consequently, if the dural flap proposed for the second operation should include these structures, the meningeal vessels may be ligatured and the sinuses mapped out with guide-threads at the completion of the first stage.

Examination of the dura mater. Considerable help may be obtained by examination of the dura mater, both with regard to the localization of the tumour and investigation as to its nature. Pulsation may be abolished or diminished, whilst the tenseness of the membrane is increased in direct proportion to the size and site of the tumour. The membrane also may be œdematous or adherent, anæmic in colour from pressure exercised by an underlying tumour, reddened from vascularization, grey-brown from the immediate presence of a malignant mass, plum-coloured from the adjacency of a subdural hæmorrhage, opaque from the presence of an arachnoid cyst.

Some evidence as to the nature of the tumour may be obtained by palpation—fluctuation suggesting cyst formation, solidity pointing to more definite formation.

Opening the dura mater. The membrane can be opened either by crucial incision or by flap formation. The latter method is to be preferred. All meningeal vessels that cross the line proposed for dural section must be underrun on either side of that line. The dural incision should always fall short of the margins of the gap in the skull by at least ½ inch, in order to allow of accurate approximation at the termination of the operation.

The following points with respect to the opening of the dura mater, though already enumerated in Chapter II, should be noted. The membrane is lightly incised with the scalpel, and, so soon as the pia-arachnoid is exposed, the section completed with the blunt-pointed scissors, or on a grooved director. The dural flap is then turned down and the brain laid bare. It is most essential that every precaution should be taken to avoid injury to superficial cerebral veins—the cortex is probably under high tension, firmly compressed against the dura mater and bulging out forcibly so soon as tension is relieved.

Examination of the brain. In the event of the exposure of the tumour, its removal can at once be attempted. If, however, the tumour be subcortical in position, its position and boundaries may be estimated by electrical stimulation, palpation and exploration.

Electrical stimulation will evidence whether the area exposed corresponds to the symptoms evinced by the patient. With respect to the actual technique, one pole is placed on the patient's extremity—it matters not which, though preferably on the homo-lateral side—the other over the exposed brain. The current should be just strong enough to contract exposed muscle—some of the fibres of the temporal muscle are generally available for the purpose. If there is much pia-arachnoid œdema, some of the fluid should be evacuated—by gentle scratching of the membranes—and the bare brain stimulated. In the event of complete degeneration of the pyramidal tracts there is little or no response to such stimulation. Under other circumstances the results are quite definite.

Palpation may reveal the nature of the tumour, whether fluid or solid.

Exploration of the brain should only be undertaken in the light of a reasonably certain diagnosis, and every precaution must be taken to avoid needless damage to the cerebral substance. The exploration should invariably be preceded by incision with the brain-knife or scalpel, introduced in such a manner as to avoid injury to all visible vessels and directed at right angles to the surface of the brain, so as to cause the least possible damage to the corona radiata, &c.

Extirpation of the tumour. The proportion of brain tumours surgically removable is small, and even when the tumour is fully exposed considerable experience is required in estimating the possibility of removal.

When the tumour is circumscribed, whether meningeal, cortical, or subcortical, it may be shelled out of its bed with greater or lesser ease according to its nature and position. This shelling out process is carried out with an ordinary tea-spoon or scoop. Hæmorrhage may be severe though generally readily controlled by lightly packing with dry gauze. More rarely one or more of the superficial vessels will require to be underrun with a small needle threaded with the finest catgut. Muscle grafts (see p. 18) may be of considerable assistance.

If a cyst be found it may be possible to shell it out entire, failing which the parietal wall is freely dissected away, and the cavity drained for two or three days.

If the tumour be extensive and ill-defined in margin, no attempt should be made at removal, the surgeon remaining content with the second desideratum of brain tumours in general—the production of a general decrease of intracranial pressure. This might be readily effected by leaving the dura open and by removing at the same time the osseous portion of the osteoplastic flap. The bone is readily dissected away and free decompression would be permitted. In such cases, however, the hernial protrusion is usually excessive, and insomuch as an osteoplastic flap is more often than not framed over the Rolandic region, the protrusion would include the motor area with disastrous results on the contra-lateral extremities. This course, therefore, should never be adopted. In such cases it is infinitely preferable to follow Cushing's method of combined exploration and decompression. This is done as follows: 'From under the portion of temporal muscle which has been turned back with the flap, a roughly semicircular area of bone is cut away with heavy rongeurs, which remove bone without jar, and so without risk of stripping the remainder of the resected bone from the soft parts. This accomplished, a similar area is rongeured away from the side of the skull well down the temporal fossa under the tourniquet, the temporal

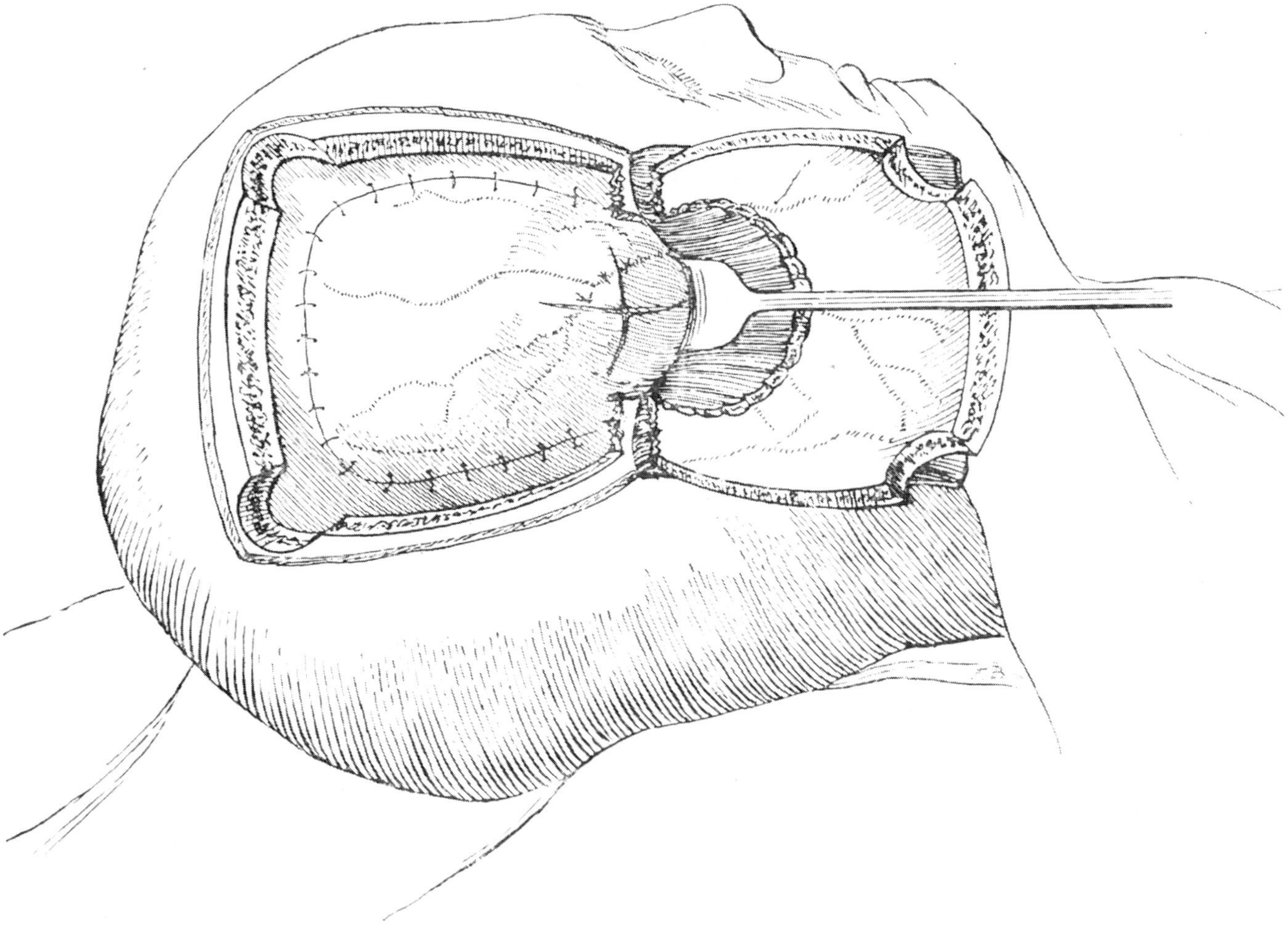

FIG. 72. COMBINED FLAP FORMATION AND DECOMPRESSION. After osteoplastic resection, the tumour has been found irremovable. The dura mater is therefore sewn back in position, after which a portion of the bone is nibbled away from the bone-flap—as depicted in the illustration—and the underlying dura mater freely incised.

muscle being held away by a retractor. If the base of the bone has been made sufficiently broad, a margin possibly a centimetre in width can be left on each side as a support for the flap after its replacement. A subtemporal bone defect is thus secured with even less difficulty than is experienced in making the usual subtemporal opening from without through a split muscle incision. The dura is then carefully opened and incised in a stellate fashion to the margin of what promises to be a sufficient circle of denuded cortex for a generous decompression.'

Closure of the dura and reposition of the flap. Whether the tumour has been exposed and removed, is deemed irremovable, or has not been found, the dural flap should be approximated and carefully sutured in position. In many cases, however, this dural approximation is exceedingly difficult to accomplish, by reason of the outward bulging of the diseased or œdematous brain. This difficulty may be overcome by adopting one or more of the following methods :—

Elevation of the head, thus reducing the amount of blood in the brain.

Lumbar puncture, a method that presents some danger when the surgeon has to deal with a subtentorial tumour, but which bears in its train excellent results from the point of view of reduction of intracranial pressure. The danger arises from the fact that the sudden escape of cerebro-spinal fluid may cause the brain-stem to be engaged in the foramen magnum, with disastrous results on the medullary centres.

Ventricular puncture, when the ventricles are dilated. A blunt-pointed aspirating needle is introduced into the lateral ventricle through the most prominent portion of the exposed brain, and a sufficient quantity of cerebro-spinal fluid evacuated.

'Milking' the pia-arachnoid, the pia-arachnoid being pricked with a needle in several places and the contained fluid squeezed out.

Subtemporal decompression—the final resource. When all other measures fail, a subtemporal decompression may be conducted on the opposite side of the brain.

The dura should be accurately sutured with numerous interrupted silk sutures. It is very important that every precaution should be taken to prevent the continued escape of cerebro-spinal fluid, and, for this and other obvious reasons, it is necessary to avoid drainage whenever possible. If such a course should be necessary—by reason of hæmorrhage—a cigarette drain may be brought out at the most dependent and convenient angle of the dural flap, and through one of the trephine holes or gap purposely cut in the bone-flap.

In any case, the bone-flap is replaced, resting on its shelf and anchored by means of numerous deep sutures, each of which picks up the aponeurosis or muscle both along the upper border of the flap and the two downward vertical prolongations. These sutures will also control bleeding from the divided scalp-vessels. The tourniquet is removed, dressings applied, and the whole maintained firmly in position by a gauze bandage applied circumferentially. These dressings are supported by bandages and the patient sent back to bed.

If the tumour has been exposed by *craniectomy*, the gap in the skull will probably require protection. This procedure (see Chapter VI) can be carried out at the termination of the main operation or at a later date. This latter course is to be preferred.

Radical operation for cerebellar tumours. Craniectomy may be regarded as the operation of choice in the exposure and removal of cerebellar tumours. The formation of an osteoplastic flap is contra-indicated (see p. 29). The operative procedures vary according as to whether it is desired to expose the one or both cerebellar hemispheres. Bilateral exposure, though presenting the great advantage of offering a larger field for exploration, is by far the more serious of the two operations.

Unilateral cerebellar exposure. The patient being placed in the semi-prone or face-down position, the incision starts at the posterior border of the apex of the mastoid process, curves inwards along the superior curved line of the occipital bone to the occipital protuberance, and then passes straight down the middle line of the neck for 2 to 3 inches. If the incision is deepened at once to the bone, hæmorrhage is severe. The incision should first involve the skin and then the muscles attached to the occipital bone. Each vessel as encountered is clipped and tied. The flap must be turned down right up to the posterior margin of the foramen magnum.

The flap being held aside, the pin of the trephine is placed in such a manner that the disk to be removed will correspond to the thin central portion of the cerebellar fossa. The trephine, placed low down, is directed more or less towards the anterior fontanelle.

The disk being removed, the bone is freely cut away with rongeur forceps—outwards to the posterior border of the mastoid process, upwards to the curved line, inwards to near the middle line, and downwards to the posterior margin of the foramen magnum.

This generally completes the first stage of the operation, for, in cerebellar tumours, it is usually advisable to complete the operation in two stages. The scalp-flap is replaced, lightly sewn into position, and the patient sent back to bed.

A few days later the flap is again turned down, the dura incised, and turned down as a flap the convexity of which corresponds to but falls short of the line of the lateral sinus. The cerebellar substance is then examined and the tumour removed after the lines enumerated in dealing with cerebral tumours. Greater difficulty, however, is experienced in the attempted removal of cerebellar tumours, for the operator is working in a very confined space, and because the cerebellum tends to herniate through the adventitious hole in dura and bone. Two other factors must be taken into consideration: (1) the danger incident to all cerebellar operations of respiratory failure,[1] and (2) the friability of the cerebellar substance. Every care must be taken to avoid unnecessary damage of the brain-matter.

When the tumour is situated in the cerebello-pontine angle, a somewhat favourite site for tumour formation, 'lateral displacement' of the cerebellum towards the middle line will aid considerably in the exposure. A flat retractor, bent to a suitable curve, is introduced between the dura and the cerebellum, and the brain-matter gently but firmly retracted towards the middle line. As the brain yields to the pressure the tip of the retractor is insinuated towards the posterior surface of the petrous bone. With the aid of a head-lamp a good view may usually be obtained of the region involved, and, as the tumour is but lightly attached, its removal can be undertaken.

The dura is then carefully sutured and the scalp-flap accurately replaced, deep sutures for the muscles and a few surface sutures for the skin. Drainage should be avoided whenever possible—the discharge of cerebro-spinal fluid is fraught with considerable danger. The gap in the skull requires no other protection than that afforded by the mass of neck muscles.

[1] In the event of cessation of respiration during trephining, the skull should be opened and the dura incised with the utmost expedition. The relief of tension so afforded often allows of respiratory recovery—with or without artificial respiration.

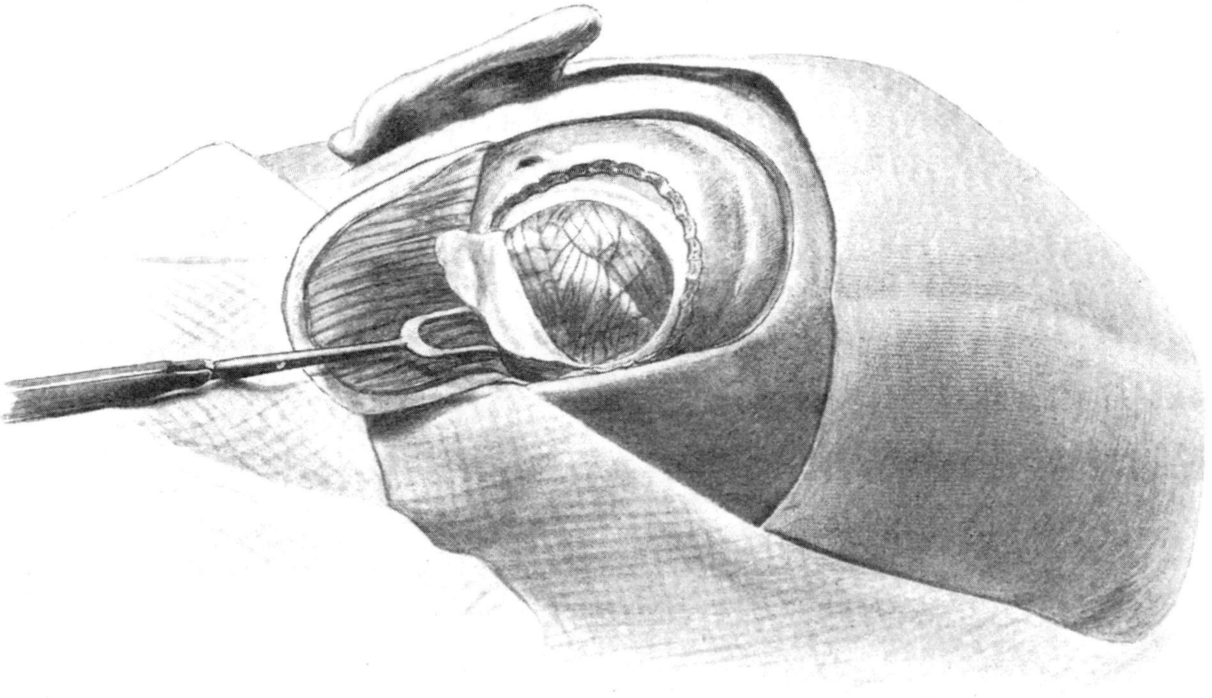

FIG. 73 A. UNILATERAL EXPOSURE OF THE LEFT HALF OF THE CEREBELLUM BY CRANIECTOMY. The scalp-flap has been turned down and is fully retracted. The cerebellum has been exposed by means of a crescentic dural flap.

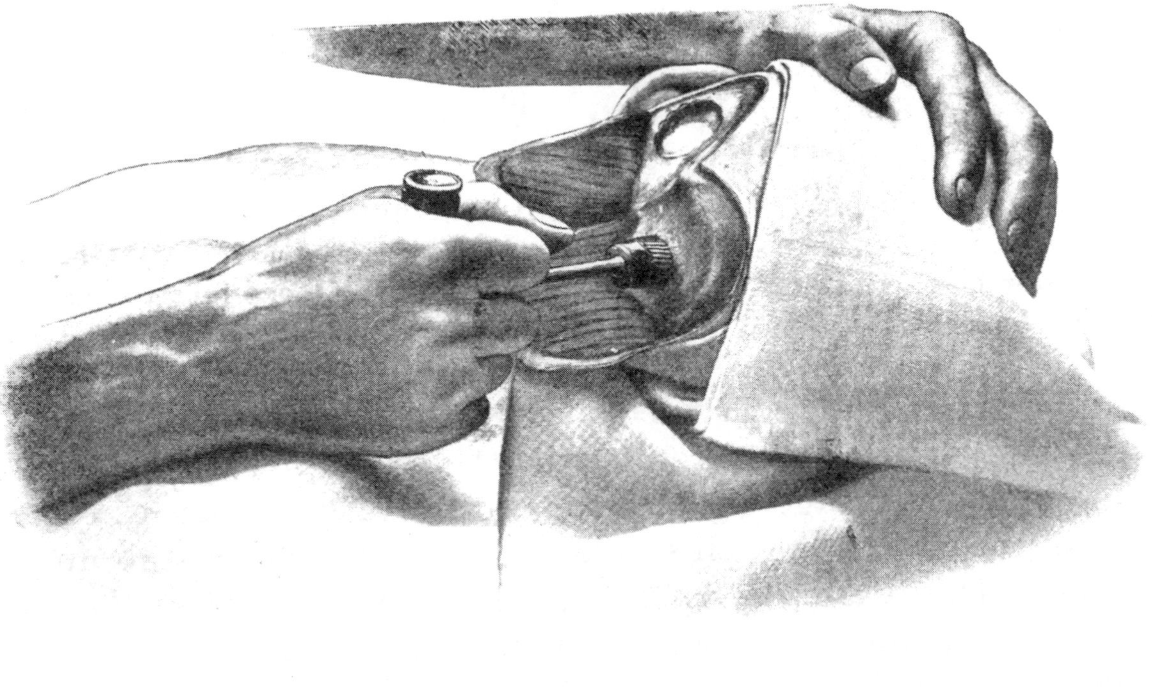

FIG. 73 B. BILATERAL EXPOSURE OF THE CEREBELLUM BY CRANIECTOMY. The left half of the cerebellum has been exposed. The trephine is being applied over the right cerebellar region. Note the position of the trephine and the direction in which it is being applied.

Bilateral cerebellar exposure. This operation is also done in two stages. In the fiıst, each cerebellar fossa is exposed in turn, the scalp-flap being framed and the trephining and cutting away of the bone carried out in the manner previously described for unilateral exposure. The osseous bridge which separates the two

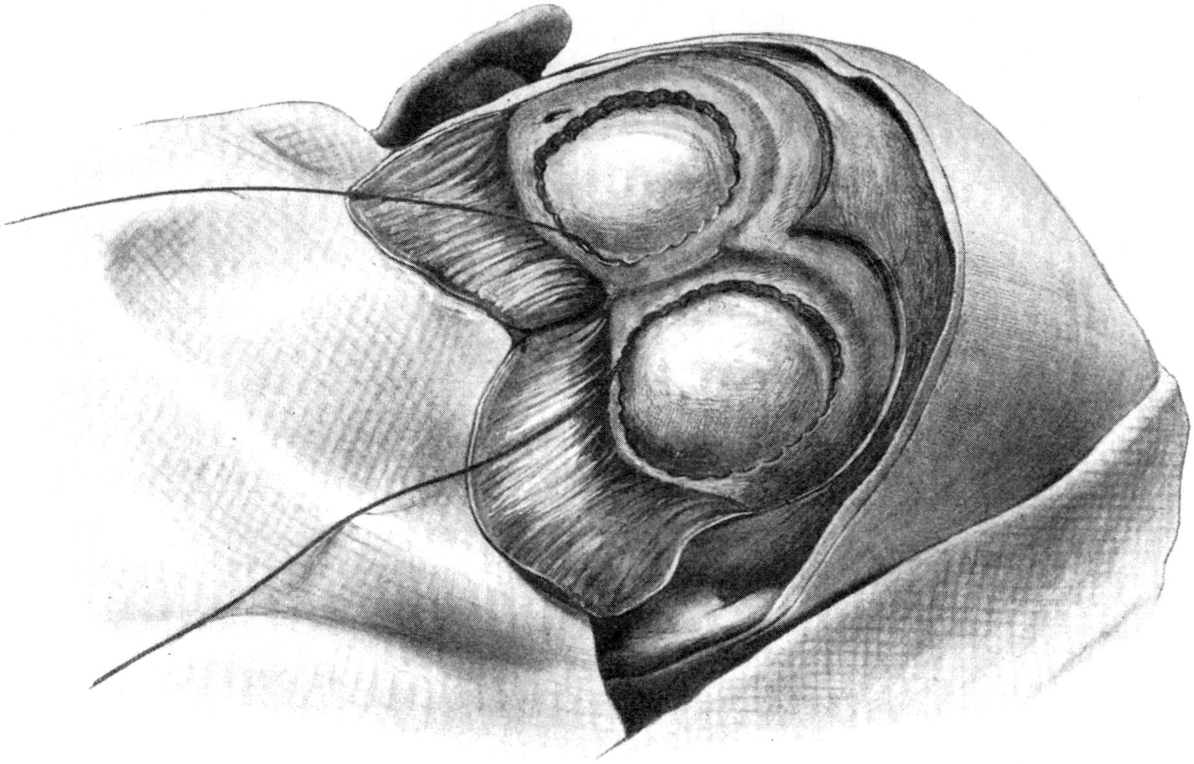

FIG. 73 C. BILATERAL EXPOSURE OF THE CEREBELLUM BY CRANIECTOMY. The walls of both cerebellar fossæ have been cut away, exposing the bulging dura mater. The Gigli saw is in position for removal of the bridge of bone intervening between the two cerebellar fossæ.

openings in the skull is divided above and below with Gigli's saw, and the intermediate part removed. This completes stage one.

In the second stage, again carried out a few days later, two dural flaps are turned down, each similar to the one described in unilateral exposure. This leaves a central portion of dura, that part which encloses the occipital sinus and to which the falx cerebelli is attached. By means of an aneurysm needle, threaded with catgut, passed through or around the falx, the occipital sinus is ligatured above and below, the ligatures being applied as high and as low as circumstances permit. The falx is then divided between the two ligatures and the two flaps thrown upwards and downwards respectively.

The extra space so afforded not only allows of the exposure of both hemispheres, but also permits of the further dislocation of the one lobe towards the opposite side, thus facilitating the examination

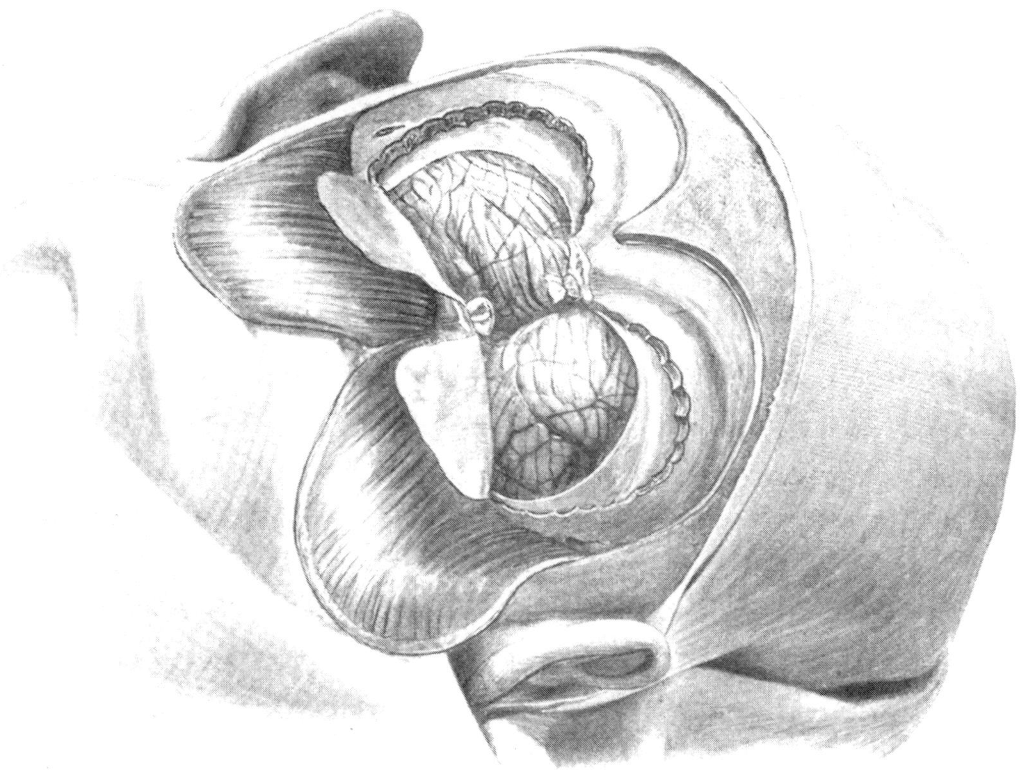

FIG. 73 D. BILATERAL EXPOSURE OF THE CEREBELLUM BY CRANIECTOMY. The bridge of bone has been removed, two crescentic flaps of dura mater have been turned down, and the falx cerebelli has been ligatured in two places and divided.

of the lateral aspect of the cerebellum and of the cerebello-pontine angle.

This bilateral method is a serious operation. Hæmorrhage may be severe, and the attendant risks of respiratory failure are not inconsiderable. It should only be adopted (1) when a tumour is so situated or so extensive that more space is required than supplied by unilateral exposure, and (2) when bilateral cerebello-pontine tumours are suspected.

Palliative operations for cerebral and cerebellar tumours. A primary palliative operation may be conducted over the region of the tumour itself, in the cerebellar region, or over the temporal lobe—one of the so-called 'silent' areas of the brain.

It is obvious that the greatest degree of pressure relief will be obtained by craniectomy conducted over the region of the tumour itself. To this course, however, there are two great objections: (1) the exposed cortex most commonly includes the motor area, herniation of which will lead to disastrous effects on the extremities of the contra-lateral side—spasticity, paralysis, aphasia, &c.; and (2) the herniation of brain-matter including, or closely related to, an irremovable tumour tends to lead to œdema of the brain tissues and softening of and hæmorrhage into the growth, with subsequent rapid development of the outwardly protruded mass.

With respect to cerebellar decompression operations, I must confess that I have formed a most unfavourable opinion. The sub-tentorial pressure can undoubtedly be relieved most effectually by such methods, but the immediate results are not infrequently disastrous, the patient dying within a few days as a result of the complete upset of medullary centres.

In the event of the surgeon deciding to confine his attempts to palliative treatment—alleviation of symptoms only—the *subtemporal operation* of Cushing is certainly the method of choice. The technique of the operation and its general advantages have already been discussed. It merely remains to add that, when the operation is conducted for tumour relief and not for injury as discussed in Chapter IV, no attempt is made to explore the temporo-sphenoidal lobe and drainage is contra-indicated. The dura, widely incised, is left open, the temporal muscle and fascia accurately sutured, and the scalp-flap secured with fine silk sutures.

With regard to the side on which this subtemporal decompression operation is to be conducted, the best results are obtained by operating on that side on which the tumour is situated. In the event of doubt, the right side is chosen, so avoiding any possibility of including, in the hernial protrusion, the motor speech area of Broca. The cranial defect should be made as large as possible, and in the event of failure in bringing about adequate decompression, a similar operation is conducted at a later date on the opposite side of the skull.

After subtemporal decompression there should be no mortality.

The immediate results are eminently satisfactory—headache is relieved, optic neuritis steadily diminishes, vomiting ceases, and the general condition of the patient is immensely improved.

The expectancy of life after such decompression operations requires careful consideration. So much depends on the nature of the tumour that it is difficult to make more than a general observation. In many cases life has been prolonged for one to two years, whilst instances are recorded in which the patient has lived for five to six years—not in a miserable condition as might be imagined, but in comparative comfort.

It might be added that, as the tumour grows, a one-sided subtemporal decompression may gradually become insufficient. In such cases, recrudescence of symptoms—redevelopment of optic neuritis, &c.—may be met by further decompression on the opposite side of the head.

Operations for tumours of the pituitary body. The pituitary body may be approached by the frontal, temporal, and nasal routes. The *temporal route*, advocated by Caton and Paul [1] and Horsley, possesses the disadvantage that the surgeon, whilst utilizing an approach similar to that used in the Hartley-Krause operation for trigeminal neuralgia, encounters on his way the structures laterally situated to the pituitary body, the internal carotid, the cavernous sinus, the third, fourth, and sixth nerves, and the ophthalmic division of the fifth. The anatomical difficulties are therefore considerable. Added to this, the tumour, in its hollowing out of the central portion of the sella turcica, may leave such lateral osseous walls that an approach from the side is impossible.

The *frontal route* is strongly advocated by Krause.[2] He states that, 'an osteoplastic flap is framed in the frontal region, immediately to one side of the middle line, so as to avoid the superior longitudinal sinus and frontal air sinus, and turned upwards. It is essential that the operator should approach the tumour along the floor of the anterior fossa, and, for this purpose, it may be deemed necessary to chip away the bone in the region of the supra-orbital ridge. Some days later, the final stages of the operation are conducted. The dura mater

[1] *Brit. Med. Journ.*, 1893, p. 1421.

[2] *Surgery of the Brain*, vol. i, p. 117.

covering the frontal lobe is stripped away from the bone and traction applied to the dura by means of broad flat spatulæ. When the lesser wing of the sphenoid is exposed, the dura mater is opened in the vertical direction on a line with the lower median angle of the wound at a depth of 5 to 5½ centimetres, as measured from the anterior surface of the frontal bone. If the incision is made at a deeper point there is danger of injury to the optic nerve, which is covered with dura mater in this situation. Laterally the dura is opened parallel to the posterior border of the lesser wing of the sphenoid, about ½ cm. in front of it, to avoid the sinus which lies immediately in contact with the edge of the bone. This exposes the optic nerve, coming from the chiasma and the internal carotid. The pituitary body is located beneath the anterior edge of the chiasma. The diaphragm of the sella turcica is now carefully incised with a small hook-shaped scapel, and the hypophysis is readily removed.'

The *nasal route*, advocated by Bruns and successfully carried out by Schloffer[1] and Cushing, seems to offer the greatest advantages and give the most successful results. The general details of the operation are as follows: starting either beneath the upper lip or externally at the base of the septum, the mucous membrane is peeled away from each side of the vomer, and, by gradual piecemeal removal of that bone, the advance is carried out towards the base of the skull in what may be called an intra-mucous space. By the introduction of suitable instruments into this space the cavity is gradually enlarged, at the expense of the turbinated bones which are compressed by the dilating instruments. By this means—gradual removal of the septum—the operator approaches the base of the skull, always working between the two layers of mucous membrane, and always avoiding, with the greatest care, any laceration of the same. Laceration at once converts the more or less aseptic operation into an infected one. When the base of the skull is laid bare in the region of the sphenoidal sinus, the bone is there chiselled away and the under surface of the pituitary body exposed. It can then be removed piecemeal.

The general details of the operation as enumerated above may require amendment as our knowledge increases. Sufficient has been

[1] *Wien. klin. Wochensch.*, No. 21, 1907.

said, however, to point out the various methods of approach and the advantages claimed for the nasal route.

Results of operation on brain tumours. Statistics are always fallacious, and this is especially the case with regard to operations on tumours of the brain. Few surgeons have operated on a sufficient number of cases to compile satisfactory statistical tables. These tables are generally made up from the combined experience of many operators, all using their own methods. The following, however, will serve to give an approximate idea as to mortality, &c.

Mortality. From earlier records the immediate mortality was estimated at 30–40 per cent. Duret, however, records 400 cases with a mortality of 19·5 per cent., 58 cases dying from shock, 10 from hyperpyrexia, and 10 from hæmorrhage. In my own practice, the mortality may be estimated at a much lower figure. Perhaps I may be too conservative, but I hold the view that, unless the tumour is readily exposed and equally readily removable, it is inadvisable to carry out further measures for its eradication. Moreover, the general technique of brain surgery has advanced with rapid strides, and the question of early and accurate localization has received equal attention. The mortality has diminished proportionately, and may be estimated at less than 20 per cent. So much depends on the surgeon and on the nature of the tumour, its position and localization, that it is impossible to make any absolute statement as to the risk to life attendant on operation. If all tumours were fibromata, cortically situated, and accurately diagnosed, the operation, in the hands of a skilled neurological surgeon, should present but a very low mortality. So long, however, as surgeons will persist in burrowing into the brain substance for a supposed subcortical tumour, so long will the mortality remain high. The great secret in operating on a brain tumour lies in knowing when to terminate the attempt at removal of the tumour and when to rest content with a pure ‘ decompression ’.

It is obvious, therefore, that cortical tumours—more especially such as give rise to early localizing symptoms, e.g. Rolandic tumours —offer a better prognosis than when the surgeon has to deal with subcortical, central, and basal tumour formation.

The mortality according to the region affected. The following table, from a series collected by Knapp, supplies valuable information as to the regional mortality.

Frontal tumours	32 cases	. . .	Mortality, 25 per cent.
Central ,,	231 ,,	. . .	,, 23 ,,
Parietal ,,	29 ,,	. . .	,, 41 ,,
Temporal ,,	17 ,,	. . .	,, 29 ,,
Occipital ,,	10 ,,	. . .	,, 20 ,,
Cerebellar ,,	54 ,,	. . .	,, 45 ,,

Sir Victor Horsley draws attention to this question in the following manner: 'If a line be drawn from the frontal eminences to the occipital protuberance, it is obvious that more shock results from operations below that line than from above, and as we proceed from the frontal to the cerebellar pole of the encephalon.'

The mortality according as to whether the tumour is found or not. According to Horsley, of 79 cases in which a correct diagnosis was made and the tumour removed, 7 died from shock; whilst in 16 cases inaccurately diagnosed, 6 died—a mortality of 9 per cent. in the first case as against 37 per cent. in the second.

The added danger resulting from unsuccessful attempts at finding the tumour must not be advanced as an argument against the palliative operations, for the failure to find and remove the tumour implies diligent search for the neoplasm, with necessary prolongation of operative procedures, and perhaps extensive manipulation of the brain substance. Statistics and experience both afford conclusive evidence that accurate localization is essential for the success of the operation.

CHAPTER VIII

THE INFECTIVE DISEASES OF THE BRAIN AND MENINGES: ABSCESS OF THE BRAIN, MENINGITIS, LATERAL AND CAVERNOUS SINUS THROMBOSIS, HERNIA CEREBRI

ABSCESS OF THE BRAIN

Abscess of the brain may be considered under the following headings :—

Multiple abscess.

Acute traumatic abscess.

Chronic abscess.

Multiple abscess. Multiple abscess results from the lodgement of infected emboli which, derived from an acute infective osteomyelitis, endocarditis, gangrene of the lung, &c., are carried by the blood-stream to the brain. Multiple abscess of the brain may therefore be considered as part of a general infection. On account of the symptoms dependent on the primary infection and on the secondary pyæmic developments, a diagnosis can seldom be determined, and, even in those rather hypothetical cases in which suspicion may be aroused, surgical interference is quite useless and the prognosis hopeless. It is, therefore, quite unnecessary to discuss the matter further.

Acute traumatic abscess. Acute traumatic abscess of the brain most commonly arises in connexion with an infected compound fracture of the skull. In the event of laceration of the dura mater, infective organisms have a ready means of access both to the meninges and to the brain itself, meningitis or cerebritis resulting. This liability to meningeal and brain infection is increased when hair, portions of clothing, bullets, or other foreign bodies are embedded amongst the comminuted fragments of bone, or driven into the brain substance. In the event of the dura mater remaining intact, meningitis or cerebritis may still develop if, as the result of scalp suppuration, the diploic vessels become thrombosed and plugged with bacteria, some of which may be carried inwards by the reversed blood-stream, and perhaps by lymphatic connexions.

The infection may remain localized to the adjacent brain substance, an acute traumatic cerebral abscess resulting, or may become more widely diffused—diffuse cerebritis—a condition usually associated with general meningeal infection.

An acute traumatic cerebral abscess is almost necessarily situated immediately beneath the site of osseous and membranous lesion, being, in fact, more a meningo-cortical abscess than a brain abscess proper. The boundaries are but ill-defined, the walls ragged, and the contents of a brown-red colour. The surrounding brain is in a condition of red softening, that is to say, extensively infiltrated with leucocytes, the vessels thrombosed and teeming with bacteria, whilst minute extravasations of blood lead to the characteristic colour both of the contents of the abscess and of the surrounding tissue.

In the more chronic cases, the surrounding area shows some attempt at repair, dense armies of leucocytes barring the way to the spread of the infection, and, in the more favourable cases, allowing of the formation of a definite fibrous barrier.

Symptomatology. The symptoms resulting from an acute traumatic cerebral abscess are largely dependent on the site of the abscess. In the earlier stages of development suspicion may be aroused by the presence of persistent headache—frequently localized to the region primarily affected—by mental and bodily irritability, restlessness, and pyrexia. All these symptoms may, however, be produced by the unhealthy condition of the scalp-wound—free suppuration, bare bone, and extra-dural suppuration.

On or about the third day, the condition of the patient becomes more grave, the change for the worse being usually of rapid development, and preceded by severe rigors and general convulsions. The patient shows further signs of mental irritation, being delirious, restless, and occasionally actually maniacal.

The temperature is high and rigors are frequent. The pulse is small and rapid, the respiration increased in frequency, irregular, and often partaking of the Cheyne-Stokes type. The face is livid, the skin hot and burning. Vaso-motor disturbance is evidenced by profuse sweating and well-marked *tache cérébrale.*

Prognosis and treatment. The prognosis is almost hopeless unless radical measures are adopted in the early stages. The scalp-wound should be enlarged and comminuted fragments of bone removed, or the skull trephined over the region of the suspected abscess. The lacerated dura mater is freely opened up and the surface of the brain exposed. Purulent material is gently removed, and the wound closed in such a manner as to allow of free drainage.

Even under the most favourable local conditions the prognosis is bad.

Chronic abscess. As a preliminary statement it must be pointed out that breaking down new growths, softening gummata, caseating tuberculous masses, actinomycotic and hydatid cysts, are regarded in the light of tumour formation and are discussed elsewhere.

Of 52 cases of brain abscess admitted of recent years into St. Bartholomew's Hospital, 41 partook of the chronic type, 30 being dependent on otitic disease, 3 on frontal sinus suppuration, 5 resulting from lung disease, and 2 of uncertain origin. The 11 acute cases were either traumatic or pyæmic.

From these and other statistics it may be regarded as generally accepted that the majority of brain abscesses are secondary to chronic disease of neighbouring bone, and more especially middle ear disease. This being the case, it might naturally be inferred—on anatomical grounds—that the temporo-sphenoidal lobe of the cerebrum and the cerebellum are more liable to infection than any other part of the brain. From 100 cases treated at my hospital the temporo-sphenoidal lobe and cerebellum were involved in the proportion of about 2 to 1. Körner,[1] reporting on another 100 cases, gives the following data :—

Abscess of the cerebrum	62 cases
,, ,, cerebellum	32 ,,
,, in both situations	6 ,,

Hunter Tod,[2] reporting on 100 cases treated at the London Hospital, found that in children under 10 years of age temporo-sphenoidal abscess occurred in 87 per cent. cases, and cerebellar in 13 per cent., whereas in adults cerebral abscess occurred in 65 per cent.

1 *Archiv für Ohrenheilkunde*, vol. xxix, p. 17.

2 *Diseases of the Ear*, Oxford Medical Publications, p. 257.

and cerebellar in 35 per cent. The development of temporo-sphenoidal and cerebellar abscesses in the same case was observed in 5 per cent. cases.

Pathology. Insomuch as chronic middle ear disease forms the main predisposing factor in the development of abscess of the brain, the pathology of brain abscess in general may be considered by discussing the main features peculiar to otitic abscess in particular.

As the result of chronic middle ear disease, the mucous lining of the middle ear and its accessory cavities becomes destroyed, the antrum filled with cholesteatomata, and the middle and external ears with granulations. The discharge of pus, previously free, is obstructed, partial or complete blockage occurring. The destruction of the mucous lining allows of invasion of the surrounding bone, the veins become thrombosed and filled with bacteria, and the cancellous spaces blocked with granulations. Further erosion of the bone results, both in the upward direction towards the tegmen tympani and in the backward towards the lateral sinus groove and cerebellum. The veins of the tegmen communicate freely with those of the temporo-sphenoidal lobe, whilst those ramifying in the mastoid region either communicate with the lateral sinus itself or with the anterior cerebellar venous system. Infection may therefore spread (1) *upwards* to the temporo-sphenoidal lobe, or (2) *backwards* to the lateral sinus and cerebellum. In the former case, meningitis or temporo-sphenoidal abscess develops: in the latter instance, meningitis, lateral sinus thrombosis, or cerebellar abscess.

For the formation of a brain abscess it is, of course, essential that the brain membranes overlying the main site of osseous erosion should be sealed off in such a manner as to prevent a general infection of the meningeal region, the dura becoming adherent to the eroded tegmen, &c. It is œdematous and throws out granulations, both on its parietal and visceral aspects. The parietal granulations aid in the further erosion of the bone, whilst the visceral may, according to Macewen,[1] even indent the brain. By means of thrombosed veins, perivascular lymphatics, and minute arterioles, a channel of infection is now opened up between the site of osseous erosion and the temporo-sphenoidal and cerebellar lobes.

[1] *Pyogenic Diseases of the Brain and Spinal Cord.*

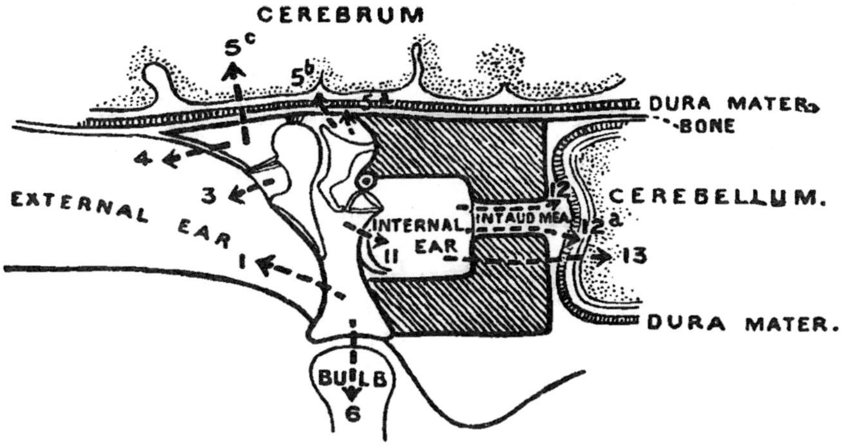

FIG. 74 A. DIAGRAM TO SHOW EXTENSION OF DISEASE FROM TYMPANIC CAVITY, IN MIDDLE EAR SUPPURATION. 1, Perforation through tympanic membrane ; 3, Perforation through Shrapnell's membrane ; 4, Fistula through outer wall of attic (roof of external meatus) ; 5 *a*, Extradural abscess ; 5 *b*, Meningitis ; 5 *c*, Temporo-sphenoidal abscess ; 6, Bulb of jugular (thrombosis) ; 11, Internal ear ; 12, 12 *a*, 13, Route of infection through internal ear giving rise to extradural abscess, meningitis, and cerebellar abscess. (After Hunter Tod.)

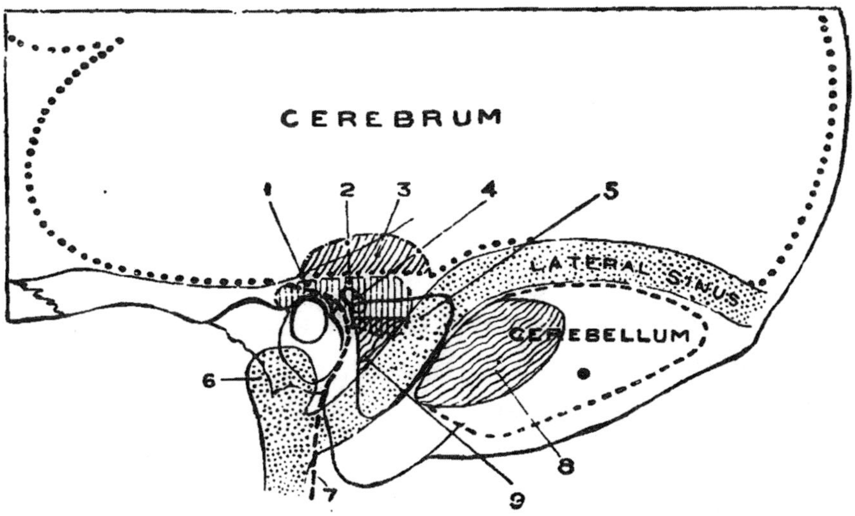

FIG. 74 B. DIAGRAM TO SHOW SURGICAL ANATOMY FOR OPERATIONS FOR OTITIC INTRACRANIAL LESIONS. 1, Attic ; 2, Antrum ; 3, Point for opening temporo-sphenoidal abscess (just above and along the tegmen tympani) ; 4, External semi-circular canal ; 5, Lateral sinus ; also shows area of bone removed in mastoid operation ; 6, Bulb of jugular vein ; 7, Facial nerve ; 8, Point for opening cerebellum behind lateral sinus ; 9, Point for opening cerebellum in front of lateral sinus (between sinus behind and external semicircular canal in front). (After Hunter Tod.)

In any case the abscess usually develops in the white substance of the brain, just beneath the grey matter, and in close relation to the primary source of infection.

The wall of the abscess. In an abscess of rapid development the walls are ragged and but ill-defined from the surrounding brain substance. In the more chronic cases the cavity is shut off from the brain by a capsule of varying density—usually not more than one-sixteenth of an inch in thickness, but occasionally of much greater development (see Fig. 86 A). Sometimes—more especially in cerebellar cases—two cavities may be superimposed, the two abscesses communicating with one another by means of a narrow, and often tortuous, channel. Successful drainage of the one cavity may be inadequate to drain its companion. This two-saced abscess will be again alluded to at a later period.

Contents of the abscess. The pus is usually of a greenish hue, odourless, and acid in reaction. Though often sterile the following bacteria may be cultivated—*staphylococcus pyogenes aureus* and *albus*, *pneumococcus*, *bacillus pyocyaneus*, and the *streptococcus pyogenes.* The pus is usually of such viscidity that it cannot be evacuated through the lumen of an ordinary aspirating needle.

The size of the abscess. In size the abscess varies greatly, seldom, however, containing more than 5 or 6 drachms of pus.

The neck of the abscess. It was first pointed out by Ballance[1] that most brain abscesses secondary to disease of the bones of the skull are 'mushroom-shaped', the narrow portion or stem being attached to the dura mater at the original site of infection. The stalked form of abscess is 'quite comparable, as to its mode of formation, to the superficial cervical abscess connected by a narrow track to a focus of disease beneath the deep fascia'.

Course pursued by an untreated brain abscess. The abscess enlarges at the expense of the surrounding tissues, either bursting into the ventricles of the brain or coming to the surface, there rupturing and leading to a diffuse meningeal infection. Some few cases have been reported in which the abscess has established a more or less efficient natural means of drainage, either along the 'stalk' of the abscess or by means of a new channel to the

[1] *Some Points in the Surgery of the Brain*, p. 95.

exterior. In one or two cases, spontaneous recovery has apparently taken place.

Mode of healing after successful operation. Previous to successful evacuation, the brain immediately surrounding the abscess cavity is compressed and anæmic. As soon as drainage is supplied, it swells out like a sponge, more or less obliterating the cavity. The closure of a cavity by means of the formation of granulation tissue probably never occurs, and, if the falling together of the surrounding brain is insufficient to obliterate the cavity, final closure is completed by the in-dragging of the overlying tissues—scalp, membranes, and brain becoming intimately fused together.

Symptomatology. The symptoms must be considered under the following headings :—

The symptoms peculiar to the INITIAL stage of the abscess
,, ,, ,, ,, LATENT ,, ,, ,,
,, ,, ,, ,, MANIFEST ,, ,, ,,
,, ,, ,, ,, TERMINAL ,, ,, ,,

The INITIAL stage. If a patient suffering from brain abscess is capable of answering questions, it will usually be found that he dates his illness from some particular day when he was sick, experienced a shivering attack, or suffered from a severe attack of headache. Further inquiry, however, will almost always elucidate the fact that, for some days or weeks previously, he was not feeling well, suffering from insomnia and loss of appetite, and experiencing occasional attacks of headache. Friends and relatives may volunteer information as to general irritability, alteration of manner, incapability of mental concentration, and worry over family and financial matters.

At this stage the headache is commonly referred to the frontal region, less frequently localized to the region of the brain involved. The patient sleeps badly, and there is often a slight rise of temperature towards the evening. Occasionally he may vomit, independently of the ingestion of food.

The LATENT stage. Mental depression becomes more marked, headache is more persistent and now shows a definite tendency to localization, food is distasteful, and bodily wasting becomes evident. The evening rise of temperature becomes more constant, sickness more frequent, and vertigo and giddiness may be noticeable features.

The MANIFEST stage. The symptoms arising during the manifest stage must be considered as follows :—

(*a*) Symptoms dependent on the general increase in the intracranial pressure.

(*b*) Symptoms dependent on the localization of the abscess.

Symptoms pointing to a general increase of intracranial pressure

General mental condition. In the latent and early manifest stages the patient will answer questions more or less correctly, but with hesitation—as if from delayed comprehension and from prolongation of the latent period. Answers are often inappropriate to the question, and given with some confusion of mind and thought—the state of ' slow-cerebration '.

The patient either lies listless and apathetic—mentally dulled—or exhibits general irritability, lying curled up in bed, intolerant of all interrogation and examination. More rarely, cerebral irritation progresses to actual mania, the patient tossing about in bed, muttering and delirious. Forcible restraint is often required. In the later manifest stages the patient lies comatose.

Headache. Headache is an almost constant feature, varying greatly in intensity, but often so severe that the patient is incapacitated from all attempts at conversation and movement. Exacerbations are frequent, the sufferer crying out in his agony. The pain may be localized or diffuse. Localization of the pain to some special region is of considerable aid to the regional diagnosis of the abscess—more especially so when it is accentuated by palpation and percussion over the suspected region.

Vomiting. Vomiting is another frequent symptom, probably dependent on stimulation of the medullary vomiting centre. It is of the so-called ' cerebral ' type, bearing no relation to the ingestion of food and unaccompanied by previous nausea and retching. The vomited material is propelled outwards with considerable force. There appears to be some relation between the exacerbations of headache and the time at which vomiting occurs. Vomiting is most constantly observed when the abscess is subtentorial in position.

Optic neuritis. It is exceedingly difficult to determine the frequency with which optic neuritis develops in cases of brain abscess. Much depends on the site of the abscess and the duration of its existence. Optic neuritis is seldom absent in the more chronic cases and is most constant when the purulent collection is subtentorial in position. The non-appearance of optic neuritis—even in chronic cases—does not confute a diagnosis of abscess formation.

When once present, the swelling of the disk may increase rapidly. In a case of cerebellar abscess recently under my care the swelling reached 6D. in three days. Whatever the localizing value of unilateral neuritis in tumour formation (see p. 216), I am strongly of opinion that in the cases under discussion, optic neuritis, when confined to or more marked on the one side, implies that the abscess is situated on that side.

The pulse and temperature. It is commonly stated that, in typical cases of brain abscess, the pulse-rate is slowed—40 to 60 per minute—and that the temperature is subnormal. Slowing of the pulse results from stimulation of the medullary centre, the lowering of temperature to less determinate causes. In the consideration of pulse and temperature—and the two must invariably be considered together—it will, however, frequently be found that the temperature is raised and the pulse-rate but little altered. Thus, in one case the pulse was 88 and the temperature 103·4 degrees, in another the pulse was 74 and the temperature 102, in a third case the pulse was 89 and the temperature 102·8 degrees. These cases are very significant, and show that the greatest attention should be paid to a comparison between pulse-rate and temperature, a *relative* slowing of the pulse being more constant than an actual retardation.

The elevation of temperature results from the fact that the great majority of cases of brain abscess are secondary to some highly infective purulent collection, as, for instance, a mastoid empyema. In such a case, if the mastoid region be cleared out, the temperature will fall and the typical clinical picture of subnormal temperature and slowed pulse-rate will be depicted.

The respiration. The increase of intracranial pressure may lead to some slowing and deepening of respiration. Irregularity is, however, the more common condition, deepening, in the later stages, to definite Cheyne-Stokes respiration. Under anæsthesia—more especially in cerebellar cases—there is considerable risk of respiratory failure (see foot-note, p. 238).

Vaso-motor changes. Vaso-motor changes are fairly constant, evidenced by sweats and flushings, *tache cérébrale*, &c.

Reflexes. In the earlier stages of the trouble the reflexes may be increased and Babinski's sign present. In the later stages, all reflexes are abolished.

Other more general symptoms. Obstinate constipation, foul tongue and breath, anorexia, deficient urine, loss of bladder and rectal

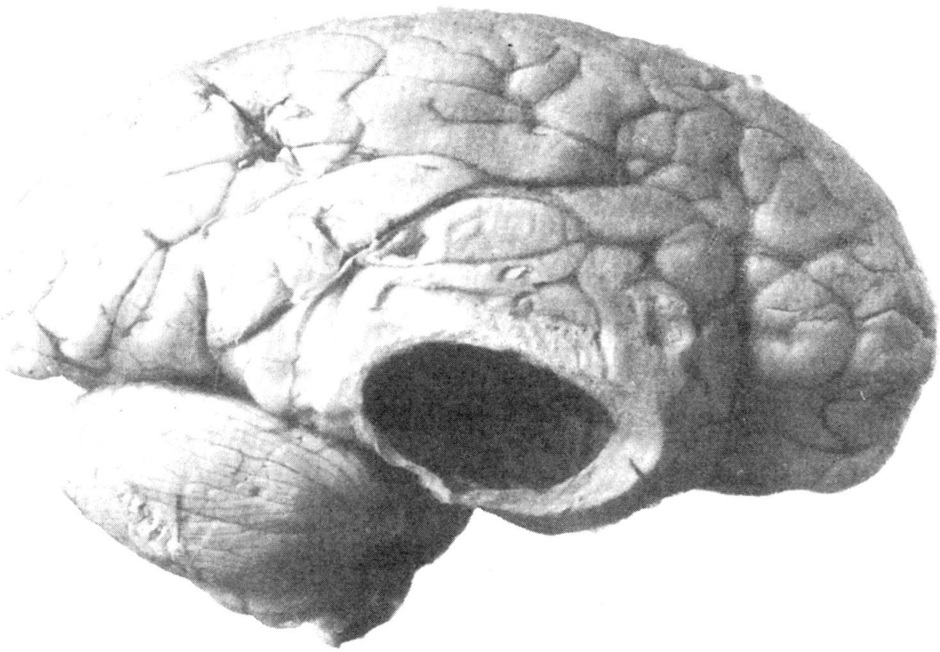

FIG. 75. A LARGE RIGHT-SIDED TEMPORO-SPHENOIDAL ABSCESS.

control, are all noticeable features. A well-marked leucocytosis is generally to be observed.

Symptoms dependent on the localization of the abscess

(*a*) **Temporo-sphenoidal abscess.** The abscess occupies one of the so-called 'silent' areas of the brain, an area merely exercising a word-hearing faculty (see p. 163). Insomuch, however, as auditory power is already impaired or lost from the disease existent in the middle ear, it follows that a temporo-sphenoidal abscess may not give rise to any localizing symptoms whatever. Definite motor symptoms will only be observed when an abscess of considerable size exercises an upward pressure on the lower motor areas, or an inward pressure on the internal capsule. Thus, (1) when the pressure effects are exercised in the *upward* direction the lower motor areas will suffer with resultant paresis or paralysis of the muscles of the contra-lateral face and upper

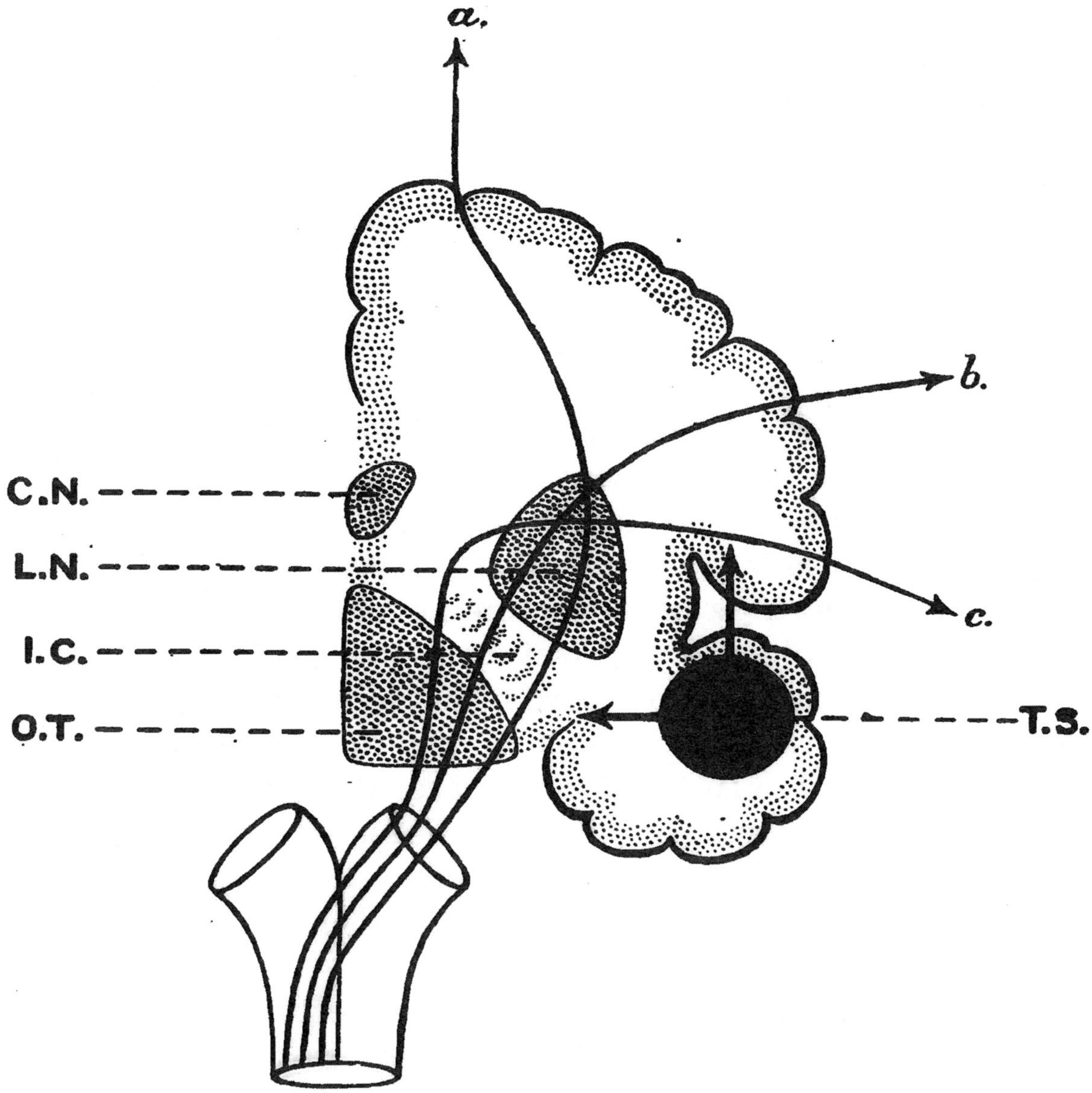

FIG. 76. TO ILLUSTRATE THE PRESSURE EFFECTS OF A TEMPORO-SPHENOIDAL ABSCESS :—(1) *upward* pressure on the lower cortical motor area, and (2) *inward* pressure on the internal capsule. T.S., Temporo-sphenoidal abscess ; *a.*, Cortical area for lower extremity ; *b.*, Cortical area for upper extremity ; *c.*, Cortical area for face ; C.N., Caudate nucleus ; L.N., Lenticular nucleus ; I.C., Internal capsule ; O.T., Optic thalamus.

extremity, and, if the abscess be situated on the left side, aphasia may also be present. And (2) when the pressure is exerted mainly in the *inward* direction so as to interfere with the internal capsule the motor areas are affected in the reverse order, lower extremity first and face last.

Aphasia will partake of the motor or sensory type according to the situation of the abscess. Thus, motor aphasia indicates pressure on Broca's area, sensory points to the involvement of the region of the angular gyrus (see p. 163). According to Schmiegelow, some type of aphasia was present in 23 out of 54 cases of otitic temporo-sphenoidal abscess.

Facial paralysis, whether due to inward or upward pressure, is of the incomplete or cortical type, the upper face-muscles escaping or being but slightly affected. No difficulty need be experienced in differentiating between the ipso-lateral paralysis which results from destruction of the facial nerve in the aqueductus Fallopii and the contra-lateral palsy dependent on the cortical lesion.

Pressure may also be exercised on the post-Rolandic sensory areas and on the tracts that evolve therefrom, but the general condition of the patient seldom allows of any accurate diagnosis with respect to sensory involvement in general.

When the abscess is of considerable size, both *third* and *sixth* nerves may be involved. For instance, the third nerve, emerging from the brain at the anterior border of the pons, and passing along the inner border of the temporo-sphenoidal lobe, is liable to irritation or pressure paralysis. In the former case, the pupil on the affected side will be contracted, in the latter instance dilated. When *ipso-lateral* third nerve paralysis coexists with paralysis of the opposite face and upper extremity, a condition of crossed paralysis results.

When the sixth nerve is involved the external rectus on the side of the lesion is paralyzed with resultant internal squint. Conjugate deviation of the eyes towards the side opposite to the lesion and secondary lateral nystagmus have both been observed.

Further assistance in the localization may be obtained by careful observation as to the position of the headache, by palpation and percussion of the skull, and by a comparison of the intensity of optic neuritis in the two disks.

(*b*) **Cerebellar abscess.** Many of the symptoms previously described when dealing with brain abscess in general are intensified when the focus of suppuration is situated in the confined space beneath the tentorium cerebelli. Thus, headache is exceptionally severe and more or less localized to the occipital and cerebellar regions. Again, optic neuritis may develop rapidly and reach a high grade of intensity, vomiting is early in onset and of frequent occurrence, whilst certain other symptoms dependent on the increased intracranial pressure—slowing of the pulse, alterations in respiratory rhythm—are correspondingly accentuated.

The more typical *localizing* symptoms are as follows :—

Vertigo is a prominent symptom, most evident on sudden alteration of position on the part of the patient. He complains, for

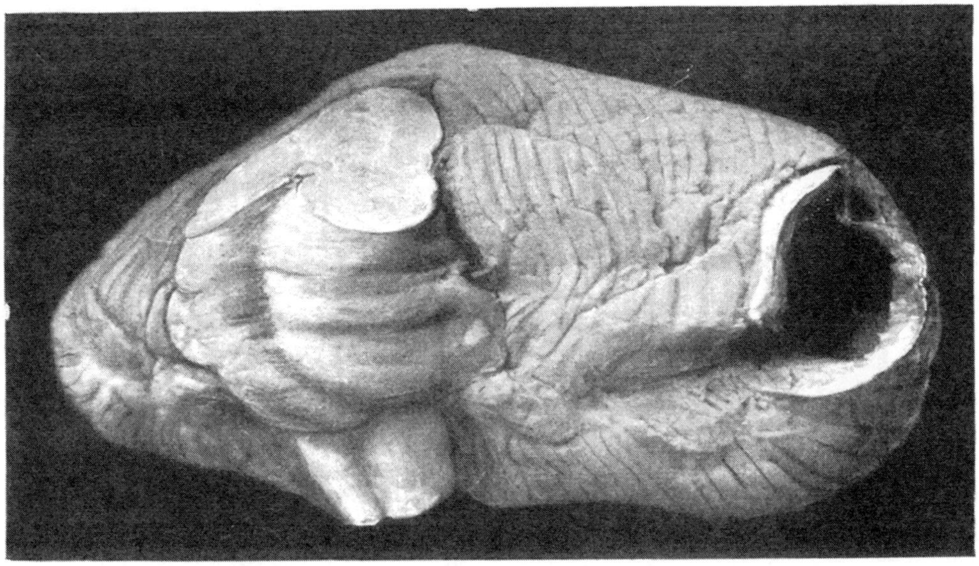

FIG. 77. A CEREBELLAR ABSCESS.

instance, of great giddiness on sitting up in bed. The sensation of movement may be of self or of objects.

When standing, he tends, when unsupported, to fall or lurch in some particular direction, more commonly, in my experience, towards that side on which the abscess is situated. On this point, however, there is some difference of opinion and, by itself, it cannot be accepted as having any great localizing value.

In some rare cases Dana's symptom may be noticed—a sudden unexpected attack of vertigo, roaring in the head, relaxation of limbs, and falling to the ground in an unconscious state. This symptom is said to be almost pathognomonic of an abscess (or tumour) situated in the region of the cerebello-pontine angle.

The *cerebellar gait* can of course only be demonstrated when the patient is in a fit condition to walk. He shows, by the position of the feet, a desire to obtain a wide base of support and staggers on, in his desire to carry out his instructions, usually inclining towards the side on which the lesion is situated. This inclination is probably dependent on the weakness of the muscles of the ipso-lateral side (see below). Another important feature may be observed in the tendency on the part of the patient to turn the head in such a way that he faces somewhat in the opposite direction, the chin being directed towards the opposite shoulder.

Disturbances of co-ordination may be demonstrated by telling the patient to touch the tip of his nose with his finger, or to strike at an object held a foot or two in front of him. Such attempts are characterized by uncertainty and irregularity of movement, accompanied by considerable tremor.

Paresis or paralysis of the limbs on the ipso-lateral side. The abscess usually occupies the antero-external aspect of the lateral lobe of the cerebellum, and is so situated that no direct pressure is exercised on the pyramidal fibres. Some weakness—perhaps paralysis—of the muscles of the extremities on the same side as the lesion can, however, usually be demonstrated. According to Luciani, this is explained in the following manner :—between the cortex of the one side and the cerebellum of the other there are certain 'associated' fibres, the strength of the impulses sent out from the cortex depending in part on the integrity of these reinforcing cerebellar fibres. In cases of cerebellar abscess these reinforcements are cut off with consequent paresis, or even paralysis, of the muscles of the face, arm, and leg on the same side as the lesion. Associated with this muscular weakness there is usually some increase in the deep reflexes. Some of the pyramidal fibres do not decussate, and, consequently, an ipso-lateral paralysis may be associated with a contra-lateral paresis.

The same lessening of cortical impulses accounts for a weakening in the external rectus of the same side, which muscle, acting with the internal rectus of the sound side, allows of a conjugate deviation of the eyes towards the opposite side, with well-marked *nystagmus*—of a coarse type—on attempting to correct this deviation.

Retraction of the head and neck. Retraction of the head and neck, stiffness of the nuchal muscles, and even opisthotonos, may be observed. The existence of these symptoms is always suggestive of meningeal infection, but an abscess of considerable size, even when

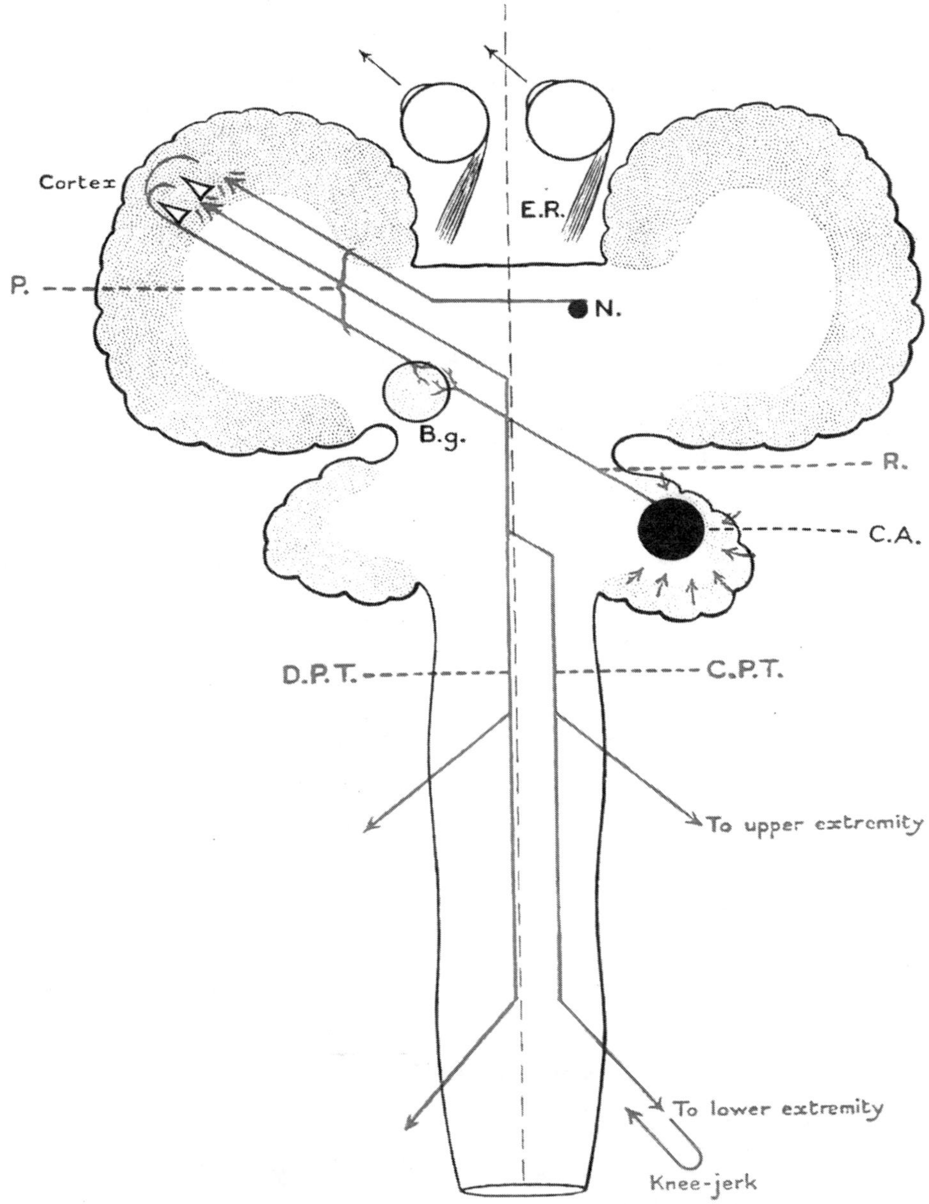

FIG. 78. A DIAGRAMMATIC ILLUSTRATION (AFTER LUCIANI) TO EXPLAIN THE SYMPTOMS OBSERVED IN CEREBELLAR ABSCESS FORMATION. P., Pyramidal fibres; C.A., Right cerebellar abscess; R., Reinforcing fibres from right cerebellum to left cortex; B.g., Basal ganglia; E.R., External rectus; N., Nucleus for sixth nerve; D.P.T., Direct pyramidal tract; C.P.T., Crossed pyramidal tract.

situated in the anterior part of the lateral lobe of the cerebellum, may so exercise pressure in the downward direction as to cork up that part of the cerebellum which normally extends into the mouth of the foramen magnum. The neighbouring upper cervical nerves may then be irritated or compressed.

Yawning. Frequent purposeless yawning is said to be pathognomonic of cerebellar disease (see p. 165).

Attitude in bed. More commonly the patient lies curled up in bed in the position of cerebral irritation, perhaps more frequently with the sound side upwards.

(c) **Frontal abscess.** The abscess is usually dependent on long-continued suppuration in the frontal sinus, with deficient drainage and spread of disease to the surrounding bone. The abscess may be situated in close relation to the focus of the disease, but, more commonly, it occupies a more posterior position, so much so that direct pressure is exercised on the corona radiata proceeding from the pre-Rolandic or motor area. It would appear also that definite localizing symptoms do not arise until the abscess has attained considerable size. The *general symptoms* peculiar to all cases of brain abscess are perhaps less definite when the abscess is frontal in position. Thus, although headache may be localized to the frontal region, and although optic neuritis may be present, yet vomiting, alterations in pulse-rate and in respiratory rhythm are less marked than usual.

The *localizing symptoms* are often reasonably definite, so much so that but little difficulty may be experienced in arriving at a diagnosis.

In the earlier stages of the abscess formation motor irritation may predominate, with the development of *fits of the Jacksonian type*, the lower and more anterior motor areas being first and mainly affected. More commonly, however, attention will be directed towards the nature of the trouble by *paresis or paralysis of the opposite side of the body*. In this case also the lower motor areas—those responsible for the opposite side of the face and upper extremity (also the motor speech-area on the left side of the brain)—are first and chiefly involved. In some cases—more especially when the abscess is of considerable size—definite hemiplegia may result.

In cases of frontal abscess, the *mental condition* of the patient demands special consideration. Some definite degree of moral perversion will usually be noticed, the patient—presuming that he is in a conscious condition—making himself as objectionable as possible.

He will upset his food, disarrange his bedclothes, disobey orders, and even pass his urine and fæces in his bed though well aware of his wrong-doing. When questioned he answers with suspicion, when examined he demands to know the why and the wherefore of the various details of the investigation. An ophthalmoscopic examination is especially difficult to carry out in a satisfactory manner. In a case recently under my care—one in which a frontal abscess was drained three times before a cure was obtained—these curious mental perversions were observed each time, and the patient subsequently acknowledged that he had performed the various acts wittingly, but was unable to deny himself the opportunity of irritating those around him.

It has been stated that these mental changes are only to be observed when the abscess involves the *left* frontal lobe. In my own experience no such lateral differentiation has been noticed.

Anosmia may be present if the patient is in a condition to respond to the tests requisite to prove the defect. In most cases, however, considerable difficulty will be experienced in applying the tests, and the results obtained are too variable. Anosmia will be associated with impaired power of taste.

Pupillary changes. 'If the abscess is of large size, the pupil on the same side is in a state of stabile mydriasis ; if small, it may be sluggish and contracted.'[1]

The TERMINAL stage. In *fatal* cases death results from the pressure exercised by the expanding abscess on the bulbar centres, or from the bursting of the abscess into the ventricular or meningeal spaces. During this terminal stage the pulse becomes very rapid, the respiration irregular and Cheyne-Stokes in character, whilst the temperature rises rapidly, reaching 105–110 degrees F. Invasion of the lateral ventricle is evidenced by violent convulsions, rigidity of the extremities, opisthotonos, retraction of the head, trepidation, and prostration. The pupils become widely dilated, and remain in that condition till death ensues.

Treatment. In the operative treatment of *otitic temporo-sphenoidal and cerebellar abscess* two courses are available :—(1) to trephine directly over the abscess through the squamous or cerebellar

[1] Macewen, *Pyogenic Diseases of the Brain and Spinal Cord.*

regions, postponing mastoid exploration till a later date (the two-stage operation); and (2) to carry out the complete mastoid operation, searching for the 'stalk' of the abscess, and draining the abscess into the now-united middle ear and antrum (the one-stage operation).

The former course is advocated by many general surgeons, the latter is the one usually pursued by the aural surgeon. The advantages claimed for the former method—the direct trephining method—are as follows:—

(1) The general condition of the patient is often of so serious a nature as to prohibit the more prolonged procedures essential to the mastoid exploration.

(2) When the exploration is conducted from the infected middle ear, an unsuccessful attempt to find the abscess carries with it an appreciable risk of meningeal and brain infection. Unsuccessful exploration through the 'clean' squamous and cerebellar regions presents no such disadvantages.

(3) The drainage as supplied through the trephine hole is often superior to that provided by dilating up the 'stalk' of the abscess into the middle ear.

(4) Many general surgeons do not possess that intimate acquaintance with the anatomy of the ear which is necessary to carry out a complicated aural operation.

Each case must be considered on its own merits, but I am inclined to advocate the two-stage method when the diagnosis is reasonably clear that the patient is suffering from temporo-sphenoidal or cerebellar abscess, mastoid exploration being carried out as soon as the patient has recovered from the first operation. When, however, considerable doubt exists as to the position of the abscess—or the nature of the complication in general—it is then advisable to start by exploration of the mastoid and aural regions, further measures being adopted according to the conditions found at the time of operation.

1. The two-stage operation.

Trephining for temporo-sphenoidal abscess. A point is chosen on the scalp which lies between 1½ and 2 inches above the centre of the external auditory meatus, and a bradawl is there introduced so as to indent the external table of the skull. A small scalp-flap is framed, one presenting an upward convexity, and all bleeding controlled. The pin of the trephine is applied to the spot previously indicated on the bone and the disk removed. On account of the absence of diploic tissue and consequent approximation of the two tables of

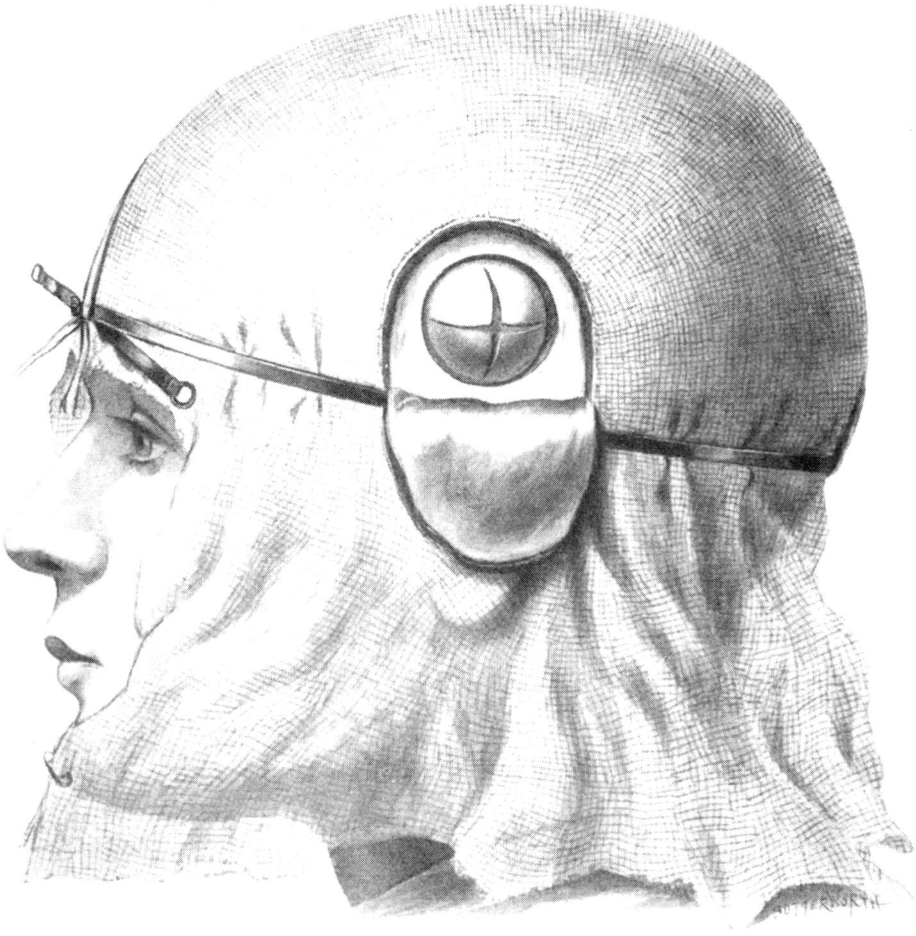

FIG. 79. THE EXPOSURE OF A TEMPORO-SPHENOIDAL ABSCESS.

the skull, care must be taken to avoid injury to the posterior branch of the middle meningeal artery and to the bulging dura mater.

The dura is then inspected and palpated; absence of pulsation, loss of lustre and tenseness, indicate the probable adjacency of the abscess cavity. The membrane should be crucially incised, all meningeal vessels that cross the line proposed for section being first under-run on either side of that line. The scalpel is lightly applied to the membrane and, as soon as the pia-arachnoid is exposed, the section completed with the blunt-pointed scissors.

The four dural flaps are turned aside and the cortex exposed. At the very apex of the bulging brain, and avoiding all visible vessels, a large blunt-pointed trocar and cannula or, preferably, Horsley's pus-evacuator is introduced and passed, for not more than $1\frac{1}{2}$ inches, in a direction inwards and slightly forwards, parallel to the roof of the middle ear. The blades of the evacuator must be opened 'once for each quarter of an inch of brain substance penetrated' (Macewen). If the trocar and cannula be utilized, similar precautions must be adopted.

In the event of failure to find pus at the first attempt, the evacuator is withdrawn, introduced at the same site, but now passed in other directions—directly inwards, slightly upwards, and finally, slightly backwards, in each case for not more than $1\frac{1}{2}$ inches.

By wide separation of the blades of the evacuator the pus is allowed to escape, to be immediately wiped away by the assistant. Irrigation of the cavity should never be attempted, not so much because of the difficulties attendant on that process, but because of the danger of infecting the neighbouring meningeal regions.

Previous to withdrawal of the evacuator, a small rubber or cigarette drainage-tube is introduced, projecting into the abscess cavity at the one end, and brought out through the scalp-flap at the other. It is advisable to stitch the tube in position.

The dural flaps are replaced in their proper position, but no attempt is made at sewing them together. The scalp-flap is sutured with the aid of a few salmon-gut stitches and the dressings applied. The tube may be shortened daily, and dispensed with after seven to ten days, according to the progress of the case.

Trephining for cerebellar abscess. The abscess usually occupies the antero-external aspect of the lateral lobe of the cerebellum. It can be drained with advantage below the level of the lateral sinus and behind the posterior border of the mastoid process.

The patient should be in the semi-prone position, the head as forwardly flexed as the administration of the anæsthetic allows.

The incision starts below the external occipital protuberance, and, following the line of the occipital crest, curves downwards along the posterior border of the mastoid process, terminating at the apex of that prominence. The cutaneo-muscular flap is turned down, every precaution being taken to diminish hæmorrhage, insomuch as severe bleeding may take place from occipital vessels, and from the mastoid and other emissary veins. Hæmorrhage from the former source is controlled with forceps, that from the emissary veins by the introduction of the end of a blunt probe into the orifice of the foramen. More permanent occlusion can be obtained by plugging the foramen with catgut, with a sterilized wooden match, or by means of special ivory, bone, and wooden pegs.

The trephine is applied in such a manner that its circle falls well below the lower level of the lateral sinus and behind the mastoid process. After removal of the disk, the dura mater is cautiously opened by crucial incision and the evacuating instrument introduced, the cerebellum being explored in the forward and slightly inward direction—towards the posterior aspect of the petrous bone. The abscess should be reached within 1½ inches from the opening in the bone. A drainage tube is introduced, stitched in position, in the manner described when dealing with temporo-sphenoidal abscess. This tube should be shortened daily and dispensed with after seven to ten days.

Trephining for frontal abscess. An abscess of the frontal lobe is generally situated so far back, and connected with the source of the trouble (the frontal sinus) by so long a 'stalk' of infection, that considerable difficulty may be experienced in attempting drainage from the frontal or nasal regions. Moreover, operations conducted through the frontal region are apt to result in considerable deformity. The operation may therefore be conducted with advantage from the temporo-frontal region. In this situation, the bone is thin, the operation can be conducted between the split fibres of the temporal muscle, excellent drainage is supplied, and the scar is inconspicuous.

For a general description of the intermusculo-temporal operation, the reader is referred to p. 121. In this instance, the field of operation is shifted further forwards, otherwise the details are very similar. The skin incision commences above and in front of the external angular frontal process, curves along the temporal crest, and terminates well in front of the ear. The temporal fascia is turned down and the muscle split in the general direction of its fibres, and well retracted on either side. The trephine is applied, the dura mater incised, and the abscess evacuated and drained in the manner previously described. The tube may be removed after seven to ten days.

The treatment of a chronic encapsuled abscess, wherever situated. In attempting to evacuate a chronic encapsuled abscess, both the trocar and cannula and the evacuator merely impinge against, and tend to push aside, the dense enclosing wall of the abscess cavity. When such obstruction is suspected, a director should be introduced in the direction of the abscess, and the brain explored till the resistance of the abscess-wall is encountered. With the aid of two narrow spatulæ, or other suitable instrument, the passage through the brain is gently enlarged till the wall of the abscess becomes visible. The margins of the passage through the brain are gently retracted and the abscess-wall freely incised with the knife. After the evacuation of the pus, a drainage tube can be introduced, but, as such a method seldom permits of a permanent cure—the abscess filling up again as soon as the tube is withdrawn—it is generally advisable to attempt the entire removal of the abscess-wall. The cut edges of the capsular incision are seized with narrow-bladed forceps, gentle traction applied, and the surrounding brain substance carefully peeled away. As a rule, there is no great difficulty attendant on this process and the hæmorrhage is seldom severe. The cavity that remains in the brain substance is *lightly* packed with gauze, this packing being allowed to remain for twenty-four to thirty-six hours, after which it is withdrawn and a little fresh gauze introduced, if necessary. The cavity fills up with extraordinary rapidity, mainly as a result of the expansion and falling together of the surrounding brain (see Figs. 86 and 86 *a*).

2. The one-stage operation.

Preliminary exploration of the mastoid operation, followed by an investigation of the middle and posterior fossæ of the skull. To expose the mastoid antrum, the incision commences immediately above and behind the ear, and, carried down to the bone throughout, terminates near the tip of the mastoid process. The soft tissues are peeled away in the forward direction and the cartilaginous ear detached from the posterior and upper boundaries of the bony auditory meatus.

Macewen's suprameatal triangle and the supramastoid crest are identified, the former landmark being taken as a guide to the communication between the mastoid antrum and the middle ear, the latter representing the uppermost limit of the field of operation.

With the aid of the hammer and chisel the bone is chipped away till the antrum is exposed—on an average this will be situated about three-fifths of an inch deep from the surface. The opening necessarily

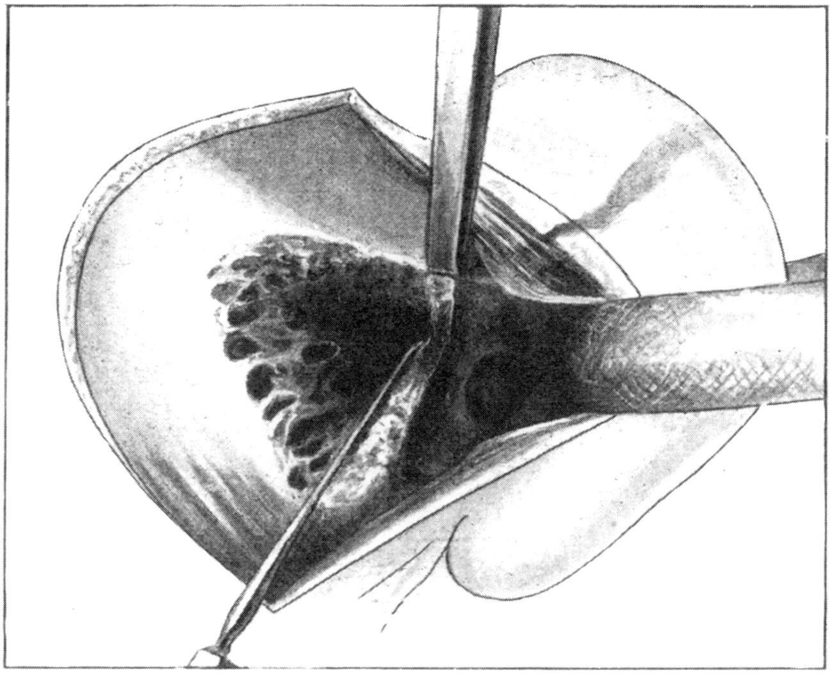

FIG. 80. THE 'RADICAL' MASTOID OPERATION. To show removal of the 'bridge' from above. The seeker, inserted into the aditus, acts as a protector to the underlying external semicircular canal and facial nerve. (After Hunter Tod.)

becomes funnel-shaped, but it should be made as complete as circumstances permit.

As soon as the antrum is exposed, the seeker or nerve-protector should be introduced into the aditus, acting as a protector to the underlying external semicircular canal and facial nerve, and the 'bridge' of bone, which now intervenes between the antrum and the middle ear, chiselled away, in the manner indicated in Fig. 80.

The field of operation is now carefully cleansed, cholesteatomata, bone-debris, and ossicles being gently removed, and—with the aid of a head-lamp—a careful search instituted for fistulous tracts, carious bone, &c. This search must be carried out with the greatest gentleness for fear of inducing further complications.

Subsequent procedures vary according to the nature of the conditions found. Thus :—

1. When the diagnosis is uncertain and when the boundaries of the cavity appear fairly healthy, the operation may terminate at this point, a post-meatal flap being formed and the cavity lightly plugged with gauze. The proximal end of the gauze plug is brought

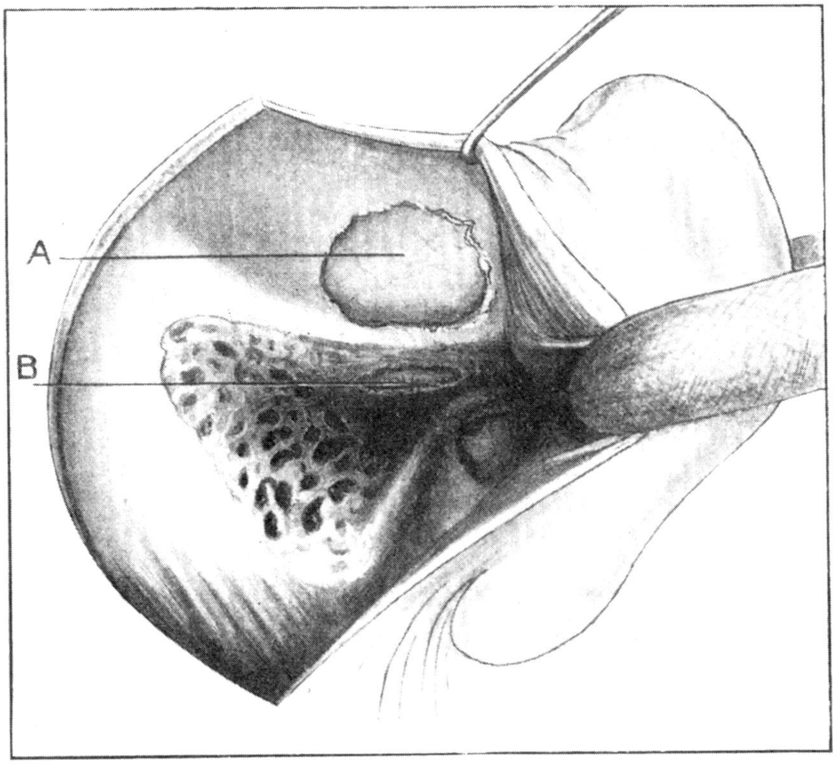

FIG. 81. EXPLORATION FOR A TEMPORO-SPHENOIDAL ABSCESS. A, Above the tegmen tympani; B, Through the tegmen tympani. Occasionally these methods are combined; the bone between the openings being also removed. (After Hunter Tod.)

out through the enlarged auditory meatus and the ear-flap sewn back with a few salmon-gut sutures.

2. When the evidence points to implication of the *middle* fossa, the scalp incision is prolonged upwards for about 1 inch and the soft parts retracted. The supra-tegmental extra-dural space can be exposed either by chiselling away the osseous roof of antrum and middle ear, or by means of a separate opening above the level of the supramastoid crest. In the event of the discovery of an *extra-dural* collection of pus, the purulent material is gently wiped away, free drainage supplied, and the wound closed.

In both this and the preceding case, the progress of the case during the ensuing twenty-four to forty-eight hours will prove whether adequate measures have been adopted.

When the symptoms are suggestive of *brain abscess*, when no extra-dural collection is discovered, and when the dura mater is tense and discoloured, then it becomes necessary to explore the brain.

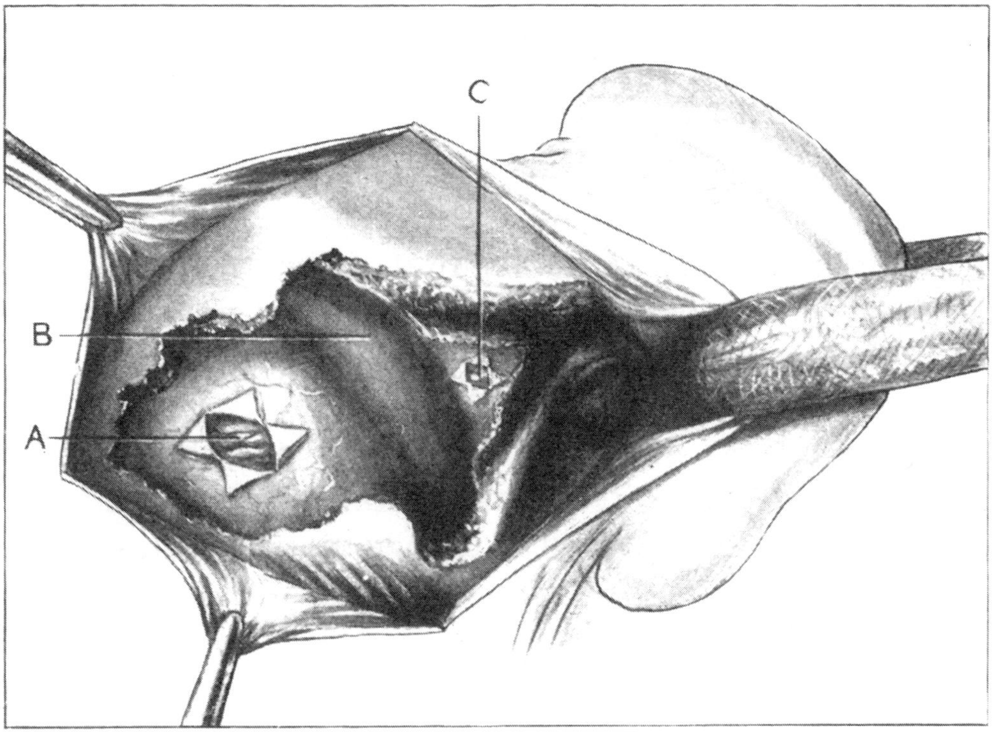

FIG. 82. EXPLORATION FOR A CEREBELLAR ABSCESS. A behind, and C in front of the lateral sinus ; B, Lateral sinus. (After Hunter Tod.)

This can be carried out through an opening made in the tegmen or above the level of the supramastoid crest. Which route should be utilized depends on the local conditions. As a general rule, it is advisable to explore through the tegmen when a sinus exists in that situation, and above the supramastoid crest under all other circumstances.

In the latter case, the dura mater is incised crucially and the bulging brain explored in the manner indicated on p. 266. The mastoid region should first be cleansed and packed with gauze, but, even with such precautions, it is obvious that there is some risk of contaminating membranes and brain in the event of failure to discover the abscess cavity—an argument in favour of exploring through the 'clean' squamous region (see p. 264).

3. When the evidence points to implication of the *posterior* fossa, an incision is carried backwards, from the mid-point of the post-aural incision, for about 2 inches, and the soft parts retracted upwards and downwards. With the chisel (or gouge) and hammer, the bone is freely cut away so as to expose (1) the lateral sinus, and (2) the dura mater below and behind the curve of the sinus. As soon as the sinus is exposed, the dura mater may be separated from the bone and the subsinus region exposed with the aid of craniectomy forceps.

The extra-dural space between the posterior aspect of the petrous bone and the lateral sinus region is first inspected, and, in the event of the discovery of a collection of pus, this is gently wiped away and further exploration postponed till the occasion should prove the necessity.

When the indications are of such a nature as to demand *exploration of the cerebellum*, the mastoid region is first cleansed and packed with gauze, after which the dura mater is incised either in front or behind the sinus according to the probable situation of the abscess cavity. After the evacuation of the abscess, a drainage tube is stitched in position in the manner previously indicated.

Difficulties and dangers attendant on the process of trephining for brain abscess.

Failure to find the abscess is usually dependent on one of the following causes:—

(*a*) The abscess may be missed if the localizing features are misleading, if the abscess be small, and if the exploring instrument be passed in a faulty direction or to an insufficient depth.

(*b*) The abscess may be traversed but not tapped if unsuitable exploring instruments be used—an aspirating syringe, for instance, through which the thick pus will not pass. Even when suitable instruments are used, the attempt to evacuate the abscess may fail if the operator does not carry out what may be called a system of progressive exploration, that is to say, if he does not periodically open the blades of the evacuator (see p. 266).

(*c*) The abscess may be encountered but not penetrated if the surgeon has to deal with a chronic abscess, the wall of which is merely pushed aside by the advancing instrument (see chronic abscess of the brain, p. 268).

Complications arising during and after the evacuation of the abscess are as follows :—

1. Leaking into the pia-arachnoid and the development of general meningeal infection.
2. Perforation of the ventricular spaces.
3. Hæmorrhage.
4. Respiratory failure.
5. Osteomyelitis of the neighbouring diploic tissue.

General meningeal infection will bring about a fatal result. Fortunately, the general rise of intracranial pressure and the formation of adhesions between the brain and the overlying membranes tend to prevent its development.

Perforation of the ventricular spaces may occur under two conditions: (1) when the abscess is associated with internal hydrocephalus, and (2) when the exploring instrument is passed too far.

Hæmorrhage is seldom serious when the operation is carried out with a light hand, all visible vessels being carefully avoided. In the event of its occurrence, it may be controlled by lightly packing the cavity with gauze.

Respiratory failure is most liable to occur when the surgeon is operating for cerebellar abscess. In the event of its occurrence the surgeon should complete his trephining with the utmost expedition, thus relieving the intracranial pressure. Under favourable circumstances, the respiratory rhythm is soon restored. In the more serious cases, artificial respiration should be attempted whilst the surgeon carries on his manipulations, opening the skull as rapidly as possible.

MENINGITIS

Previous to entering into the question of general meningeal infection, some allusion must be made to the rarer forms of meningitis.

Serous meningitis. Quincke demonstrated in 1895 the existence of a serous form of meningitis, one characterized by a serofibrinous exudate. He showed that, just as we have to deal with a serous or purulent pleurisy, so we have to consider the possibility of a serous or purulent form of meningitis.

The exudate appears at first sight to differ but slightly from normal cerebro-spinal fluid, being clear, yielding the normal chemical reactions of that fluid, and occupying the subarachnoid region. Later on it becomes slightly turbid, contains a fair quantity of albumen, and is proportionately rich in cellular elements—lymphocytes and polymorphonuclear leucocytes. The membranes are swollen, the vessels dilated, whilst occasionally many minute hæmorrhages may so allow of the escape of red blood-corpuscles as to impart to the exudate a yellowish-red coloration. At a still later stage the exudate becomes flocculent as a result of the deposition of a fibrinous coagulation, a gum-like material forming over the surface of the brain.

Pachymeningitis externa. Pachymeningitis externa is almost necessarily dependent on disease of the middle ear, on suppuration in the accessory sinuses of the nose, and on infected fractures of the vault and base. The inflammatory changes primarily involve the external aspect of the dura mater, the external surface of which is injected, roughened with fibrinous exudate, and, in the more chronic cases, covered with granulations. In itself the process seldom gives rise to symptoms, but so soon as the inner surface of the dura shares in the affection (meningitis), or the infection spreads to the venous sinuses (sinus thrombosis), or to the brain (brain abscess), definite symptoms arise pointing to the nature and character of the change.

Pachymeningitis interna and pachymeningitis interna hæmorrhagica. As the direct result of alcoholic excess, of syphilitic infection, and of trauma, the inner surface of the dura mater loses its shiny appearance, becomes opaque and thickened, especially in the region of the falx cerebri and over the convexity of the brain. The sodden and œdematous condition of the dura gives rise to a fibrinous and membranous exudate, terminating in the formation of false membranes—one of the factors in the formation of so-called ‘arachnoid cysts’ (see p. 203). These membranes are seen to be attached to the dura mater by means of newly-formed vessels, some of which may rupture, giving origin to blood exudate sufficing to impart to the membranes a brownish-red coloration. In the more marked cases, especially in those of a recurrent nature, the membranes partake of a lamellated type. Occasionally, the hæmorrhages are more excessive, giving rise to the formation of subdural hæmatomata from the partial absorption of which the various types of pachymeningitis hæmorrhagica arise.

These rarer forms of meningitis seldom give rise to such definite symptoms as to allow the surgeon to carry out surgical procedures in their earlier stages. Later on, by reason of the development of cystic accumulations of fluid or other complication, operation may be carried out with a reasonable degree of success. The operative technique adapted to the individual case is discussed under appropriate headings—Jacksonian epilepsy, meningeal cysts, &c.

It is possible that some criticism may be aroused with regard to the non-inclusion of tuberculous meningitis. Insomuch, however, as I have operated on a considerable number of cases of tuberculous meningitis—some intentionally from a decompression point of view, others by reason of doubtful diagnosis—and have never brought about more than some temporary alleviation, I have come to regard such cases as beyond the realms of surgery.

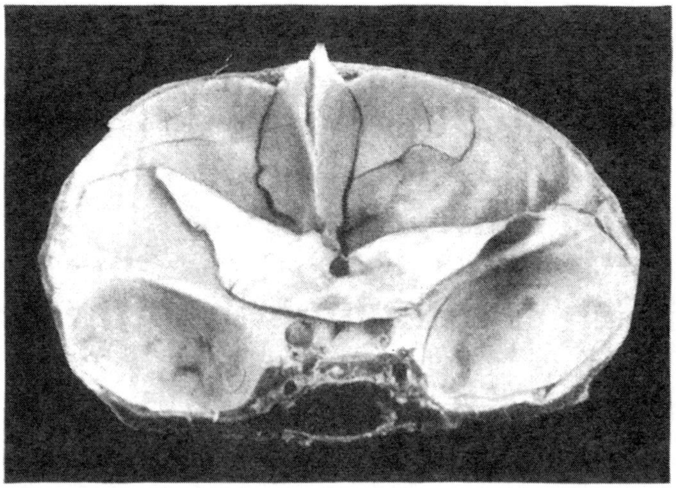

FIG. 83. A FRACTURE OF THE ANTERIOR FOSSA WHICH WAS FOLLOWED BY THE DEVELOPMENT OF MENINGITIS.

Acute lepto-meningitis. This condition will be considered under the more familiar, though less correct, designation—*meningitis.*

Attempts have been made to classify the various forms of meningitis on a bacterial basis. When, however, it is realized that almost any known form of organism may be present in the exudate, and that the symptoms dependent on these various infections closely resemble one another, merely differing in their acuteness and intensity, it would appear that some other form of classification is preferable.

The following method of classification will suffice :—

1. Meningitis of traumatic origin. The organisms either obtain direct entrance to the meningeal space by means of a compound fracture of the vault or base of the skull, or reach their destination along the course of the numerous emissary and diploic veins that bring the extra- and intra-cranial channels into communication.

2. Meningitis secondary to disease of neighbouring regions.

(1) The accessory sinuses of the nose and ear.

(2) The bones of the skull.

(3) The soft parts—scalp, orbit, nose, and face.

3. Meningitis secondary to disease of more distant regions. Through the medium of the blood-stream bacteria may be carried to the meningeal region in many acute infections—more especially in diseases of the lung.

Some anatomical considerations of meningitis. The *pia* is closely applied to the surface of the brain, dipping down into all the fissures, both major and minor. The *arachnoid* is only reflected into the greater fissures—the mesial longitudinal fissure, the fissure of Sylvius, Rolando, &c. The pia and arachnoid are therefore separated from one another by a potential space over the convolutions themselves, and by an actual space in the region of many of the cortical fissures.

On the under aspect of the brain the two membranes are so disposed and so separated from one another as to form three great basins or cisternæ, three great spaces acting as a water-bed for the brain. These are the *cisterna magna*, the arachnoid bridging over the wide interval between the back part of the under surface of the cerebellum and the medulla, the *cisterna pontis*, the angular space between the pons, medulla, and cerebellum, and the *cisterna basalis*, the arachnoid there covering in the structure situated in the interpeduncular space, including the Circle of Willis.

The subarachnoid space, both cortical and basal, is traversed by numerous trabeculæ which, passing from one membrane to the other, break up the space into innumerable small compartments, all containing cerebro-spinal fluid and all intercommunicating. The cerebral vessels ramify in the space, the tributaries being supported by the framework and bathed in the fluid.

All cranial nerves carry with them in their emergence from the skull a process of both pia and arachnoid, variable in extent, but so arranged that the nerve trunk is surrounded for some distance by a funnel-shaped process of membrane, the cerebral cerebro-spinal fluid being thus brought into connexion with the cervical lymphatic spaces.

With respect to the origin of the cerebro-spinal fluid and its wave of flow, the researches of Leonard Hill tend to prove that it is formed from the lining ependyma and choroid plexuses of the three main ventricles of the brain, passing thence into the spinal cerebrospinal region and, by means of the foramina of Majendie, Key, and Retzius—apertures in the roof of the fourth ventricle—on to the surface of the brain. From this latter region there appears to be

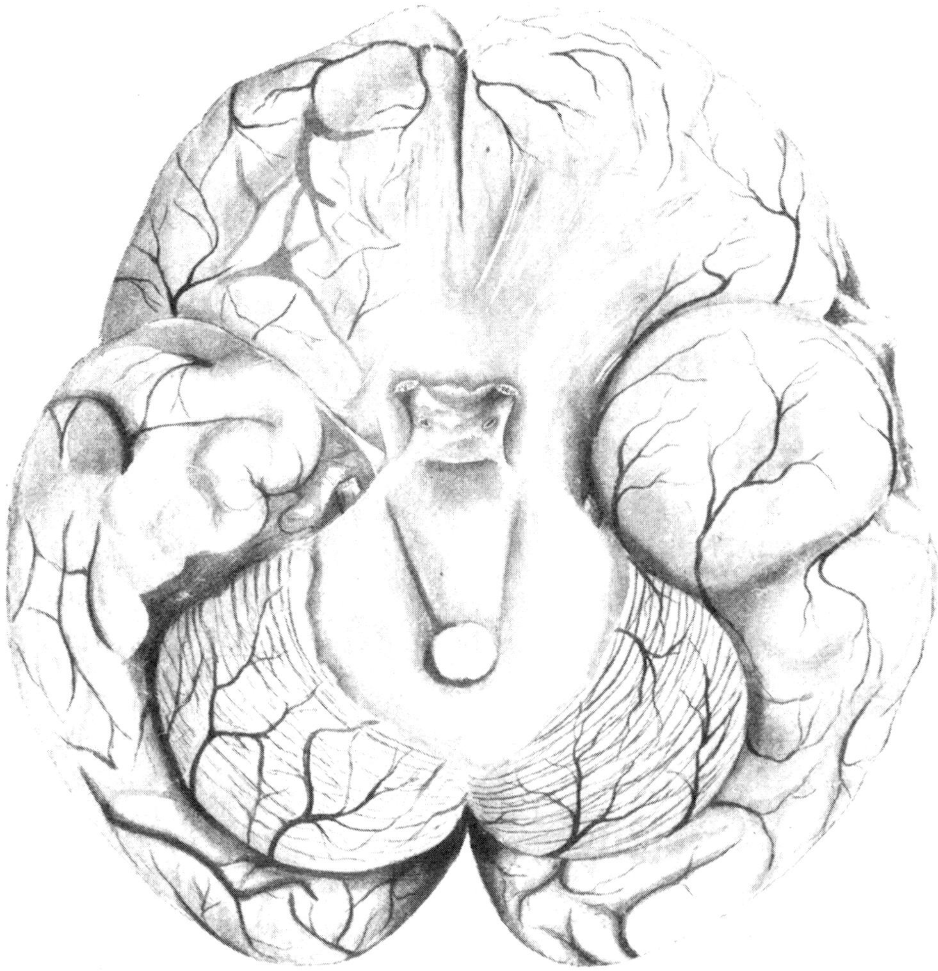

FIG. 84. BASAL MENINGITIS SECONDARY TO TEMPORO-SPHENOIDAL ABSCESS.

a general tendency for the fluid to pass upwards from the basal aspect of the brain towards the superior longitudinal sinus where it is again absorbed, probably through the medium of the Pacchionian bodies and lacunæ laterales of the venous sinus.

From these few anatomical facts it is manifest (1) that a sub-arachnoid purulent effusion has every opportunity of spreading widely over the surface of the brain, and (2) that inflammation and its results in the immediate neighbourhood of the roof of the fourth ventricle will tend to impede the normal flow of cerebro-spinal fluid through the foramina in that region, thus inducing a degree of internal hydrocephalus directly proportionate to the degree of obstruction.

Furthermore, it is obvious that the anatomical arrangements are entirely opposed to the possibility of providing adequate drainage in cases of general meningeal infection. It has been suggested that trephine holes should be made on either side of the skull, and that the intervening meningeal space should be washed out between the two apertures. It is, however, impossible to attain such a result, not only because of the futility of attempting to wash through the subarachnoid meshwork, but also on account of the outward bulging of the brain substance through the trephine holes and the corking up of those apertures.

The pus rapidly spreads over the surface of the cerebrum and over the base of the brain, along the sheaths of the emerging cranial nerves, and down the spinal canal. Associated with vascular dilatation there is extensive leucocyte extravasation into the perivascular spaces, the course of the line of the attack being mapped out by white and yellow lines and areas of exudation. Insomuch, also, as the meningeal vessels are in direct continuity with those of the cortex itself, it follows that a well-developed case of meningitis implies a corresponding degree of cerebritis, with red or white softening of the brain substance according to the degree of hæmorrhagic extravasation.

Symptomatology. Meningitis is generally sudden in onset and ushered in by a rigor, frequently of a most intense character. Headache is always a marked feature, commonly diffuse, but sometimes localized to the region primarily and mainly affected. The headache is intense and exacerbations are marked, the patient crying out in his agony. There is great mental irritability and all attempts at clinical examination are strenuously resisted.

After the initial rigor the temperature remains high, with occasional remissions during the early hours of the morning. Vomiting may be frequent and violent, but, according to my observations, this has not been a conspicuous feature.

The pulse-rate is increased, whilst, in the early stages, the volume is full and the tension high. The skin is burning hot and dry, except during the post-rigor periods when sweating predominates.

The face is flushed, often turgid, and the eyes are bright. General restlessness is a marked feature.

The more *localizing* features may be arranged in three groups: intellectual, motor, and sensory.

Intellectual symptoms. The condition of the patient is one of great restlessness, increasing sometimes to actual violence and mania. Attendants are usually required to restrain his movements, and, tossing about in bed, crying out in his pain, muttering and wandering in his delirium, he offers a typical clinical picture of cerebral irritation.

Motor symptoms. The motor symptoms vary according to the region mainly involved, cortex or base. In the *former* case, excitation results in twitchings and convulsions of the regions supplied by the cortical areas involved. Convulsions may be general or confined to a certain group of muscles, the former condition usually present in children, the latter more often observed in adults and occasionally partaking of the Jacksonian type. Convulsions may be associated with contractures of the limbs, the flexors mainly affected in such a manner that an attitude of general flexion may be assumed. The patient appears to suffer pain when attempts are made to straighten the limbs. In any case, such attempts are resisted.

Implication of the *base of the brain.* This is evidenced by symptoms sufficiently definite. Thus, the following symptoms may be observed :—

Optic neuritis.

Myosis and squints, from involvement of the third, fourth, and sixth nerves.

Trismus, from implication of the third division of the fifth nerve.

Facial paralysis, from implication of the seventh nerve.

Deafness, from involvement of the eighth nerve.

Dysphagia and dyspnœa, from involvement of the ninth and tenth nerves.

Rigidity of the neck and torticollis, from involvement of the eleventh nerve.

Retraction of the head and neck, from involvement of the posterior divisions of the upper cervical nerves.

Opisthotonos, from the involvement of the posterior divisions of the upper cervical nerves, sometimes of so excessive a nature that the body is bent backwards to such a degree that the head and heels are almost brought into contact. More rarely, pleurosthotonos or lateral flexion is observed.

Sensory and other phenomena. Amongst such symptoms may be mentioned cutaneous hyperæsthesis, photophobia, and vaso-motor changes—the last-named evidenced by flushings, sweats, and *tâche cérèbrale.*

Rapid emaciation, anorexia, and distaste for all nourishment are the rule, whilst retention of urine, albuminuria, and glycosuria have been observed.

The reflexes, both deep and superficial, are often increased. Kernig's sign is generally present.

The period of depression. The acute stage seldom persists more than two or three days, the period of excitation giving place to that of depression. The transition is usually of a rapid nature. The depression stage is dependent on exhaustion of the cortical and basal centres.

The temperature remains high, rising towards the evening and falling a degree or more in the early hours of the morn. Death usually takes place when the temperature is at its highest.

The pulse may become slower as the intracranial pressure increases, but, more commonly, as the result of toxic poisoning, the rate increases whilst the rhythm becomes irregular and the tension lowered.

Respiration may partake of the Cheyne-Stokes type, whilst the impaired æration of the blood and the weak action of the heart are evidenced by cyanosis of the face, œdema of the lower extremities, &c.

Death, primarily due to respiratory failure, is often preceded by general twitchings or convulsions.

The whole course of the illness seldom lasts more than a week, the more acute cases terminating within two or three days.

Treatment. Whether threatening, developing, or obviously present, the patient should be treated with urotropin (see p. 116). In its early stages of development immediate operation affords some hope of cure, such treatment having as its basis the supply of adequate drainage. The source of the infection must be removed—so far as circumstances permit—the dura mater freely incised, and the pia-arachnoid region so opened up as to allow of the escape of some of the purulent or semi-purulent fluid. The wound is largely allowed to remain open, packed with gauze. The predominant organism may be isolated and, if time allows, suitable vaccine treatment instituted. In the meantime, 20 to 40 cc. of pyogenes serum should be administered.

From the point of view of diagnosis, *lumbar puncture* should never be omitted. The fluid escapes at high tension, is turbid and contains many polymorphonuclear leucocytes and organisms, the latter verified with the greatest advantage after centrifugalization. Repeated lumbar punctures are also said to be of some benefit with respect to *treatment.*

SINUS THROMBOSIS

Lateral sinus thrombosis. Soon after entering on its course across the mastoid process the lateral sinus presents a well-marked S-shaped curve. This sigmoid sinus bulges markedly forwards—especially on the right side—towards the region of the mastoid cells and antrum, so much so that a mere shell of bone intervenes between the sinus on the one hand and the antral region on the other. Indeed, the relations are so intimate that one would expect a more frequent occurrence of lateral sinus thrombosis. Furthermore, the sinus receives numerous venous communications from the mastoid cells, antrum, and other parts of the temporal bone, conspicuous amongst the last-named group of vessels being the mastoid emissary vein which, passing inwards at the upper and posterior border of the mastoid process, connects the posterior auricular and occipital veins with the lateral sinus.

From these considerations it is obvious that any acute or chronic infective process originating either in the aural region or in the neighbourhood can readily infect the sinus by direct propagation of organisms along one or more of these inter-communicating vessels (thrombo-phlebitis).

The sinus may also become infected in middle-ear disease by the more gradual process of mining and sapping, the osseous barrier between the antrum and sinus being progressively destroyed by the backward progress of the aural disease. The sinus may erect an additional barrier by throwing out granulations (external pachy-meningitis) against the invading host, but, in the event of the attack overcoming the defence, sinus thrombosis may result, at first perhaps of a non-infective type but soon becoming definitely septic, the clot softening and disintegrating (osteo-phlebitis).

There can be no question that middle-ear disease is responsible for the very great majority of cases of lateral sinus thrombosis, and whether the infection takes place by extension of thrombus along the connecting veins (thrombo-phlebitis), or after destruction of the osseous barrier (osteo-thrombosis), the results are more or less identical.

Thrombosis first occurs in that part of the sinus which is in closest relation to the primary cause of the infection, the clot rapidly increasing in size until the lumen of the sinus is entirely obliterated. In its early stages the thrombus is of a chocolate colour, softening at a later date and breaking down into a purulent material. Many varieties of bacteria may be present though the infection is mainly dependent on the presence of the streptococcus pyogenes.

Two changes may now occur :—(1) the central portion of the thrombus, having softened into a purulent material, may be limited by the firmer thrombus in front and behind; and (2) the thrombus may extend into the neighbouring and connecting venous channels *downwards* along the course of the internal jugular vein, *backwards* along the course of the lateral sinus, *inwards* along the course of the superior petrosal sinus, *outwards* along the line of the mastoid emissary vein, *downwards* through the posterior condyloid foramen, and *inwards* along meningeal veins.

The **symptomatology** may be considered as follows :—

(1) Symptoms dependent on the extension of the thrombus to neighbouring venous and lymphatic channels.

(2) Symptoms resulting from toxic absorption or dependent on the transmission of infected material to other parts of the body.

1. *Symptoms dependent on the extension of the thrombus to neighbouring venous and lymphatic channels.* When the thrombus spreads *downwards* along the course of the *internal jugular vein,* there is swelling and tenderness along the line of the vein. The vessel, though thrombosed in its upper part—perhaps throughout its whole extent—is itself seldom palpable, the cervical swelling usually being dependent on associated lymphadenitis and lymphangitis. In those few cases where the thrombosed vein can be felt, resembling a 'buried lead pencil', the thrombus is sometimes of the non-infective type.

The combined venous and lymphatic involvement causes œdema of the tissues, pain, and rigidity on attempted movement. The anterior and external jugular veins may become engorged from the extra strain thrown upon them. Subsequently, the inflamed parts may break down and extensive cervical suppuration result.

When the thrombus spreads *backwards* along the course of the *lateral sinus,* the coagulation process may extend as far as the torcula and even further. Evidence as to the nature and extent of the process is not always apparent, though one expects to find some œdema of the overlying scalp tissues.

When the process spreads *inwards* along the course of the *superior petrosal sinus* there is considerable risk of involvement of the corresponding cavernous sinus, possibly of the opposite sinus also (see p. 288).

When the process spreads *outwards* along the course of the *mastoid emissary vein,* œdema, and dilatation of veins in the post-auricular region are observed, associated with tenderness on palpation. This is most apparent at the upper and posterior border of the mastoid process.

When the thrombus spreads *downwards* along the course of the *posterior condyloid vein,* there may be some œdema and pain on pressure in the upper part of the posterior triangle of the neck, associated with glandular enlargement in the region. These symptoms are dependent on the connexion established by the posterior condyloid vein between the sigmoid sinus and the deep veins of the neck.

When the thrombus extends *inwards* along the meningeal veins, meningitis, meningo-cerebritis, and cerebral abscess result.

2. *Symptoms resulting from toxic absorption or dependent on the transmission of infected material to other parts of the body.*

Optic neuritis is present, according to Hunter Tod, in about 50 per cent. cases. It develops rapidly and attains a high degree of intensity.

Headache is usually intense in character, persistent, but little remedied by drugs and presenting marked exacerbations. It is often most acute over the affected region.

The *mental condition* of the patient is subject to variation. In the average case mental symptoms are quite disproportionate to the severity of the disease. Sometimes the patient is cheerful, perhaps rather excited, retaining his faculties to the last, in other cases—as the result of excessive toxic poisoning—he lies in a stuporose, typhoid-like state. When the thrombus is associated with meningitis, meningeal symptoms predominate.

Vomiting is often a conspicuous feature, generally of the so-called 'cerebral' type, a regurgitation without nausea and retching.

The *pulse* is rapid, the rhythm irregular, and the tension lowered.

The *temperature.* The formation of the thrombus is usually notified by the advent of one or more severe rigors, the temperature rising to 103° or more. During the height of the illness the temperature is high but remittent, and rigors are frequent. The occurrence of a series of rigors is almost certainly indicative of sinus thrombosis. Any marked remission of temperature is succeeded by profuse sweating, but, with this exception, the skin remains dry and burning.

Each rigor implies the extension of the thrombus to other venous channels or the transference of infected particles, by means of the blood-stream, to other parts of the body. In the young general convulsions are often observed.

The tongue is brown and dry, the breath foul and diarrhœa of common occurrence. The skin may be jaundiced, and septic rashes are prone to develop. The liver and spleen may be enlarged and tender. Cough and foul sputum point to pulmonary infarction.

Treatment. The mastoid antrum is rapidly exposed and the conditions investigated. The bone is then chiselled away in the backward direction, with the hammer and gouge, so as to expose the lateral sinus. The question then arises as to the condition of the sinus. This is a matter that may require considerable experience. The surgeon should be guided, not so much by exploratory puncture as by the surroundings and general appearance of the sinus. Thus, the absence of bleeding from the mastoid emissary vein during the process of exposure is very significant of sinus thrombosis. Again, whilst the normal sinus pulsates, is of dark blue colour and presents a shining surface, the thrombosed channel may be covered with pale granulations or obscured by fibrinous deposit, it does not pulsate, and appears of a yellow or deep purple colour. Between it and the bone there may be a collection of purulent matter. In the event of doubt, the surrounding regions should be carefully protected with gauze, after which the sinus may be punctured with a needle. The absence of fluid blood is conclusive of thrombosis.

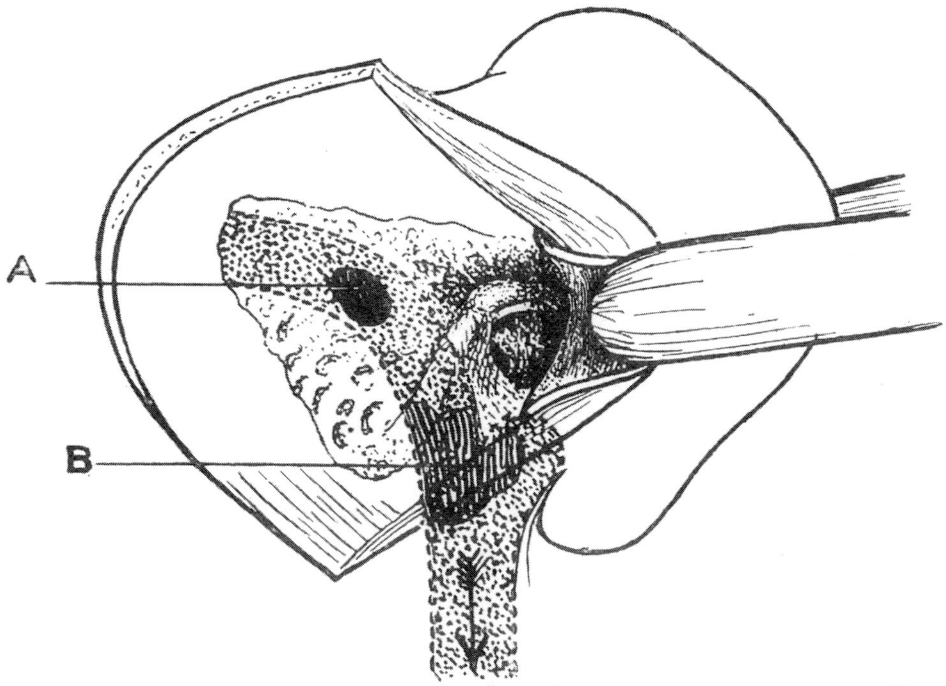

FIG. 85 A. DIAGRAM TO SHOW THE USUAL POINTS AT WHICH THE LATERAL SINUS IS PRIMARILY INFECTED. A, High up; from the posterior mastoid cells. In this case it may not be necessary to tie the jugular vein. B, Low down; involving the jugular bulb. This necessitates ligature of the vein. (After Hunter Tod.)

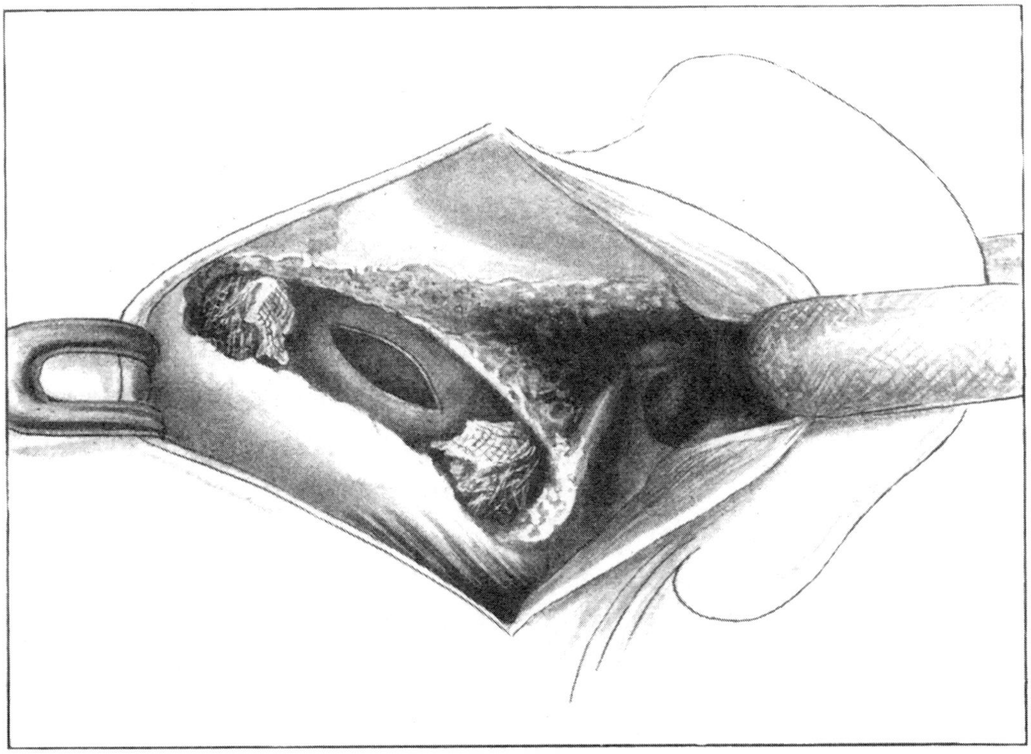

FIG. 85 B. THE LATERAL SINUS EXPOSED AND OPENED. The lumen of the sinus is obliterated above and below the region of the infected thrombus by plugs of ribbon gauze pressed in between the sinus wall and the overlying bone. In this case it is not necessary to tie the jugular vein. (After Hunter Tod.)

In the event of the surgeon concluding that thrombosis is present, subsequent procedures vary according to the extent of the thrombus. Thus, *when the clot appears to terminate above the jugular bulb*, a strip of gauze is inserted between the bone and the parietal wall of the sinus so as to obliterate the lumen of the sinus on the cardiac side of the clot.

The danger of further extension of the clot being thus obviated, the bone is nibbled away in the backward direction till at least half an inch of healthy vessel is exposed on the occipital side of the thrombus. A second gauze plug is then introduced so as to obliterate the sinus lumen in that region also.

In the interval between the two plugs the sinus is freely laid open, all clot and granulations being gently curetted and washed away. Some bleeding may take place during these procedures, from the mouths of certain vessels entering the sinus between the two compressed regions. This is in itself a favourable symptom, insomuch as it proves that the thrombotic process has not extended in those directions. This hæmorrhage may be controlled with gauze plugs. The parietal sinus wall in direct relation to the thrombus is freely cut away, after which the whole field is lightly packed with gauze and the ear sewn back into position. The main portion of the wound is left open, the sinus plugs being brought to the surface whilst those inserted into the combined middle ear and antrum emerge from the external auditory meatus.

All gauze-plugs may be withdrawn after twenty-four to thirty-six hours, the wound cleansed and lightly repacked. This process is continued daily till all is healed.

When the clot extends into the jugular bulb, and when the jugular vein appears to be involved, it is necessary to expose and ligature the vein in the neck, thus preventing further extension of coagulation and diminishing the risk of general infection. This measure should be carried out before the lateral sinus is laid open. With fresh gloves and another set of instruments, the vein is exposed so as to allow the application of two ligatures, and the division of the vessel between those two ligatures. If possible, the ligatures should be applied above the level of the entrance of the common facial vein. In all cases, however, the application must be carried out, if possible, below the lower limit of the thrombus. After the vein has been divided, the upper end may be dissected in such a manner as to allow of its being brought to the surface of the wound and there anchored.

Elsewhere the neck-incision is sewn up and protected with collodion gauze. The surgeon then returns to the mastoid and sinus regions, completing the exposure of the sinus and laying it open freely to the surface At the termination of these procedures, an attempt may be made, by irrigation between the open sinus above and jugular vein below, to wash away all thrombus contained in the intervening portion of the vessel.

Finally, both sinus and aural regions are packed with gauze, in a manner similar to that described above. Dressings are reapplied as circumstances demand, and the wounds allowed to heal by granulation.

The great frequency of a streptococcus pyogenes infection justifies one in the early administration of anti-streptococcic serum (20 to 40 c.c. of Burroughs Wellcome's 'Pyogenes') followed by an autogenous vaccine as soon as that can be prepared.

MAIN POINTS IN THE DIFFERENTIAL DIAGNOSIS BETWEEN

	BRAIN ABSCESS	MENINGITIS	LATERAL SINUS THROMBOSIS
Onset	Insidious.	Acute.	Acute.
Temperature	Subnormal (see p. 255).	First a rigor, then high and continuous temperature, usually intermittent.	First a rigor, then high and continuous temperature, usually remittent. Frequent rigors.
Pulse	Slow (see p. 255).	Rapid.	Rapid.
Mental condition	Often apathetic. In the later stages, stupor and loss of consciousness.	Very restless and delirious. Sometimes maniacal. Coma towards the end.	In the early stages, the mind is clear. This condition may persist till near the end when delirium and coma become evident.
Special symptoms	Paresis or paralysis, according to the site of the lesion.	Squints, retraction of the head and neck. Irregular palsies.	Œdema over mastoid, pain along course of internal jugular vein. Enlarged cervical glands.
Blood and cerebro-spinal examination	Progressive leucocytosis. Increased leucocytes in cerebro-spinal fluid.	Increased leucocyte count and organisms in fluid withdrawn by lumbar puncture.	Blood infection frequent.

In typical cases no great difficulty will be experienced in diagnosing between brain abscess, meningitis, and lateral sinus thrombosis. In many cases, however, two or more of these conditions may be co-existent. Thus, both brain abscess and lateral sinus thrombosis are often complicated by the presence of a meningeal infection. Again, the undue prominence of abdominal, cardiac, or pulmonary symptoms—more especially in cases of lateral sinus thrombosis—demand the full consideration of enteric fever, endocarditis, and pneumonia. Thus, in a case recently under my care at the hospital, and in which I had the benefit of the wide experience of my Aural colleague, Mr. West, operative procedures were carried out on the mastoid region, the patient dying some days later from enteric fever. Again, the question of differential diagnosis between tuberculous meningitis, brain tumour and brain abscess is always cropping up. Thus, a short time ago, I explored both temporo-sphenoidal lobes in a boy suffering from double otitis media and presenting well-marked general cerebral symptoms, only to find that he was a subject of tuberculous meningitis.

The diagnosis is often difficult, and no trouble must be spared in the complete investigation of the case. *Lumbar puncture* should invariably be carried out, the fluid being examined both cytologically and bacteriologically. In all cases of doubt one would be wise to call in further advice before undertaking exploratory operation.

Cavernous sinus thrombosis. Thrombosis of the cavernous sinus arises either as an osteo-phlebitis or as a thrombo-phlebitis. In the former case, the thrombus is dependent on disease of the bones related to the sinus—arising more especially as the result of prolonged sphenoidal sinusitis—whilst, in the latter instance, the sinus becomes infected through one of the many vascular communications connecting it with other neighbouring regions. Thus the radicles of the ophthalmic vein, by means of their communication with orbital, ethmoidal, and upper nasal vessels, and their connexion at the inner canthus of the eye with radicles of the angular vein, afford the most ready means of infection. Again, infection may spread from the auditory region along the superior petrosal sinus, and from the tonsillar and pharyngeal regions along the various emissary veins connecting the cavernous sinus on the one hand with the deep cervical vascular system on the other.

The two cavernous sinuses intercommunicate by means of the circular sinus, and consequently thrombosis of the one sinus is liable to involve its fellow. According to Macewen,[1] bilateral trouble occurs in 50 per cent. cases, the infection often spreading from one sinus to the other within twenty-four to thirty-six hours.

Thrombosis of the cavernous sinus is often associated with meningeal infection or brain-abscess.

Symptomatology. (*a*) *Symptoms dependent on the formation of the thrombus and its extension to neighbouring venous and lymphatic channels.* The presence of the thrombus and its extension into ophthalmic, angular, and retinal veins leads to proptosis, paresis of the ocular muscles, disturbances of vision, and œdema. *Proptosis* is of rapid development, frequently reaching its maximum within a few hours, the globe being protruded in the downward and outward direction. With respect to *ocular palsies*, the movements of the globe are greatly restricted with squints, ptosis, and perhaps complete ophthalmoplegia. The pupil may be contracted during the earlier stages, becoming fully dilated and insensitive at a later date. The *vision* suffers in proportion to the degree of paralysis of ocular muscles and associated retinal hæmorrhages and thrombosis. The veins of the lids, conjunctivæ, and upper part of the face and forehead are engorged, with corresponding œdema of the soft parts. The conjunctivæ may be chemotic.

The spread of the thrombus to the opposite sinus results in the development of bilateral symptoms, whilst the involvement of the petrosal sinus may bring about thrombosis of the lateral and sigmoid sinuses, with corresponding developments.

In other cases the meningeal veins are affected at an early date, in which case the symptoms dependent on the cavernous thrombus are obscured by those resulting from the meningeal infection.

(*b*) *Symptoms dependent on toxic absorption or resulting from the transference of infected particles to other parts of the body.* These more general symptoms closely resemble those enumerated when discussing lateral sinus thrombosis (see p. 283). Headache, however, is of the most intense type, and pain, of a severe neuralgic character, is referred along the course and distribution of the first and second divisions of the fifth nerve.

[1] *Pyogenic Diseases of the Brain and Spinal Cord*, p. 247.

Treatment. It has been suggested that exploration could be carried out, the thrombus evacuated, and the cavernous sinus region drained from the naso-ethmoidal region or by approach along the floor of the middle fossa of the skull—an exaggerated Gasserian ganglion operation. Both these methods have been tried, but the difficulties encountered and the want of success tended to show that cavernous sinus thrombosis was beyond the reach of the surgeon. However, of recent date, more hopeful views have been entertained, it being suggested that the globe should be removed, the sinus explored, and the orbital cavity packed with gauze. It is doubtful, however, whether the end justifies the means.

The prognosis in brain abscess, meningitis, and sinus thrombosis. A patient may be expected to recover from *brain abscess,* whether temporo-sphenoidal, cerebellar, or frontal, if an early diagnosis be made, if the case be uncomplicated by meningeal infection or sinus thrombosis, and if the evacuation be carried out without any great difficulty. As Sir William Macewen[1] pointed out, 'an uncomplicated brain abscess may be regarded as the most hopeful of all cerebral affections.' In fatal cases, death results from general meningeal infection or from the bursting of the abscess into the lateral ventricles.

In *meningitis* the prognosis is bad, more especially when the process is widespread. Early exposure of the affected region and the supply of adequate drainage offer the only hope of recovery. This, even under the most favourable circumstances, is a desperate remedy.

The prognosis in *lateral sinus thrombosis* hinges to a large extent on the time at which operative procedures are carried out. When the case is seen and operated on at an early date in the history of the disease, recovery may be anticipated in about 50 per cent. cases. Hunter Tod states that, when all cases are considered of whatever grade, about one-third recover. Death results from pyæmia, septicæmia, meningitis, or brain abscess.

Cavernous sinus thrombosis of the infective variety almost necessarily terminates fatally. Death results from causes similar to those observed in cases of lateral sinus thrombosis.

[1] *Pyogenic Diseases of the Brain and Spinal Cord.*

HERNIA CEREBRI

The term Hernia cerebri was formerly used as inclusive of all those conditions in which the brain protruded through some aperture in the skull, whether such opening was congenital, traumatic, or post-operative.

Owing to the recent advances in cranio-cerebral surgery, especially with reference to the frequent adoption of decompression operations, it is advisable that the cases should be classified into two groups :—

1. **Cases of hernial protrusion,** including cephaloceles (see Chapter I), protrusions intentionally produced by the surgeon in a decompression operation, and those which follow after unsuccessful operations for tumour removal. It will be observed that, in all these cases, the projecting brain, though bulging through its osseous barrier, is still protected by a more or less normal scalp-covering.

2. **Cases of hernia cerebri.** Here, as the result of injury to scalp, bone, dura, and brain, the cerebral substance bulges through a deficiency in the vault and presents on the surface, uncovered by integument. Hernia cerebri *can* develop under non-infective conditions, the congested state of the bruised or lacerated brain bringing about that degree of intracranial tension which can only be relieved by the outward projection of the brain. Still it must be accepted that Hernia cerebri almost invariably implies some bacterial infection.

Hernial protrusions are dealt with elsewhere. *Hernia cerebri* requires some consideration. Its development, by reason of its usual bacterial agency, must always be regarded as of serious import. The congested brain bulges through the aperture in the skull and presents on the surface as a purple—sometimes black—fungating mass, bleeding freely, and associated with a considerable discharge of cerebro-spinal fluid, serum, and pus.

The effects produced by this condition vary according to the extent of the cerebritis, and the question of associated meningeal infection.

When associated with meningitis those symptoms which might result from the hernial protrusion are more or less obscured by those dependent on the meningeal infection. Under other circumstances, the symptoms vary according to the extent and position of the area involved. Thus, when the infection is limited to the surface of the brain in the immediate vicinity of the aperture in the bone, the patient may merely complain of some headache and present some symptoms of cerebral irritation. More usually, the infection spreads rapidly to the surrounding brain substance, and the patient evidences the

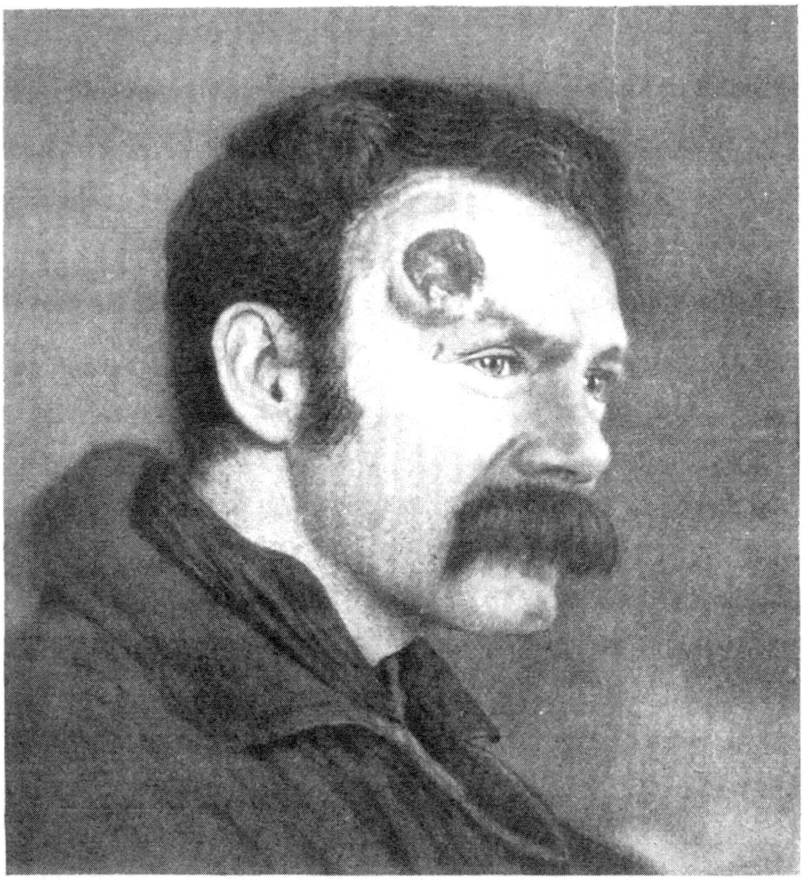

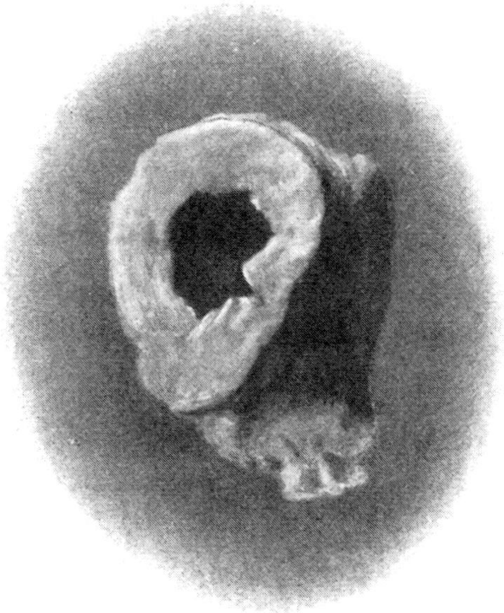

A

FIG. 86. A CASE OF HERNIA CEREBRI. A, The abscess after removal (natural size), cut so as to show the thickness of capsule.

most acute stage of cerebral irritation, passing thence rapidly into a stuporose, typhoid-like condition.

Treatment. With the object of reducing the infectivity of the protruding brain, fomentations have been advocated. From my own experience, however, it would appear that their application tends to increase the degree of protrusion, and that better results may be obtained by keeping the exposed brain as dry as possible, painting over with a $2\frac{1}{2}$ per cent. solution of iodine in rectified spirit, dusting with antiseptic powder, and protecting with dry dressings, frequently replaced.

In the event of failure to improve the condition by means of these minor remedies—a too-frequent occurrence—excision of the protruding mass may be regarded as a perfectly justifiable procedure, providing that the hernia does not include the cerebellum or motor cortical region. The protrusion is shaved away flush with the level of the skull, the raw surface of the brain lightly painted with iodine, dusted with iodoform or other antiseptic powder, and protected with gauze and wool.

The prognosis is necessarily most grave, but the most astounding recoveries have taken place under this mode of treatment.

CHAPTER IX

BULLET-WOUNDS OF THE SKULL AND BRAIN

In the consideration of bullet-wounds of the skull and brain the following factors must be taken into account :—

The velocity of the bullet.

The distance at which the bullet is fired.

The size of the bullet.

The nature of the bullet.

The angle of impact.

The position of the bullet at the moment of impact.

Before, however, noting the varying effects on the skull as produced by one or more of these factors, it will be necessary to allude briefly to the average effect on the skull as produced by bullet-wounds in general.

'When a foreign body passes through any part of the skull—it matters not what the direction may be—the aperture of exit is always greater than the aperture of entry.' Such was the law enunciated by Teevan in 1864. The explanation is as follows: 'The aperture of entry is caused by the penetrating body only, whilst the aperture of exit is larger, insomuch as it is made by the penetrating body plus the fragments of bone driven out of the proximal table and diploe.' It might also be added that the greater degree of damage will always be incurred by the unsupported table—the internal at the wound of entry, the external at that of exit.

The size and shape of the aperture of entry through the external table bears a close resemblance to the size and shape of the entering bullet. As a general rule, it is round or oval, and presents clean-cut edges with some small radiating fissures. The aperture of entry through the internal table is larger, the margins inverted towards the brain, the radiating fissures more pronounced, and small fragments of bone in-driven towards the brain.

In the event of perforation of the skull through the medium of a high-velocity bullet, the aperture of exit through the internal table closely resembles that through the external table at the site of entry, with the exception that it is influenced by any changes in position that the bullet may have undergone during its transmission through the brain. The wound of exit through the external table is again greater than that through the internal—in accordance with Teevan's law—the margins everted, the surrounding bone fissured or comminuted, whilst fragments of bone may be driven out beneath the lacerated scalp, or even blown completely away. On the other hand, when the bullet is fired at close range, the aperture of exit is often considerably larger than that of entry—due, in all probability, to superadded explosive effect.

The effect of the *velocity* of the bullet on the fracture:—The greater the velocity of the bullet the greater the resemblance of the wounds of entry and exit to the size and shape of the bullet, the 'cleaner' the holes, and vice versa.

The effect of *distance*:—When the bullet is fired from a distance, but with full effect, the hole is clean cut and presents the characteristics enumerated above. When the bullet is 'spent', the osseous injury at the point of impact is usually of a more extensive character than when the bullet possesses a higher degree of velocity. When fired at close quarters the damage incurred from the impact of the bullet is increased by the force of the forwardly driven air and gas. The skull suffers proportionately, the scalp being severely lacerated, burnt, and circumferentially ingrained with powder, the bone extensively comminuted, and the brain severely lacerated.

The effect of *size and shape* of the bullet:—The effects produced on the skull in relation to the size and shape of the bullet are so obvious as to require no description. The nature of the bullet must also be taken into consideration, whether of the soft-nosed variety, expansile, &c.

The effect of the *angle of impact*:—The lesion produced by the bullet varies according as to whether the bullet glances across the vault or strikes the bone at right angles. In the former case a 'gutter' fracture may result, varying in degree and associated brain complication according to the angle of impact. In the latter case the skull is penetrated or perforated.

The effect of the *position of the bullet* at the moment of impact :—The bullet, at the moment of impact, may be so changed in position—head-over-heels, ricochet, &c.—that the skull may be struck by its long axis instead of by its nose. In such cases, the wound of entry will be more extensive than under ordinary circumstances.

It is obvious, therefore, that many factors require consideration in estimating the extent of the osseous lesion and the nature of the complications existent in any given case. Due allowance must also be paid to other factors entering into the case, more especially in relation to the weapon used—pistol, revolver, gun, &c.

Injury to the bone. The various injuries to bone may be classified as follows :—

Fractures limited to the external table.
Fractures limited to the internal table.
Gutter fractures.
The complete fractures produced by a penetrating wound.
The complete fractures produced by a perforating wound.

Fractures limited to the external table. Fractures of this nature are of exceedingly rare occurrence. They are produced by a bullet which strikes the skull in such an oblique direction that the scalp and external table are torn away ('gutter' fractures), or by a bullet which, directed against the outer wall of the frontal sinus, possesses sufficient force to comminute the outer wall of that sinus, but, from loss of momentum, is incapable of penetrating further.

Fractures limited to the internal table. These fractures are even more rare than those described above. Their occurrence is probably only possible when the bullet strikes the skull in a markedly oblique direction, and with greatly diminished velocity—'spent' bullets. I believe I am correct in stating that only one instance of this particular variety of fracture was observed in the South African War. In any case, they are of such infrequent occurrence that they may be practically disregarded.

Gutter fractures. Gutter fractures are almost invariably dependent on the impact of a glancing bullet. They may be arranged in three groups, according to the extent of the osseous lesion.

1. Where the external table is blown away, leaving the internal table exposed, perhaps comminuted.

2. Where the internal table is driven in the inward direction, pressing on, irritating, and perhaps lacerating the dura mater.

3. Where the whole thickness of the bone is blown away, leaving a gaping wound from which brain-matter may protrude.

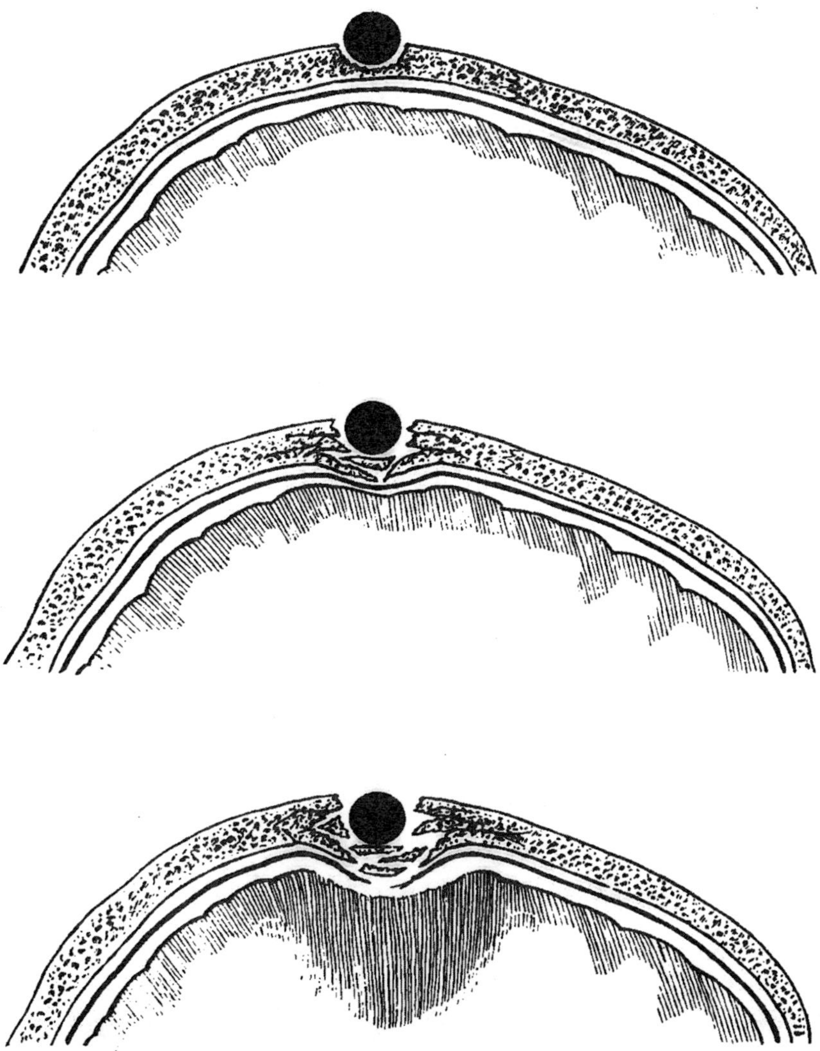

FIG. 87. DIAGRAMMATIC ILLUSTRATION OF THE THREE FORMS OF 'GUTTER' FRACTURE. (For further description, see text.)

The complete fractures produced by penetrating and perforating wounds. The general effects as produced by penetrating and perforating bullet-wounds of the skull and brain are depicted in Fig. 88, and described in the text associated with that figure.

Injury to the brain. Brain lesions vary 'from a single track with small points of extravasation in neighbouring areas to a condition of hæmorrhagic pulp, which latter condition is the result of injury from the projectile associated with bleeding, often extensive, into neighbouring areas, disintegrating and pulping the brain-substance. These latter cases are generally fatal, and are accompanied not infrequently with meningeal and ventricular hæmorrhage' (Bowlby).[1]

The worst degrees of brain-injury arise when the injury is inflicted at close range, more especially at the site of emergence of a perforating bullet, the damage to the soft parts being there magnified by the waves and vibrations set up by the bullet during its passage across the brain. In many cases also the brain is dashed as a whole against the opposing osseous barrier (laceration by contre-coup).

The general effects produced on the skull and brain by a perforating bullet of high velocity are shown in Fig. 88.

Symptomatology. It is unnecessary to enter into details with regard to the symptoms arising from bullet-wounds of the skull and brain, for they closely resemble those previously enumerated in the chapters dealing with fractures of the skull and injury to the brain. There are, however, a few special points to which attention should be directed.

1. External hæmorrhages are seldom profuse.

2. The escape of cerebro-spinal fluid is of infrequent occurrence, probably due to the fact that the apertures of entry and exit are blocked up with scalp, fragments of bone, and pulped and swollen brain.

3. Concussion and irritation are prominent symptoms, compression is rarely seen in its typical form. As Spencer[2] says, 'The dominant feature is usually concussion. The extent of the paralysis depends on the region injured, and there is often at first extensive temporary paralysis from vibratory concussion of the brain substance suspending its functions over a wide area around the bullet-track.' Cerebral irritation and Jacksonian fits are frequently observed.

Indications for operation. There is a great uniformity of opinion with regard to the indications for operation as expressed by those who have had considerable experience in wounds of this nature. One has only to glance through the works of recognized authorities—

[1] *A Civilian War Hospital.*

[2] *Gunshot Wounds*, p. 170.

Spencer,[1] Bowlby,[2] Makins,[3] Lawford Knaggs,[4] &c.—to see that it is an accepted rule that all bullet-wounds of the skull and brain call for early operative interference, it being granted that the condition of the patient is compatible with such treatment.

Operation. The operative details may be considered under two headings :—

(*a*) The exploration of the wounds of entry and exit.

(*b*) The search for and removal of the bullet.

The exploration of the wounds of entry and exit. Whether the skull be penetrated or perforated, the wounds are investigated after

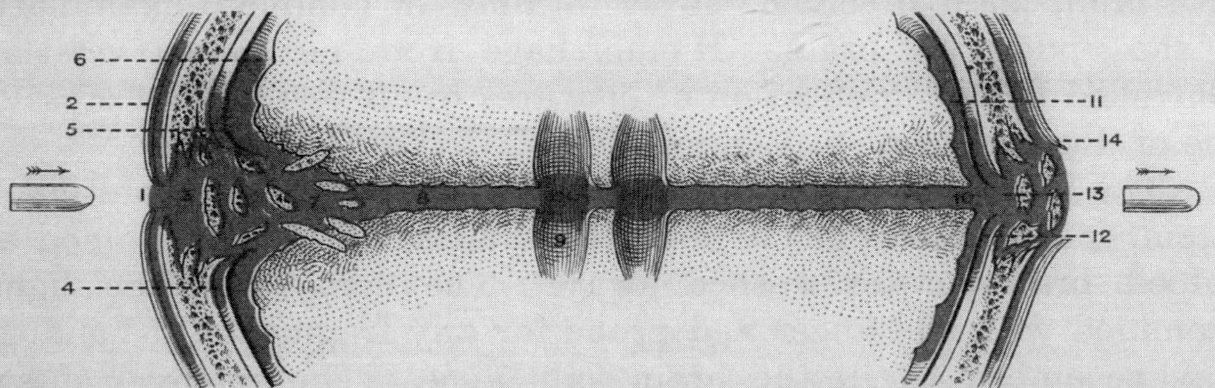

FIG. 88. TO ILLUSTRATE THE EFFECTS PRODUCED BY A PERFORATING BULLET-WOUND. 1, The inverted scalp at wound of entry ; 2, Subaponeurotic hæmorrhage ; 3, The wound of entry into the skull ; 4, Extra-dural hæmorrhage ; 5, Lacerated dura mater ; 6, Subdural hæmorrhage ; 7, In-driven fragments of bone ; 8, The passage through the brain-substance ; 9, Ventricular hæmorrhage ; 10, The wound of exit through the brain ; 11, Subdural hæmorrhage ; 12, The wound of exit through the dura mater ; 13, The wound of exit through the skull ; 14, The wound of exit through the scalp.

similar general principles. After careful shaving and cleansing of the whole scalp, and after application of the scalp-tourniquet, a scalp-flap is turned down, the centre corresponding as far as possible to the site of entrance or emergence of the bullet. The under aspect of the flap is examined for loose fragments of bone, hair, portions of headgear, &c. These are removed and the flap cleansed. The bone is next examined. All loose fragments are removed, both large and small. The smaller are discarded, the larger are boiled (for ten minutes)

[1] *Gunshot Wounds.* [2] *A Civilian War Hospital*, p. 228.

[3] *Surgical Experiences in South Africa*, p. 293. [4] *Lancet*, March 3, 1906.

and preserved in hot saline solution for replacement at the termination of the operation, if such a course should be deemed advisable (see p. 132). Those fragments of bone which retain their pericranial attachments are merely elevated and turned aside, to be again placed in position at the proper time.

Trephining is seldom necessary, the hole in the bone usually allowing of the application of craniectomy forceps, if any enlargement should be requisite.

A good view of the dura mater can now be obtained. If that membrane be merely punctured or incised, the tear must be enlarged with blunt-pointed scissors so as to allow of complete examination of the underlying brain. Hæmorrhage from meningeal vessels is controlled by the application of ligatures to all vessels that cross the line of dural section.

The lacerated brain is *gently* irrigated with saline solution (at a temperature between 110° and 115° Fahrenheit), and all blood and pulped brain matter washed away. The cortex is then lightly examined with the finger and probe for any fragments of bone that may be embedded in the brain substance. The removal of such fragments should be conducted with all possible gentleness. The surgeon should be satisfied that no foreign body remains. The bullet, when encountered, is removed. Needless to say, the presence of a bullet and the existence of in-driven fragments of bone should be investigated previous to the adoption of operative measures by means of X-ray photography.

If the brain be penetrated or perforated a drainage tube is introduced through scalp-flap and dura mater in such a manner that its distal end lies in relation to the track through the brain or flush with its lacerated surface. Elsewhere the dura is sewn up (fine catgut sutures) and the scalp-flap replaced, the drainage tube being anchored to the scalp with a single suture. The tube should be allowed to remain *in situ* for at least forty-eight hours and longer if necessary, the surgeon being guided by the amount of discharge and by the general progress of the case. In all cases of doubt the surgeon should err on the side of leaving the tube in position for a longer period of time, merely shortening it daily. Premature removal may lead to disastrous results. There can be no question that ultimate success hinges to a large extent on primary or early healing of the wound.

The search for and removal of the bullet. In the event of a wound of entry only, it may be presumed that the bullet is within the skull. Bullets, however, pursue such unexpected and devious courses within the skull, and possess such a tendency to gravitate towards the base of the brain, that no attempt should be made at removal except after full X-ray investigation, stereoscopic if possible.

To this rule there are two exceptions :—(1) where the bullet lies superficial in the brain substance, and (2) where there exists, at the opposite side of the skull, what may be termed an area of attempted exit, that is to say, an area of bone elevation and blood extravasation, suggesting that the bullet has penetrated through the brain and impinged against the opposite side of the skull. In both these instances operative measures are not only justifiable but often definitely indicated. On the other hand, it cannot be urged too forcibly that hasty and ill-determined explorations usually terminate in failure. Even under the most promising circumstances it by no means follows that the bullet will be found at the site of counter-trephining, as it may have rebounded to some more distant region of the brain, necessitating an operation conducted over a totally different region. Thus, in a case recently under my care, the bullet entered at the right temporal region, penetrated the brain and produced on the left side of the head a well-defined wound of attempted exit. The bullet, however, on striking the opposing side of the skull rebounded, and was subsequently found in the apex of the descending cornu of the right lateral ventricle. This case affords a good example of the uncertain course pursued by bullets entering the cranial cavity.

However, in certain cases of emergency and in others of expediency an immediate search should be made for the bullet. The operation should be carried out with a light hand and not unduly prolonged.

In order to find and remove the bullet various probes and extractors have been invented. Perhaps the best of these is Sheen's bullet-forceps, probe, and telephone-detector.

'The forceps are so constructed that they may be attached directly to the telephone-detector and used as a combined probe and forceps, or they may be used in combination with the specially designed graduated probe attached to the detector in the following manner: The bullet having been located with the probe, the forceps are introduced along the probe, the jaws of the forceps being provided with an oblique groove for this purpose. In both methods of use the telephone-detector is in uninterrupted contact with the bullet during extraction, an advantage which much facilitates the operation, and ensures the least possible damage of tissue. In cases where the forceps are used as a probe and forceps combined, the connexion attached to the forceps is composed of silver wire, which can be readily sterilized, and while of sufficient rigidity to avoid risk of accidental short-circuiting with the patient's body, is flexible enough not to interfere

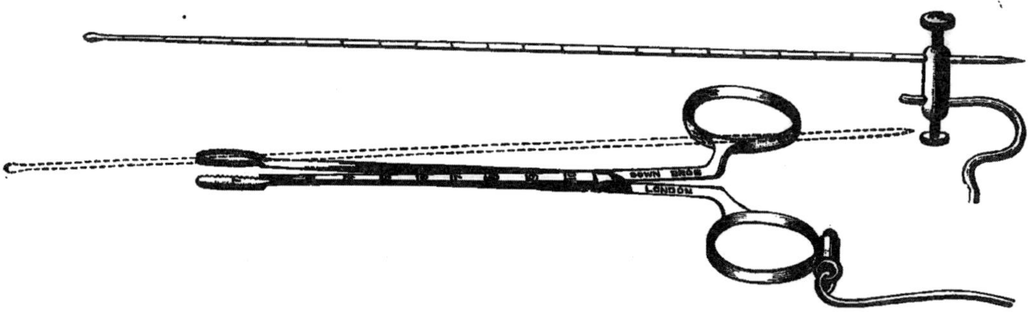

FIG. 89 A. SHEEN'S BULLET-PROBE AND FORCEPS.

with the delicacy of manipulation. The telephone-detector is placed on the head of the operator, and the flat plate on the patient's body, good contact being secured by means of a damp roll of lint, or other material, moistened with a saturated saline solution.'

'The probe is introduced, and when a metallic foreign body is touched a fall of potential occurs, and the telephone buzzes. It is necessary to point out that no mistakes can be made, as may be the case with a battery in circuit. In using the "auto-telephone probe" the body constitutes an electrolyte, the plate one pole of a voltaic circle, the probe the other; on touching a metallic body different to that of the probe, a difference of potential occurs, and the current ensuing flows through the telephone and is recorded by the diaphragm in the usual way.' [1]

If the bullet be not found it should be allowed to remain *in situ* till such time shall have elapsed as will enable the surgeon to determine whether further operative measures are indicated, time being

[1] *Army Med. Corps Journal*, April 1905.

allowed also for skiagraphy and for the evolvement of another plan of campaign. It is of course a well-known fact that bullets in certain regions of the brain—e. g. the frontal lobe—may exercise but little effect on the individual. Further measures are also indicated when the want of cleanliness of the wound and the anatomical situation of the bullet demand secondary operative procedures. All remote operations are planned according to the localizing symptoms, aided by X-ray photography.

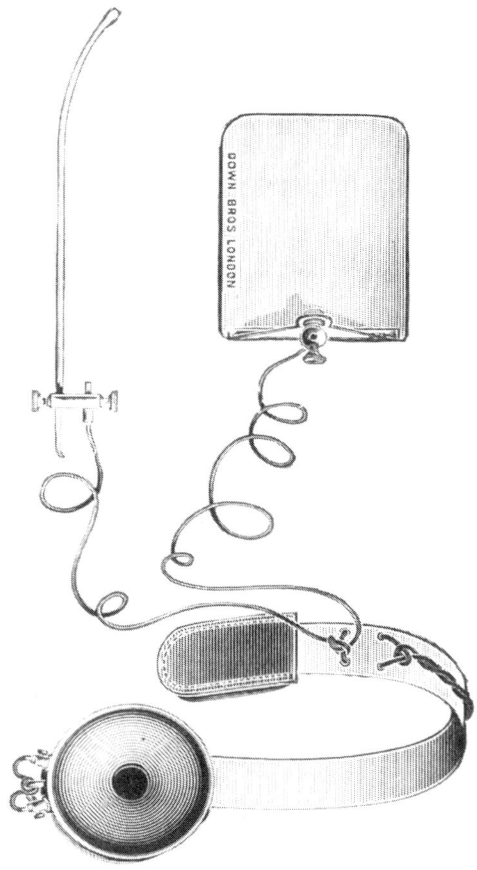

FIG. 89 B. SHEEN'S TELEPHONE BULLET-DETECTOR.

After exploration for and removal of the bullet an extensive osseous defect may remain. Opinions differ with respect to the time at which an attempt should be made to remedy the deficiency and as to the operative technique appropriate to the condition. The nature of the wound must always be taken into consideration, for the application of any plate of foreign material is doomed to failure in the event of the slightest degree of suppuration. As a general rule, it may be accepted that it is advisable to postpone such measures till after the primary or early healing of the wound. Further delay, however, tends to allow of the formation of such adhesions as will result in the development of Jacksonian epilepsy, chronic headache, traumatic insanity, &c. The operative features requisite to the interposition of plates between the bone and the scalp, and other measures, are fully detailed in Chapter VI.

'The *after treatment* consists in keeping the patient as quiet as possible, and the administration of a fluid diet. In some cases, recurring symptoms pointed to the continued presence of bone fragments; these were usually indicated by signs of irritation, or often by local inflammation, in the latter case infection taking the greatest share in the causation. Such cases needed secondary exploration, and the wonderful success of this operation, even when the wound was evidently infected, was perhaps one of the most striking experiences of surgery in general.' (Makins.)[1]

Complications. The more important early complications are meningitis, hernia cerebri, and brain abscess. For the Symptomatology and Treatment of these conditions the reader is referred to Chapter VIII.

Results. The prognosis in any given case depends on the degree of bone and brain injury, on the presence or absence of the bullet in the brain, and on the 'cleanliness' of the wound. In the American Civil War 61·2 per cent. of all fractures of the skull terminated fatally, in the Franco-German War 51·3 per cent., and in the South African War 33·1 per cent. This decreasing mortality is undoubtedly dependent on the improved methods of treatment.

When the injury is inflicted at short range the prognosis is undoubtedly less favourable. 'At short range, the characters of the wounds, and the severity of the symptoms, rendered the immediate prognosis uniformly bad, a very great majority of the patients dying, and that at the end of a few hours or days.' (Makins.)

The best results were obtained when the injury was received in the frontal region. The occipital region comes second, and the cerebellar last. Most injuries near the base of the skull were fatal. Longitudinal wounds were more serious than transverse. However, the most surprising recoveries were made, both with and without operative treatment.

The prognosis with regard to pistol wounds is absolutely bad. Phelps[2] records the following results in cases that came under his own observation.

Death occurred at once or within the first hour in 15 cases.

Death occurred within twelve hours in 7 cases.

Death occurred within fifteen hours to forty days in 10 cases.

Recovery in but 8 cases.

The more remote results are exceedingly difficult to determine, for it is impossible to obtain an accurate account of the subsequent course of events in all cases. With regard to the question of the after-

[1] *Surgical Experiences in South Africa.*

[2] *Traumatic Injuries of the Brain*, p. 387.

history, Makins [1] writes, 'I feel certain that a long roll of secondary troubles from the contraction of the cicatricial tissue, irritation from distant remaining bone fragments, as well as mental troubles from actual brain destruction, await record in the near future.' In the experience of the writer, this statement is fully justified. The hospital surgeon continually meets with cases exemplifying the more remote effects, varying from slight lesions associated with chronic headache to others showing considerable deficiency in the vault of the skull with cortical degeneration.

Some of these cases are still capable of being cured, others are hopelessly inoperable.

In the consideration of the more remote results, it must be remembered that the surgeon comes mainly into communication with those cases which require further treatment. The more favourable are lost to view. Hence the difficulty in estimating with certainty the absolute results obtained after lesions of this nature.

[1] *Surgical Experiences in South Africa.*

CHAPTER X

TRIGEMINAL NEURALGIA

Neuralgia of the fifth or trigeminal nerve is, in its varying degrees, of frequent occurrence. In its cause, manifestations, and progress, it offers so wide a field for discussion that the question must be focussed down by means of some simple form of classification such as enables one to include the majority of cases that come before one's observation.

For all practical purposes, the following types will be sufficiently inclusive :—

Neuralgia minor.
Neuralgia major.
Hysterical neuralgia.

NEURALGIA MINOR

This variety is almost invariably dependent in its development on some exciting cause. In some cases this cause is readily demonstrated, in others great difficulty may be experienced before the source is discovered.

These secondary neuralgias may be regarded as resulting from the following injuries and diseases.

Diseases of the tongue, fauces, and pharynx. For example, the pain referred to the lingual nerve in epithelioma of the tongue.

Diseases and injuries of the maxillæ. For example, the neuralgia associated with dental caries.

Injuries and diseases of the nose and its accessory cavities. For example, the infra-orbital pain experienced in empyema of the antrum.

Injuries and diseases of the bones of the skull. For example, the pain referred along the course of those nerves emerging through the basal foramina involved in a fracture of the base of the skull.

Errors of refraction. For example, neuralgia of the supra-orbital nerve.

Anæmia, influenza, alcoholism, Bright's disease, cold, worry, malaria (brow-ague), rheumatism, &c.

But slight allusion need be made to the *symptomatology* of neuralgia minor—the conditions are more or less familiar to every one. The pain, though usually most intense in that particular branch of the nerve which is most intimately related to the source of the neuralgia, is often referred to other branches of the same nerve-trunk, and sometimes to an entirely different nerve. Thus, in the case of an epithelioma of the tongue, the pain, though perhaps most acute in the region supplied by the lingual nerve, is nevertheless frequently referred to the ear along the course and distribution of the chorda tympani.

The pain is more or less continuous, often associated with exacerbations, but seldom paroxysmal. The patient frequently complains of heat and tenderness over the areas supplied by the nerve in question and, in almost every instance, there are points of special tenderness corresponding as a rule to the emergence of the nerve-trunk through some osseous foramen. Again, some relief may be obtained by the application of pressure over the site of that foramen. For example, neuralgia dependent on antral empyema is most acute in the region of the infra-orbital foramen, and relief may be experienced by pressure applied over that foramen.

In the event of failure to discover an exciting cause, some difficulty may be experienced in coming to a correct conclusion as to whether the case belongs to the minor types of neuralgia, or should be relegated to the more serious group of neuralgia major (tic doloreux). In general, however, the neuralgias minor may be distinguished from the major variety by the following features :—

(1) The presence of some detectable forms of nerve-irritation. In the neuralgias major there may be no such cause.

(2) The relief of symptoms on the successful treatment of the cause.

(3) The relative absence of those paroxysmal attacks which are so typical of neuralgia major.

(4) The infrequence of severe vaso-motor, trophic, and sensory

changes in the regions supplied by the nerve affected. Such changes are more or less constant in neuralgia major.

(5) The wide distribution of the pain and its reference to other nerves, with no clear line of demarcation from neighbouring areas supplied by totally different nerves. In neuralgia major the pain, though often involving both second and third divisions of the fifth nerve, is referred to the areas supplied by those nerves only, with a clear line of demarcation from neighbouring regions.

In cases of neuralgia of doubtful origin one can only observe the effect of treatment and be guided by the results obtained.

Treatment. The source of the neuralgia requires primary consideration. When this has been rectified the patient should be treated after general medical principles. In the event of failure at relief, we have two other strings to our bow—alcohol injections, and neurectomy of the nerve involved. Alcohol injections are dealt with later. Neurectomy—after Thiersch's method of avulsion—is greatly preferable to all the older methods of neurotomy, nerve-stretching, and nerve-division. These older methods brought about in their train but transitory alleviation of pain.

Neurectomy of the inferior dental nerve. A transverse incision is made through the skin and subcutaneous tissues at the level of junction between horizontal and vertical rami of the jaw, extending from the anterior border of the vertical ramus to the posterior border of the same. The tissues are retracted and the masseter muscle exposed. The muscle fibres are split in the vertical direction and the bone laid bare. A ½ inch trephine is applied, and a disk of bone removed so as to expose the inferior dental nerve at its entrance into the inferior dental canal. The nerve is freed from the corresponding artery, divided at the centre of exposure, and the two ends seized with forceps, twisted and avulsed in such a manner as to destroy and remove the maximum number of nerve-fibres. The disk of bone is replaced, the muscle fibres brought together with a few catgut sutures, and the margins of the skin incision approximated.

Exposure of the infra-orbital nerve. A curved incision is made through the skin and subcutaneous tissues parallel to and below the infra-orbital margin, the tissues retracted, and the small muscles overlying the infra-orbital foramen divided or retracted so as to allow exposure of the foramen. The nerve is isolated and divided. The peripheral end is seized with forceps and avulsed. The central end may be treated after similar fashion, or, preferably, again exposed in the infra-orbital groove or canal, the tissues being peeled away from the floor of the orbit and the nerve sought for as it traverses the infra-orbital canal. With this object in view, it may be necessary to gently break away the osseous roof of the canal before the nerve can be exposed. It is then lifted up with a small hook, drawn through the infra-orbital foramen, seized with forceps, and avulsed in such a manner as to be torn away somewhere in the region of the spheno-maxillary fossa. The wound is then sewn up.

Exposure of the supra-orbital nerve. The nerve is exposed through a curved incision parallel to the supra-orbital margin, and so planned as to be concealed by the eyebrow. The fibres of the orbicularis palpebrarum are separated and the foramen identified. The nerve is separated from its artery, divided, the peripheral portion avulsed, and the central portion again exposed as it courses along the roof of the orbit. For this purpose the tissues of the upper lid are detached from the supra-orbital margin, the nerve delivered with the aid of a small hook, brought out through the foramen, and avulsed in such a manner as to be torn away somewhere in the region of the sphenoidal fissure. The wound is then sewn up.

NEURALGIA MAJOR

Neuralgia major originates most commonly in the third division of the nerve, less frequently in the second, and rarely in the first. Whichever division be primarily affected, there is a very general tendency for other branches to become involved, and this in a very definite way—the pain spreading centrally from the nerve first involved, radiating to other nerve-trunks so soon as they shall be reached. Thus, pain originating in the inferior dental branch of the third division spreads to the lingual and other branches of that division and then involves the second division. Fortunately, whether the trouble originates in the third or second divisions, the ophthalmic tends to escape or to become less seriously involved—a fortunate circumstance considering the terrible conditions associated with neuritis of that nerve, the disastrous results on cornea, conjunctiva, &c.

The disease is undoubtedly of a progressive nature, originating without rhyme or reason. It seldom becomes evident before the ages of 45 to 55, affecting both rich and poor alike.

Wilfred Harris [1] collected 265 cases, and showed that the disease was slightly more common in men than in women—144 to 131. There appeared to be some predilection for the disease to involve the right side in preference to the left—179 to 80. In 6 cases the affection was bilateral.

Trigeminal neuralgia does not in itself lead to fatal results, but the continuous pain, the want of sleep, and the difficulty experienced in taking sufficient nourishment soon reduce the patient to such a miserable condition that, unless relieved by the surgeon, amelioration is sought in morphia or release in death.

Before proceeding further it will be convenient to enumerate certain points aiding in the differential diagnosis between the true and hysterical forms of trigeminal neuralgia.

True Neuralgia.	*Hysterical Neuralgia.*
Patient old, probably over 50, and more commonly of the male sex.	Patient young, more commonly of the female sex.
Pain paroxysmal.	Pain severe for long periods together.
Vaso-motor, trophic and sensory changes common.	All these changes very rare.
Pain strictly unilateral and constant in site.	Pain variable in distribution, radiating irregularly to the opposite side of the face.

The **pathology** of tic doloreux is most obscure. The parts requiring examination are the peripheral nerve-trunks, the ganglion, the sensory root, and the central nervous system. The last two regions may be excluded, not only on the ground that research has failed to show any constant structural changes, but also because the removal of the ganglion may be regarded as curative of the disease. The ganglion itself and the peripheral nerve-trunks remain for investigation.

[1] *Lancet*, November 27, 1909.

In the peripheral nerve-fibres no constant material changes have been observed. The epineurium, on the other hand, is almost invariably shrunken and sclerosed. Considerable stress might be laid on this fact unless it were also taken into consideration that the nerves were examined in patients who had suffered from major neuralgia for prolonged periods of time. Similar changes have also been observed in patients who have never exhibited neuralgic symptoms.

In the ganglion itself the following changes have been observed :—(1) arterio-sclerosis ; (2) alteration in the character of the nerve-fibres traversing the ganglion ; and (3) adhesions between the ganglion and the surrounding parts. All these changes, however, are so inconstant that but little importance can be attached to them.

At the present time there is a disposition to regard trigeminal neuralgia in the light of an ascending neuritis, originating peripherally and ascending towards the Gasserian ganglion. Sir Victor Horsley first pointed out that the ganglion acts as a barrier to the further upward spread of the affection. This is proved by the success obtained in the removal of the ganglion.

Symptomatology.

Pain. The onset of pain may be preceded by premonitory symptoms such as tinglings, throbbings, and burning sensations in the parts subsequently involved, whilst, in the earlier stages of the disease, the pain may be more or less localized to the site of emergence of the nerve from an osseous foramen.

In the earlier stages also the attacks, though severe, are paroxysmal, of short duration, perhaps not lasting more than half a minute, and definitely localized to some special nerve-trunk. During the periods of remission the patient feels quite well. Gradually the pain increases in severity, the periods of remission shorten, and the pain in its distribution becomes more widespread, the neuritis—or whatever the process may be—spreading centrally and radiating along the course and distribution of such branches of the nerve as shall be encountered.

Paroxysms are a marked feature, occasionally of so severe a nature that the patient falls to the ground as if struck by lightning, recovering after a variable period of time.

In the later stages of the disease the pain may be almost continuous, and the condition of the patient is truly miserable.

The attacks are often ushered in by the slightest stimulus—talking, mastication of food, draughts, emotion, &c.—and, in order to avoid the occurrence as far as possible, the patient abstains from talking, dreads eating, &c. Dribbling from the mouth may be observed in those cases in which the patient finds some relief in keeping the mouth open. It is also frequently seen during the height of the paroxysm. At such stages the patient is collapsed, with feeble pulse, shallow respiration, the temperature subnormal, and the skin clammy. The attacks occur both during the day and the night, sleep fails, and the body nutrition suffers.

The site at which the pain originates can often be fixed by the patient himself. Occasionally relief may be attained by pressure applied over some particular part, by heat or by cold, or by some other method discovered by the patient himself.

The attacks are often accompanied by twitchings of the muscles supplied by the facial nerve, and, according to some investigators, by fibrillary twitchings of the muscles of the region affected.

In the later stages, wasting of the muscles may be observed.

Vaso-motor and trophic changes. The skin and mucous membrane supplied by the nerve involved become hyperæmic and hyperæsthetic, and, in the more chronic cases, these changes may be associated with œdema of the subcutaneous tissues—the clinical picture now closely resembling that observed in some cases of angio-neurotic œdema.

Other symptoms of similar nature are herpes, increased salivation, furred tongue (on the side of the lesion), sweating of the skin, lacrimation, conjunctivitis, and keratitis.

General decline in health. This depends, not only on the difficulty experienced in taking sufficient nourishment, but also on the moral effect produced by the more or less continuous pain. In the more severe cases emaciation is rapid.

Treatment.

1. *Therapeutic remedies.* The following drugs have been recommended.

Quinine, in large and increasing doses.

Arsenic, given in a similar fashion.

Gelsemium, in toxic doses, every few hours until tinglings in the fingers and nausea show that the drug has been pushed far enough (Sir Victor Horsley).

Methylene blue, in three-grain doses (Sir Watson Cheyne).

Iron, antipyrin, strychnine, cannabis indica, &c.

Morphia. This drug is undoubtedly beneficial in its results, but the habitual use thereof is strongly contra-indicated, not only because of the temporary benefit received, but also because of the necessary increase in the quantity required to alleviate the pain. If persistently used the patient gradually develops the morphia habit.

Some of these remedies suffice for the neuralgias minor, but with regard to their action in cases of neuralgia major, their effect may be summed up as follows: 'True tic doloreux has been the therapeutic despair of most physicians and surgeons,'[1] and 'too often the operation is put off till the patient is addicted to the morphia habit, depleted in strength and vitality by drugs, sleepless nights, and years of intense suffering'.[2]

Until quite recently, with the exception of these medicinal remedies, the only other methods at our disposal in the treatment of trigeminal neuralgia were Gasserian ganglion removal and other intracranial operations on the three divisions of the fifth nerve. In 1906, however, Schlösser[3] of Munich advocated the injection of alcohol into the region of those foramina at the base of the skull through which the nerve trunks emerged. As the result of these injections it was stated that, although some slight degree of cutaneous anæsthesia frequently resulted, yet that it was usually of an unimportant and transient character, and that the pain subsided and finally ceased, remaining absent for a variable period of time, usually about ten months. In the event of recurrence the injection was repeated, each period of recurrent pain being less intense and less prolonged, whilst the periods of remission increased proportionately.

Whilst it is clear from the results obtained by those who have

1 Purves Stewart, *Brit. Med. Journ.*, June 11, 1910, p. 848.

2 Frazier, *Univ. of Philadelphia Bulletin*, April 1909.

3 *Berlin. Klin. Wochenschrift*, No. 3, 1908.

followed in Schlösser's footsteps, that alcohol injections are, as a rule, reasonably satisfactory, yet it must be clearly understood that beneficial results are not always observed, and that in the event of failure the more radical intracranial operations must be carried out.

The technique of alcohol injections.

Question of anæsthetic. Freezing of the skin or other method of local anæsthesia suffices to allow of the painless introduction of the needle. A general anæsthetic should be avoided wherever possible, as the burning sensation experienced by the patient when the nerve-trunk is encountered greatly assists the accuracy of introduction.

The needle. The needle should be stout—10 cm. long, 1·5 cm. in diameter, and graduated in centimetres up to 5 cm., and provided with a blunt stilette.

Introduction. The skin is cleansed, the stilette slightly withdrawn, and the needle introduced. After puncture of the skin the stilette is pushed home, all further introduction being carried out with the blunt advancing point. When in position, the stilette is withdrawn, and a glass syringe, ready filled with alcohol, fitted to the needle and the injection made.

The solution. Purves Stewart recommends the injection of 1–1·5 c.cm. of the following solution :—

Beta eucaine, 2 grains
Absolute alcohol, 6 drs.
Distilled water to the ounce.

Wilfred Harris advises 90 per cent. alcohol, preceded by a 2 per cent. solution eucaine. He urges that two or three drops should be injected slowly, and if the needle be correctly placed a sharp burning pain will instantly be felt over the area of the distribution of the nerve, lasting fifteen seconds or so and then dying away. Two or three more drops are then injected, and thus ' a few drops at a time, from 1 to 1·5 c.cm. are injected, the pain produced with each succeeding push of the syringe being less and less '.

To reach the *foramen ovale* (third division), the needle is introduced through the cheek behind the last molar tooth, at the lower border of the zygoma, at a point 2½ cm. in front of the descending root of the zygoma. The blunt needle penetrates the masseter muscle and the posterior part of the temporal muscle. It is then directed backwards and slightly upwards till it impinges on the skull at the external pterygoid plate. It is then pushed on, upwards and backwards, till it enters the foramen ovale at a depth usually of about 4 cm. from the zygoma. In case of difficulty in passing the needle through the sigmoid notch of the jaw the mouth should be widely opened.

If the needle be directed too low it may penetrate the pharyngeal wall or the Eustachian tube; if too far back, the middle meningeal artery.

To reach the *foramen rotundum* (second division)—a rather more difficult procedure—it is necessary to find the posterior border of the orbital process of the malar bone, prolonging this line downwards to the lower border of the zygoma and inserting the needle ½ cm. posterior to this point. The needle is pushed horizontally inwards and the point directed slightly upwards, the foramen being reached in the pterygo-maxillary fossa at a depth of about 3 cm. from the zygoma. The needle, for an average-sized skull, should never penetrate deeper than 5 cm. The structures pierced are the anterior fibres of the masseter and the buccinator muscles. If directed too horizontally, the needle will pass below the nerve and reach the spheno-palatine region; if too high, the sphenoidal fissure may be reached and the branches of the third nerve damaged, causing diplopia and dilatation of the pupil.

To reach the *sphenoidal fissure* (first division), the needle is introduced at the outer margin of the orbit, close within the fronto-malar articulation, and passed along the outer wall of the orbit to a depth of 3½ to 4 cm.

Needless to say, it is essential that these injections to the basal foramina should only be carried out in the first instance after experimentation on the cadaver.

In each case a single injection may suffice, but as a general rule it is advisable to repeat the process after two or three days, and again at longer intervals. It is not necessary that the nerve-trunks should be pierced, but better results are obtained by so doing. The surface area to which the particular nerve-trunk is distributed immediately becomes anæsthetic, remaining in that state till the effect of the injection shall have passed off. The masticatory muscles are paralysed. The injection may be followed by paresis of the facial muscles, by œdema of the lower lid, and by hæmatomata. These last-named results are, however, transitory.

Results. Schlösser, who injects 15 to 20 minims of an 80 per cent. solution of alcohol, reported in 1907 that he had treated 123 cases, the average period of relief from pain being ten and a half months.

Wilfred Harris[1] reported on 38 cases, 31 of which were completely relieved for periods varying from two to eleven months. In a more recent communication he reports on 86 cases, in only 3 of which was no relief obtained. In 7 cases the injection was made into the ganglion itself, in anticipation of more permanent results.

Operative procedures. Intracranial procedures for trigeminal neuralgia were formerly associated with so high a rate of mortality that they were not regarded with favour. Of recent years, however, as the result of the general improvement in technique, it has been clearly demonstrated that, in experienced hands, 'the ganglion can be readily exposed, hæmorrhage and shock need no longer be considered elements of danger: the risks of the operation are only those associated with every major operation. Recovery from the effects of the operation is rapid; the patients are frequently up and about on the third or fourth day, and the ultimate results are, to say the least, most gratifying to the patient and to the operator.'[2]

The following operations require consideration :—

1. Intracranial resection of the second and third divisions of the fifth nerve (Abbé's operation).

2. Operations for the removal of the whole or part of the Gasserian ganglion (Hartley-Krause operation and its modifications).

3. Operations on the sensory root of the ganglion (Frazier's operation).

Intracranial resection of the second and third divisions of the fifth nerve and operations on the ganglion itself resemble one another so closely in their preliminary operative stages that they may be considered together. After the usual preparatory treatment—in which

[1] *Brit. Med. Journ.*, June 11, 1910.

[2] Frazier, *Univ. of Philadelphia Bulletin*, April 1909.

the shaving process may be confined to the temporal region—the incision, commencing well above and behind the external angular frontal process, passes backwards below the level of the temporal crest and terminates immediately in front of the tragus of the ear. The front part of the incision, as depicted in Fig. 91, is prolonged too far downwards. It should not be carried further forward than the anterior margin of the hairy scalp, any further downward prolongation tending to involve that branch of the facial nerve which is distributed to the anterior belly of the occipito-frontalis muscle.

The incision, carried out methodically, first involves the skin only, pressure being applied by the surgeon on the one side and his

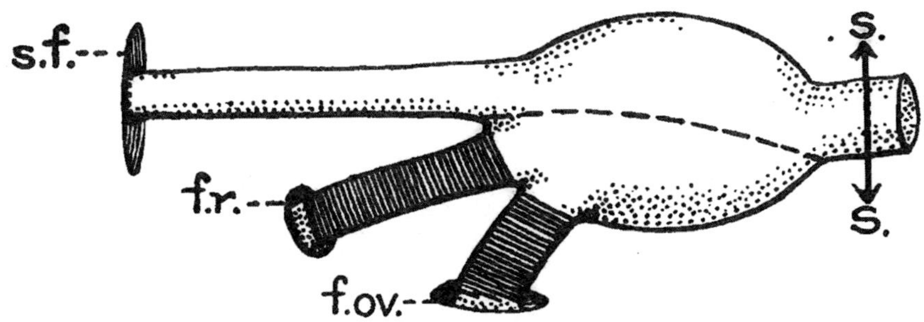

Fig. 90. To illustrate the Operations on the Gasserian Ganglion. s.f., sphenoidal fissure; f.r., foramen rotundum; f.ov., foramen ovale; s.s., Frazier's operation on the sensory root. The dotted line = the line of section in removal of the lower two-thirds of the ganglion (*Jonathan Hutchinson's operation*). The shaded portions = parts removed in intracranial resection of the second and third divisions of the nerve (*Abbé's operation*).

assistant on the other, so as to control bleeding. All divided vessels are at once clamped. The operation may be a prolonged one, and in its later stages bleeding from meningeal vessels and emissary veins may not be so readily controlled. It is essential, therefore, that the earlier stages should be as bloodless as possible.

The temporal fascia is next incised—slightly below the line of the skin incision. Finally, the temporal muscle is divided—again at a lower level than the fascial incision. Skin, fascia, and muscle are then turned down to a zygomatic base. Some surgeons split the temporal muscle in the direction of its fibres, a course, however, that tends somewhat to cramp the operative field.

The trephine is applied to the bone, the surgeon aiming at striking the angle between the anterior and posterior branches of the middle meningeal artery. The bone-disk is removed. With the aid of craniectomy forceps the bone is nibbled away, more especially in the downward direction towards the base of the skull. It is essential that the operator should get down as low as possible, for the lower the line of attack the easier the approach to the ganglion and the less the damage incurred by the brain (from retraction).

The opening in the bone, oval in shape, should present a diameter in the vertical direction of about 1 to $1\frac{1}{4}$ inches, and an antero-posterior diameter of about $1\frac{1}{2}$ inches.

The dura is stripped away from the base of the skull, partly with the fingers and partly with the blunt dissector, and a flat, slightly malleable retractor introduced along the floor of the middle fossa, the dura and overlying temporo-sphenoidal lobe being gently lifted upwards. The surgeon should take upon himself the responsibility of retracting the brain, holding that instrument with the one hand and working inwards with the other, directing his course towards the foramen spinosum (middle meningeal) and foramen ovale (third division of the fifth nerve).

During this stage hæmorrhage, derived mainly from the branches of the middle meningeal, is often troublesome. It may be controlled by the insertion of dry or wet gauze—in the latter case the gauze is soaked in saline solution or sterilized water (at a temperature of about 110° Fahrenheit)—or by the introduction of cotton-wool plugs to each of which a silk thread is attached, for the purpose of facilitating their final removal.

The middle meningeal artery acts as a guide to the foramen spinosum, a foramen that lies immediately posterior and external to the foramen ovale. In many cases the position of this artery so hampers the operator in his manipulation that ligature is demanded. For this purpose Cushing's silver 'clips' will be found most serviceable. One clip is applied to the artery immediately after its entry into the skull, the other a short distance above, the vessel being divided between the two (see Fig. 6).

The foramen ovale is then identified, the dura being stripped away from the nerve trunk by blunt dissection. The surgeon then works inwards and forwards to the second division of the nerve and its foramen, the foramen rotundum. Hæmorrhage, in this case derived from emissary veins, may again be troublesome. Considerable perseverance is required, and, although each attempt at further separation of the dura from the bone entails more oozing, the difficulties—except in the most exceptional cases—may be overcome.

The *second and third divisions may now be resected.* For this purpose it is essential that the two nerves should be exposed from the point of their exit from the skull right up to the margin of the ganglion. Their dural coat seldom requires to be incised with the knife, the membrane being readily stripped away with the blunt dissector. When fully exposed, the nerve trunks are picked up with a blunt aneurysm needle and divided in two places, flush with the basal foramina and close up against the ganglion. The intermediate parts are removed.

To prevent regeneration of nerve fibres—with consequent return of symptoms—the basal foramina are blocked up with small ivory pegs—well driven home—or with amalgam.

All gauze plugs are removed, the field of operation well dried, and dura and brain allowed to fall back into position. The wound is closed, if possible without drainage. In the event of considerable oozing a cigarette drain should be inserted for twenty-four hours. The scalp-flap is sewn up, skin, muscle, and fascia being united separately.

Removal of the Gasserian ganglion. There is some divergence of opinion as to whether it is necessary to remove the ganglion entire or whether it suffices to resect the lower two-thirds—that part through which the fibres of the second and third divisions course—the upper third being left intact. This latter course is advocated by Jonathan Hutchinson on the grounds that (1) the first division is but rarely involved in the neuralgic process, (2) its inclusion in the process of removal entails some risk to the eye—conjunctivitis, keratitis, and sloughing of the cornea, and (3) resection of the lower two-thirds of the ganglion, when carried out in suitable cases, is but rarely followed by the development of neuralgia in the first or ophthalmic trunk. Added to these facts, it must be admitted that the complete removal of the ganglion is associated with added operative risk—wounding of the cavernous sinus and injury to the third, fourth, and sixth nerves.

The Gasserian ganglion lies in the cavum Meckelii, a depression on the anterior aspect of the petrous portion of the temporal bone, and is situated between the two layers of dura mater, the stronger on the upper or cerebral side, the weaker between it and the bone. Under the pathological conditions often existent in cases of trigeminal neuralgia, considerable adhesion may be present between the ganglion and its enveloping coats. Consequently, its complete exposure is often a matter of considerable difficulty. The dura must be stripped away from the outer aspect of the ganglion, firstly by dividing the membrane along the border of the ganglion between the site of emergence of the second and third divisions, and then by blunt dissection.

The ganglion and its efferent branches being exposed, *resection of the lower two-thirds* may be carried out. The second and third nerve trunks are severed flush with the basal foramina, traction applied, and the lower portion of the ganglion resected.

During the final stages, the manipulations of the operator are again likely to be obscured by venous oozing and by the discharge of some cerebro-spinal fluid. Patience, careful application of gauze plugs, and good illumination of the field of operation are required to overcome these difficulties. In some few cases the bleeding has been so profuse that the operation has had to be abandoned for the time being, a fresh attempt being made some days later. This course should, however, rarely be necessary.

Similarly, if the operator should deem it necessary to remove the whole ganglion, this procedure may now be carried out. The posterior part of the ganglion is exposed, together with its sensory root. This root is hooked forward with a small blunt-pointed hook and then divided. Traction is applied to the ganglion and it is turned forwards, the three terminal divisions being divided one after the other with the minimum risk of injuring the cavernous sinus.

Modifications of the Hartley-Krause operation. With the object of obtaining further manipulative room, some surgeons recommend the formation of an osteoplastic flap. This method should never be adopted. It is quite unnecessary, it prolongs the operation, and entails more deformity. Others advise division of the zygoma, both in front and behind, with downward displacement of the intermediate portion. Burghard[1] recommends division and downward displacement of the zygoma together with section of the

[1] *A System of Operative Surgery*, vol. i, p. 437.

coronoid process, this process being turned upwards together with its attached temporal muscle.

From my own experience, I should regard all these modifications as quite unnecessary, the Hartley-Krause operation permitting an adequate operative field. The deformity resulting from all these

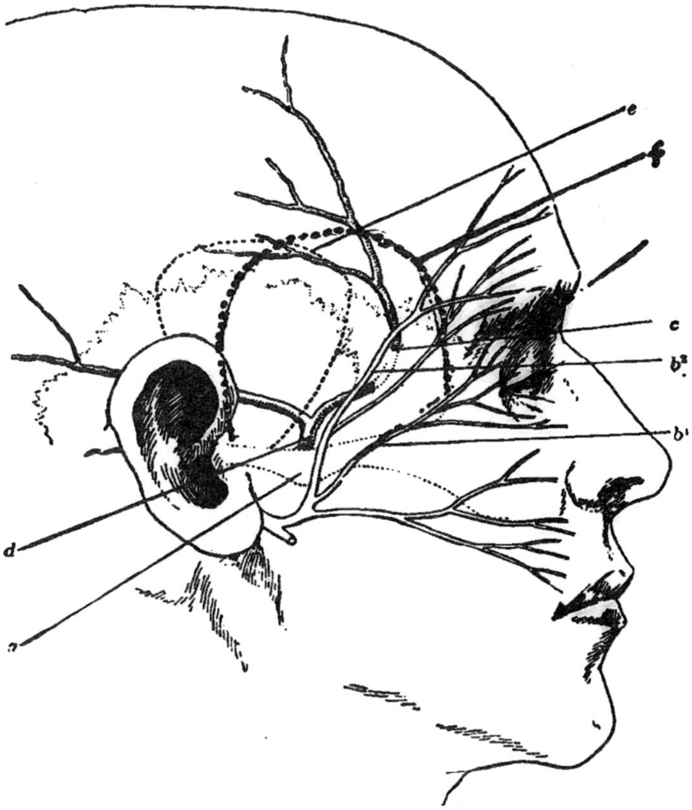

FIG. 91. TO ILLUSTRATE THE OPERATIONS FOR EXPOSURE OF THE GASSERIAN GANGLION. *e*, The incision for Frazier's operation ; *f*, The incision for the Hartley-Krause operation (in its most recent modification, the front part of this incision is not carried so far downwards, thus avoiding b^2, that branch of the facial nerve which is distributed to the anterior belly of the occipito-frontalis muscle ; *c*, The intra-osseous portion of the anterior division of the middle meningeal artery ; b^1, The branches of the facial nerve to the orbicularis palpebrarum, &c.

more extensive procedures must also be taken into consideration. The lines of incision in the Hartley-Krause operation are more or less concealed by the hairy scalp.

Operations on the sensory root (Frazier's operation). Charles Frazier advocates the 'physiologic extirpation' of the sensory root of the ganglion. The advantages claimed over other methods are as follows :—

1. *Control of hæmorrhage and avoidance of risk of injury to the*

cavernous sinus. The ganglion receives its main blood-supply from below. Division of the sensory root leaves the base of the ganglion undisturbed, and this cause of free bleeding is removed. With respect to the cavernous sinus, the operation is confined to the root of the ganglion and consequently the sinus is in no wise concerned.

2. *Simple technique.* The operation of division of the sensory root is complete before the difficulties common to extraction of the ganglion have commenced.

3. *Avoidance of injury to adjacent structures.* The cavernous sinus is not touched; the sixth nerve, which is intimately related to the ophthalmic branch, is not exposed; and the motor-fibres which, passing beneath the ganglion, join the third division outside the skull, and which are almost necessarily injured in the ganglionic operation, may, in division of the sensory root, escape implication.

4. *Reduction in the rate of mortality.* The operation is said to be more economical of time, to entail less hæmorrhage, and therefore to be less dangerous.

5. *Absence of ocular changes.* After division of the sensory root ocular changes are absent, due in part to the fact that the ocular nerves are left intact, and also to the probability that 'sympathetic fibres pass to the eye after entering the trigeminal nerve through the Gasserian ganglion' (Spiller).

In the consideration of these advantages it should be noted that they are mainly directed against procedures in which complete extirpation of the ganglion is attempted, and are of less weight when contrasted with the partial excision advocated by Hutchinson.

Frazier's operation[1] on the sensory root. 'A horse-shoe shaped incision is made, beginning at the middle of the zygoma and terminating a little below the apex of the lobe of the ear (see Fig. 91). The musculo-cutaneous flap is made purposely a little larger than the opening in the skull. An opening is made in the skull with a diameter not exceeding 3 cm. and extending down as far as the infra-temporal crest. The dura is separated from the base of the skull with a blunt retractor as far as the foramen spinosum. The middle meningeal artery is ligatured and the dura mater incised directly over the third division at the margin of the foramen ovale and separated from the

[1] *Univ. of Pennsylvania Medical Bulletin,* April 1909.

upper surface of the ganglion as far back as the sensory root. The latter is picked up with a blunt hook, grasped with forceps and divided or avulsed. It is necessary only to expose the posterior portion of the ganglion ; the second and third divisions of the fifth, the structures on the inner side of the ganglion, and the cavernous sinus, are left undisturbed.'

Choice of operation. There are both advantages and disadvantages to each of the various operations enumerated. There are also other operations. From my own experience I have come to the conclusion that the two operations of choice are resection of the second and third divisions of the fifth nerve and division of the sensory root. The former of these two operations is carried out when the general condition of the patient is not altogether satisfactory, presuming, of course, that the neuralgia is limited to those divisions of the nerve. Under more favourable circumstances excellent results are obtained by exposure and division or resection of the sensory root, with, I think, the minimum risk.

The results obtained by operation. The prevailing impression that these operations are associated with a high mortality is totally incorrect. From my own experience and from numerous recorded cases, the mortality may be estimated at not more than 5 per cent.

The extent of anæsthesia resulting varies according to the nature of the operation. Thus, if the upper part of the ganglion be spared or the operation confined to the second and third divisions, the upper lid, conjunctiva, cornea, and forehead escape. In any case, taste is but little impaired, the posterior part of the tongue being supplied by the glossopharyngeal and the tip and sides by the chorda tympani. In all cases, except perhaps in Frazier's operation, the motor fibres which accompany the third division are almost always divided, with consequent paralysis of the corresponding masseter, temporal, and pterygoid muscles. The degree of discomfort and deformity resulting from such anæsthesia and paralysis is, however, not very considerable, and in contrast with the relief from the terrible pain, of very little import. It is, as Jonathan Hutchinson says, the price which the patient has to pay for the cure of the neuralgia.

With respect to recurrence of pain, there is every reason to believe that the resection of the sensory root and the complete removal of the ganglion are never followed by recurrence of pain. With respect to Jonathan Hutchinson's and Abbé's operations, there is some divergence of opinion. There would appear to be some cases recorded in which the symptoms have recurred—often many years later. With regard to Hutchinson's operation I have no personal experience, but it is stated that in some few cases the pain has recurred in the first division. I believe, however, that I am correct in stating that this is denied by Hutchinson from the experience based on his own cases. As regards Abbé's operation, recurrence may take place if the basal foramina are not completely occluded, some few nerve fibres growing through the foramina on either side of the occluding medium. Such complications have not taken place in the cases in which I have carried out this operation.

Besides experiencing immediate and complete relief from pain, the patients sleep well, eat well, and rapidly convalesce. For some two or three days they may suffer from some headache, presumably due to the necessary manipulations of the brain, but this, besides being relieved by drugs, soon passes off. Frequently, the patients are up and about within a few days.

Whatever the nature of the operation, the greatest care must be taken to protect the eye on the affected side—the conjunctival sac is washed out daily with a mild boracic solution and the cornea guarded from exposure to air and dust by means of a glass covering fastened round the forehead. This appliance should be worn for two or three weeks.

The **main difficulties and dangers of operation** are as follows :—

1. Hæmorrhage (from middle meningeal artery and cavernous sinus).
2. Infection.
3. Shock.
4. Ocular complications.
5. Later after-results—insomnia, restlessness, impairment of memory, aphasia, and hemiplegia—all of which are dependent either on rough handling of the brain or lighter handling of an already diseased brain.

CHAPTER XI

TUMOURS OF THE SKULL-BONES

In this the last chapter of this work, I originally intended to deal with tumours of the scalp and skull-bones. With respect to tumours of the scalp there is, however, but little to say. The various conditions are well recognized, their pathology is known, and there is in general but little to relate. Tumours of the skull-bones come under a different category and require some consideration.

Tumours of the skull-bones. The more important of these tumours are as follows :—

Osteomata.
Sarcomata, primary and traumatic.
Secondary sarcomata and carcinomata.

OSTEOMATA

Exostoses of the skull, though by no means of frequent occurrence, occupy such definite positions that it would appear as if they were dependent on some local governing cause. They develop most frequently in the following positions :—

At the external angular frontal process.

At the frontal and parietal eminences.

In the region of the frontal sinus.

In the region of the external auditory meatus and mastoid process.

All pathological museums possess specimens illustrating the formation of such exostoses, tumours of a like nature in other parts of the skull being excessively rare.

In endeavouring to arrive at an explanation it would appear necessary to direct one's attention to tumours of a similar nature occurring in other parts of the body, more especially in the long bones. There, it is well recognized that their development is dependent on irregularities of growth in the region of the epiphyseal lines, regions where activity of growth is long maintained.

On referring again to the skull, similar features appear. For instance, the frontal bone, besides possessing one primary centre for the frontal eminence, has secondary centres for the external angular frontal process, for the trochlear fossa, and for the nasal spine,

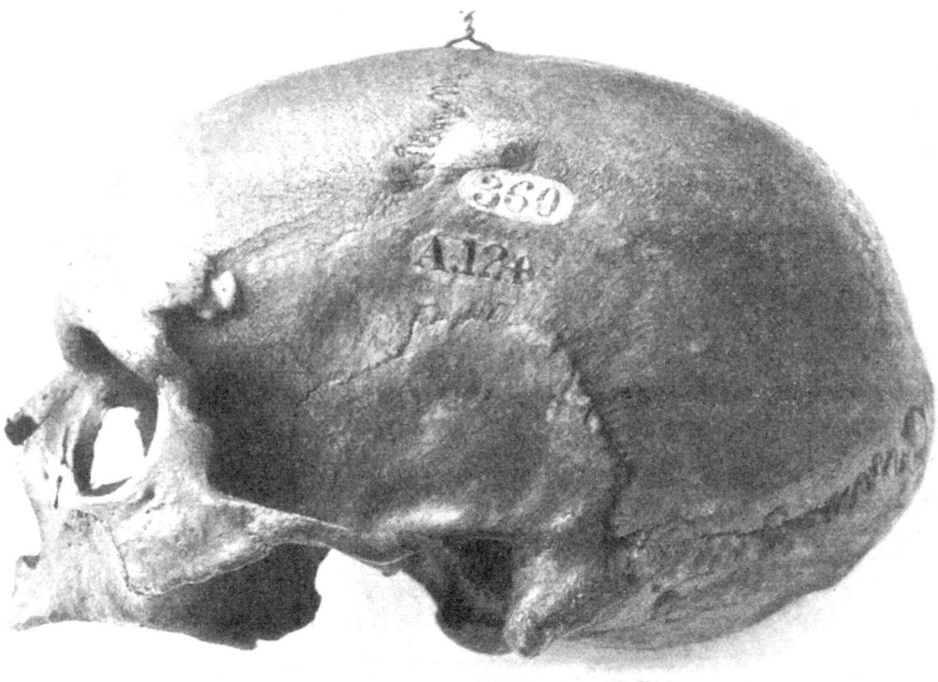

FIG. 92. IVORY EXOSTOSES OF THE SKULL.

and it is highly probable that those exostoses which develop in the region of the frontal sinus in reality arise from one or other of the secondary centres situated in that region.

Both frontal and parietal eminences are also sites of active and prolonged ossification, and the tumours there arising are to be explained on a like hypothesis.

Similar features are to be observed with respect to those bony tumours which develop in the aural region, the numerous centres of ossification for the periotic capsule accounting satisfactorily for their origin.

Whether originating in the region of the frontal sinus or in the aural area, the tumour naturally develops along the line of least resistance, filling up the frontal sinus and growing into the external auditory meatus and mastoid antrum.

More rarely, small exostoses develop on the inner aspect of the skull, chiefly from the frontal bone in the region of the crista galli. In some cases the inner aspect of the skull is studded with small bony tumours, more especially along the line of the superior longitudinal venous sinus.

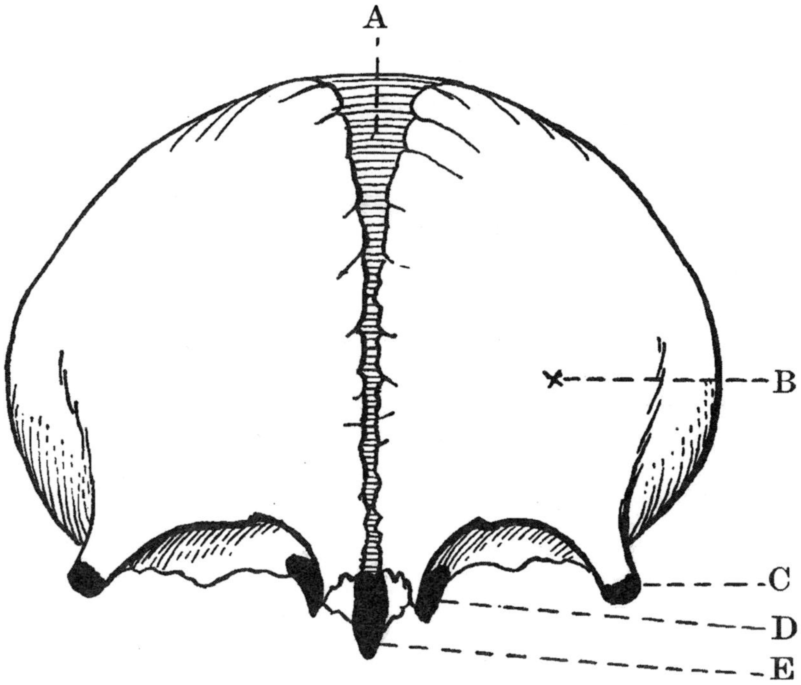

FIG. 93. THE DEVELOPMENT OF THE FRONTAL BONE. A, Metopic suture; B, Primary centre for frontal eminence; C, Secondary centre for external angular frontal process; D, Secondary centre for trochlear fossa; E, Secondary centre for nasal spine.

These internal exostoses seldom give rise to pressure symptoms, although, according to Wilks and Moxon,[1] they may push inwards the dura mater and even lead to idiocy and epilepsy. I have seen several cases of internal exostosis development, but in all cases their discovery was accidental.

Clinical characteristics. Exostoses vary greatly both in size and consistency. Some are densely hard—ivory exostoses—others possess a covering of compact bone, whilst their interior is made up of cancellous tissue continuous with that of the bone from which

[1] *Lectures in Pathological Anatomy.*

they arise. The denser variety seldom attain any considerable size, but the less compact, growing in the direction of least resistance, often attain such dimensions as to be both unsightly and dangerous. Thus, a frontal exostosis may invade the frontal air sinus and grow into the orbital cavity, obliterating the sinus, interfering greatly with ocular movements, causing protrusion of the globe and even destruction of the eye.

An aural exostosis may block up the external auditory meatus, compress the facial nerve, and lead to the development of a mastoid empyema.

It might also be added that there are a few cases on record in which a frontal exostosis, by reason of extensive inward growth, has produced cerebral symptoms—general compression and intellectual deterioration.

Treatment. In considering the question of treatment, it must be accepted that, although of slow growth, some of these exostoses are definitely progressive, tending to interfere with the character and functions of the region with which they are anatomically situated. There is also reason to believe that those secondary changes—sarcomatous, myxomatous, &c.—which are occasionally observed in the exostoses of long bones are also liable to develop in those cranially situated. The question of treatment hinges, therefore, to a large extent on the nature and position of the tumour.

When of the ivory type and growing from the flat bones of the skull, but so situated that no marked deformity or pressure symptoms are likely to ensue, they may be left alone, but when definitely progressive and situated in accessible regions, they should be removed. Their exposure is carried out by the formation of a suitable scalp-flap—designed as far as possible so as to be subsequently hidden by the hairy scalp—and the exostosis removed by the application to its base of a Gigli saw. This method is greatly superior to the older procedures whereby the tumour was chiselled away with hammer and gouge.

Occasionally the tumour is so dense and presents so wide a basal attachment that it becomes necessary to attack from a more distant line, cutting out a trench, deepened to the diploic tissue, circumferentially around the tumour and levering away the central mass.

When the tumour extends more deeply, involving nearly the whole thickness of the skull, it may be removed by the application of a small trephine immediately to one side of the tumour, followed by the use of de Vilbiss forceps circumferentially around the main mass, thus freeing it from its surroundings. The resultant gap in the skull may be protected by one or other of those measures enumerated in Chapter VI.

Frontal and mastoid exostoses often necessitate formidable operations insomuch as their size and anatomical relations present considerable difficulties (see Fig. 94).

The **indications for operation in the case of aural exostoses** are as follows[1]:—

1. If there is middle-ear suppuration and signs of retention of pus.
2. When the pressure of the exostosis produces pain which cannot otherwise be relieved.
3. If the exostosis nearly blocks up the meatus of both ears, and there is prospect of each side becoming completely blocked in the near future. Here operation is carried out on the worst side.
4. If the meatus is nearly blocked by the exostosis and the patient going to a country where he cannot be within easy reach of a competent medical man.

The **indications for operation in the case of a frontal exostosis** are as follows :—

1. When the exostosis interferes with the actions of the ocular muscles, causes proptosis and threatens the integrity of the globe.
2. When associated with pain which cannot otherwise be relieved.
3. When the exostosis leads to blockage of the accessory sinuses of the nose, more especially when such blockage is associated with pus pent up within.
4. When very unsightly.

The accompanying figure illustrates the deformity and dangers associated with large frontal exostoses. The tumour developed from the inner angle of the orbital cavity, pushing the globe forwards and outwards, with diplopia and severe neuralgia.

[1] Hunter Tod, *Diseases of the Ear*, p. 37.

It is barely possible to enter into the **operative details** suited to frontal and aural exostoses—the operations are so atypical. It is sufficient to say that the operation may be a very formidable one, that the details must be carefully thought out, and that every precaution must be adopted to avoid injuring neighbouring structures.

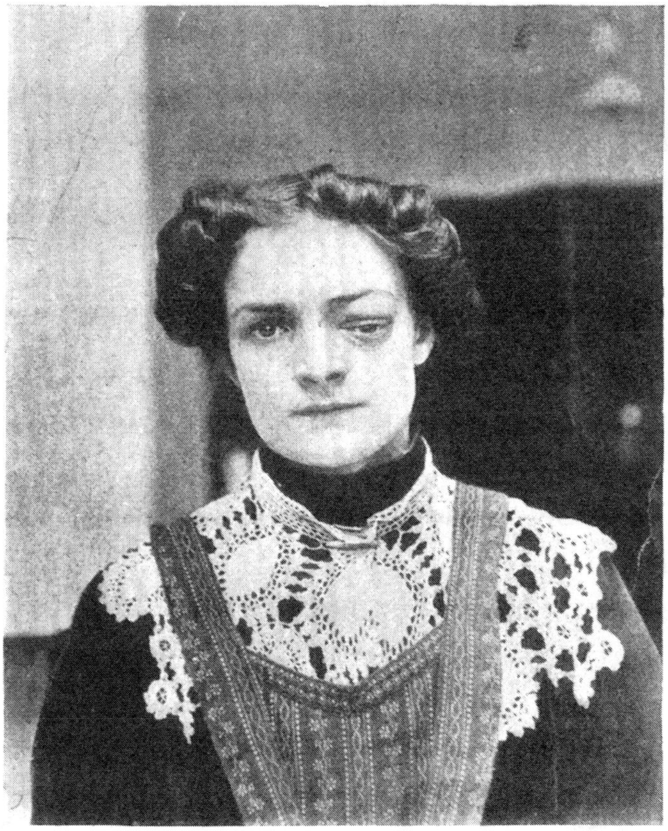

Fig. 94. An Exostosis of the Orbit.

SARCOMATA, PRIMARY AND TRAUMATIC

Primary sarcomata of the skull, when compared to sarcomata developing in other situations, is undoubtedly a rare disease. Still, many cases have been recorded, and four have come under my own personal care, one of which is depicted in the figure.

The disease is equally prevalent in the two sexes, and, excluding chloromata (see p. 334), usually develops at or after middle life. The growth may originate in the diploic tissue (as a myelogenous tumour), or may spring from the pericranium. The cellular structure varies accordingly. More commonly the cells are of the large round or spindle type, and are proportionately malignant.

As regards site of development, the temporal bone (squamous portion) is most commonly involved, next to which comes the frontal bone.

In considering the ætiology of sarcoma in general, *trauma* must always be taken into account, for it is an undoubted fact that it plays an important part in the development of this dire disease.

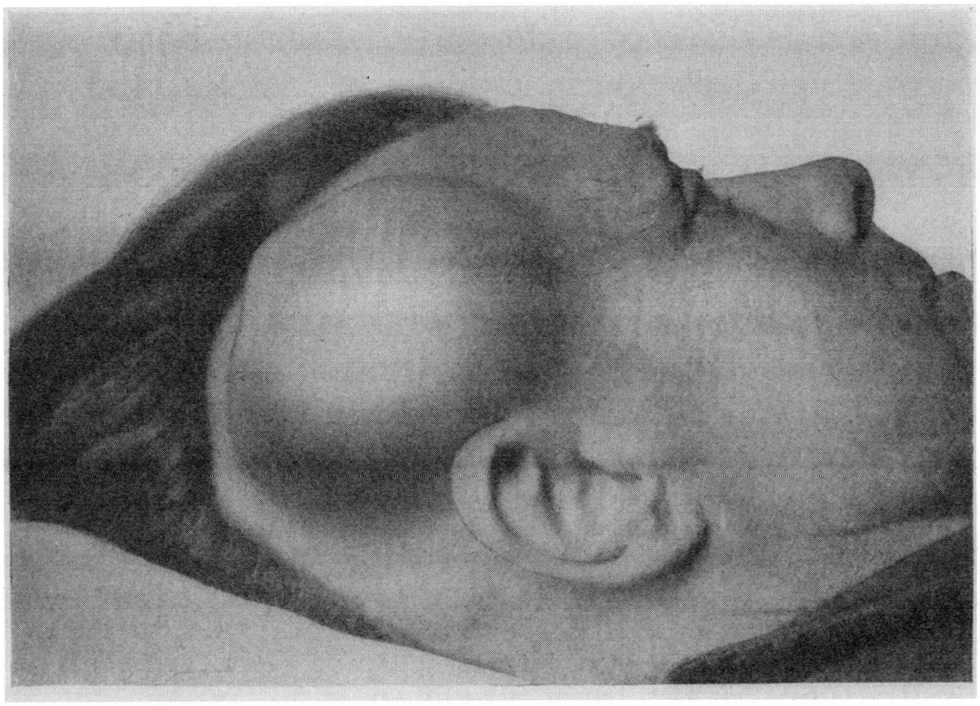

FIG. 95. AN EXTRINSIC SARCOMA OF THE SKULL.

With respect to the skull similar factors come into play. For instance, Fröhlking,[1] after collecting 48 cases of sarcoma of the skull, found a definite history of trauma in 9—21 per cent.

Ziegler [2] lays down the following essentials in establishing the traumatic origin of the tumour : It must develop directly after the trauma on the basis of the swelling or directly in the scar of the wound.

The tumour must be palpable immediately after the acute swelling has diminished.

At the site of the trauma constant or intermittent pain must be present.

1 *Sarkomen des knöchernen Schädelgewölbes*, 1895.

2 *Über die Beziehung von Träumen zu den malignen Geschwülsten*, 1895.

A considerable number of cases of sarcoma of the skull will fulfil even these arbitrary conditions. Such sarcomata may definitely be labelled ‘ traumatic ’ sarcomata.

Whether dependent on injury or not, the *symptoms* associated with sarcoma of the skull vary according to whether the tumour is extrinsic or intrinsic—whether, for instance, the growth develops in the inward direction and presses on the brain, or grows from the pericranium and is directed externally. *Intrinsic* tumours, with the exception of some local pain, œdema of tissues, and dilatation of superficial veins, give rise to symptoms closely resembling those observed in intracranial tumour formation. When *extrinsic,* the tumour varies in size, but is necessarily attached to the bone, the base being the widest part of the tumour. In the earlier stages the overlying skin, with the exception of a few dilated vessels, is more or less normal. Later on, the integument becomes adherent to the tumour, then red and inflamed, and finally ulcerated, the growth now fungating to the surface. The tumour itself is of variable consistency, first hard, then softer, and lastly semi-fluctuating.

Pain, though not very severe, is more or less constant—of a dull, aching character. The extrinsic tumours may, however, give rise to acute neuralgic pain in the event of implication of cutaneous nerves; whilst the intrinsic, in the later stages of the disease, lead to the more severe types of headache observed in intracranial tumour formation.

Secondary nodules appear in other parts of the scalp—all appertaining, in their clinical characteristics, to the primary growth; the cervical glands become infected, and death results from repeated hæmorrhages, pulmonary complications, &c., usually within one to two years from the date of primary development.

Treatment. The removal of an extrinsic tumour should only be carried out when the tumour is small and non-adherent to the tissues of the scalp. With respect to the intrinsic variety greater circumspection is required. The presence of cerebral symptoms and the inward extension of the growth—verified by symptoms and by X-ray investigation—may be regarded as implying that the conditions are beyond the reach of surgery. In both varieties of tumour, extensive glandular implication acts as a contra-indication to operation.

Under the more favourable conditions an attempt may be made at the extirpation of the growth. The operation should be rendered as bloodless as possible, for which purpose it is essential that the scalp-tourniquet should be applied as a preliminary measure. A scalp-flap is then framed, suited to requirements, and allowing of free exposure of the tumour and surrounding healthy tissues. The skull is then trephined to one side of the growth, and the disk removed. The dura is separated from the overlying bone, and by the circumferential

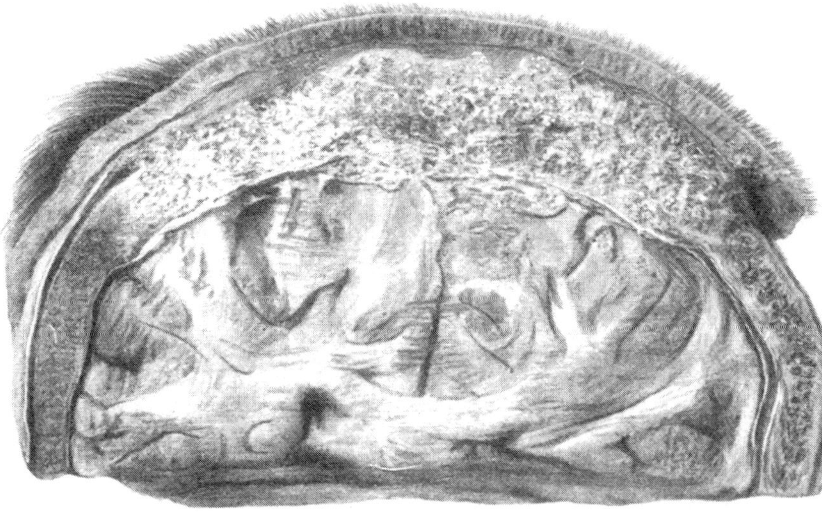

FIG. 96. AN INTRINSIC SARCOMA OF THE SKULL.

application of de Vilbiss or other craniectomy forceps the central mass is isolated and removed. During these manipulations free hæmorrhage may be experienced from the numerous dilated diploic veins. For the arrest of this the surgeon should have ready to hand, ivory pegs, bone-wax, and other aids for the control of hæmorrhage (see Chapter II). The scalp-flap is then replaced.

The gap in the bone may be covered in, at a later date, if the patient's condition is favourable.

The operation may be a formidable one, but records are to hand of 35 cases in which radical measures were adopted. Ten cases died from the operation, 13 were well for periods varying from six months to six years, and recurrence took place soon after the operation in 21 cases.

Chloromata. Chloroma, a peculiar type of sarcoma characterized by the pale green hue of the tissues, usually develops in the young. The cells are small and round, the pigment distributed in and around the cell elements. The colour, said to be dependent on the presence of a pigmented fat, is most intense immediately after the removal of the tumour, fading rapidly on exposure to light.

The tumour develops from the periosteum of bones, more especially from those which enter into the formation of the orbit and base of skull. In fact, nearly all the cases reported have originated from the temporal and orbital regions. Great rapidity of growth and early dissemination throughout the viscera are conspicuous features—no organ of the body can be said to be exempt from metastatic deposits. The meninges and brain are early involved by direct extension.

Proptosis, as the result of cavernous sinus thrombosis and orbital invasion, is a prominent and early symptom. Death results within six months. No treatment, surgical or otherwise, is of any avail.

Carcinoma can only involve the skull-bones as a metastatic deposit—more commonly in association with mammary cancer—or by direct invasion from an overlying epitheliomatous scalp ulcer. In the former instance, any radical treatment would be contrary to all surgical principles. In the latter case, presuming that the cervical glandular region is unaffected or capable of removal, the scalp ulcer should be freely excised together with the whole thickness of underlying bone. The resultant osseous gap may be covered in by means of a plastic flap derived from neighbouring healthy tissue.

INDEX